Craniofacial Dysfunction and Pain

Commissioning editor: Heidi Allen
Development editor: Myriam Brearley
Production controller: Anthony Read
Cover designer: Alan Studholme

Craniofacial Dysfunction and Pain: Manual Therapy, Assessment and Management

Edited by

Harry von Piekartz BSc Ft M App Sc PT MT

Physiotherapist, Ootmarsum, The Netherlands
Teacher, International Maitland Teacher Association, Neuro-orthopedic Institute

and

Lynn Bryden MSc MCSP SRP
Physiotherapist, London, UK

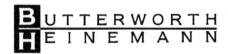

BUTTERWORTH
HEINEMANN

OXFORD AUCKLAND BOSTON JOHANNESBURG MELBOURNE NEW DELHI

Butterworth-Heinemann
Linacre House, Jordan Hill, Oxford OX2 8DP
225 Wildwood Avenue, Woburn, MA 01801-2041
A division of Reed Educational and Professional Publishing Ltd

A member of the Reed Elsevier plc group

First published 2001

Reed Educational and Professional Publishing Ltd 2001

British Library Cataloguing in Publication Data
A catalogue record for this book is available from the British Library

Library of Congress Cataloguing in Publication Data
A catalogue record for this book is available from the Library of Congress

ISBN 0 7506 2963 0

Transferred to digital printing 2006

Typeset by Bath Typesetting
Printed and bound by CPI Antony Rowe, Eastbourne

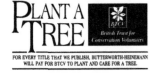

Contents

List of Contributors   vii
Foreword   ix
Preface   xiii
Acknowledgements   xvii

1 Skull growth in relation to mechanical stimulation   1
   H. A. J. Oudhof
2 Features of cranial tissue as a basis for clinical pattern recognition, 22
   examination and treatment
   H. J. M. von Piekartz
3 Primary and secondary cranial asymmetry in KISS children   46
   H. Biedermann
4 Manual therapy movements of the craniofacial region as a   63
   therapeutic approach to children with long-term ear disease
   H. E. M. Spermon-Marijnen and J. R. Spermon
5 Cervicogenic headache: a clinician's perspective   85
   P. Westerhuis
6 Cervicogenic headache: physical examination and management   100
   P. Westerhuis and H. J. M. von Piekartz
7 Neurodynamics of cranial nervous tissue (cranioneurodynamics)   116
   H. J. M. von Piekartz
8 Experience of pain and the craniofacial region   148
   D. S. Butler
9 The influence of posture and alteration of function upon the   163
   craniocervical and craniofacial regions
   L. Bryden and D. Fitzgerald
10 Clinical reasoning – a basis for examination and treatment in   188
   the cranial region
   M. Jones and H. J. M. von Piekartz

11   Pain management in patients with chronic craniofacial pain   216
     F. A. M. Winter
12   Clinimetrics for the clinician – the use of some indexes applicable
     in the craniocervical and craniofacial regions   228
     G. Aufdemkampe

     Glossary   237
     Index   241

Contributors

G. Aufdemkampe MSc PT
Senior Research Associate, Department of
Physical Therapy, Polytechnic of Utrecht,
Utrecht, The Netherlands

H. Biedermann
Physiotherapist, Antwerp, Belgium

L. Bryden MSc MCSP SRP
Physiotherapist, London, UK

D. S. Butler M App Sc MT
Teacher, Neuro-orthopedic Institute
Lecturer, University of South Australia

D. Fitzgerald
Physiotherapist, Dublin, Ireland

M. Jones BSc M App Sc
Physiotherapist
Senior Lecturer, Coordinator,
Graduate Programs in Manipulative
Physiotherapy, School of Physiotherapy,
Division of Health Sciences,
University of South Australia

H. A. J. Oudhof MD
Assistant Professor, Department of
Carielogy, Endodontology and
Pedodontology, ACTA (Academic
Centre of Dentistry)
The Netherlands

**H. J. M. von Piekartz BSc Ft M App Sc PT
MT**
Physiotherapist, Ootmarsum,
The Netherlands
Teacher, International Maitland Teacher
Association, Neuro-orthopedic Institute

J. R. Spermon M App Sc
General Practitioner
Nijmegen, The Netherlands

H. E. M. Spermon-Marijnen BSc PT MT
Physiotherapist
Berlicum, The Netherlands

P. Westerhuis BSc PT
Physiotherapist, Langendorf, Switzerland
Principal Instructor, International
Maitland Teacher Association

F. A. M. Winter PhD
Director, Pain Clinic Rehabilitation
Centre, Roessingh,
Enschede, The Netherlands

Foreword

Congratulations, a book that was needed. Normally in orthopaedics we study a body without a head, we understand the biomechanics of the spine and extremities, but the craniofacial region is usually neglected. Only recently with the introduction of osteopathic principles in orthopaedic manual therapy, many physiotherapists and kinesiologists have become extremely interested in the philosophy of cranial techniques.

For many years I have been introducing the concept of maxillofacial disorders (including TMD). It has been a difficult task, but worthwhile. Currently around the world we see manual therapists in collaboration with the dental profession and medical and other health professions, dealing with the multifactorial dilemma of head neck and orofacial pain. What has united our professions has been pain! For us as manual therapists, no pain – no patient!

Many academies throughout the world are trying to establish a consensus in diagnosis and treatment approach to a great variety of craniofacial disorders and pain. These include the Iberian Latin American Academy of Head Neck and Facial Pain, the European Academy of Craniomandibular Disorders and Facial Pain, the Asian Academy, the American Academy of Orofacial Pain and many other sister academies. All of these are working together in standardizing procedures for many of the pathologies involved, but we are still very weak in the field of intracapsular temporomandibular joint disorders. We still do not have strong well documented etiological factors for many disk pathologies (with or without pain), such as what causes a unilateral or bilateral disk luxation, or what causes a medial luxation on one side and a lateral luxation on the contralateral side, with or without anterior discotemporal luxation. Examples of these pathologies are seen in everyday practice and are common, but they remain without a protocol for clinical diagnosis and there is no protocol for treatment, either dental or in other orthopaedic practice. This remains a challenge for all of us in manual therapy as specialists in the treatment of synovial joints.

The cranial and facial bones also remain an obscure area as a source of pain. This book attempts to make life easier and increase our understanding by gathering different philosophies in relation to a variety of dysfunctions in the craniofacial region. For the most important concept, growth and development, the focus is on how soft tissues guide the patterns of growth and development. How the neuro-cranium increases in volume and develops, influences the shape, symmetry and pro-portions of the cranium and the face. The indivisible relation in function, growth and the need for normalization of the cranio-vertebral biomechanics for symmetrical growth of the head and face. A slight rotation of the atlas (C1), can be the cause of a severe craniofacial deformity during the most important phases of growth and development – the first three years of life. This asymmetry will remain until adult-hood. Early recognition and good manual skills used to detect and normalize the craniovertebral dysfunction will be the solution for proportional growth. If un-diagnosed, this might be the cause of future malocclusions, or of head or face pain of cervical origin being misdiagnosed. One specific manoeuvre for the atlas in one treatment session might be the solution. This is described with good clinical exam-ples and provides motivation to continue early intervention in orthopaedics, so the result is a well developed child.

This book has good coverage of differ-ential diagnosis. Something we urgently need. We cannot continue to practice with blind techniques. Physical examination follows a treatment approach, and is backed with good clinical case descriptions that show differentiation of the areas involved, through provocation/alleviation type testing. This leads on to conclusions from which appropriate treatment can be applied. We are reminded of the impor-tance of how the structures are held together by large amounts of highly vascu-larized and innervated connective tissue

which can be the source of pain. Any area which involves a cranial suture and altera-tion of mechanics due to cranial dysfunc-tion, with or without trauma, can be the source of pain.

The general concepts of pain are reviewed showing the difficulties in identifying the origin of the pain. Pain is classified into categories:

Nociceptive
Peripheral Neurogenic
Central Sensitization
Output mechanism
Others.

We are given guidance in identifying the different types of and approaches for treatment, making this chapter very inter-esting and easy to apply in practical situations. This provides motivation to continue to find new avenues in manual therapy with the emphasis on differential diagnosis. A good summary with a very interesting proposal for pain recognition, full of suggestions and inspiration for future research.

An excellent reference review on the controversial topic of the relation between posture, function and dysfunction of the craniocervical and craniomandibular func-tional unit. Great emphasis is placed on the importance of the deep pre- and para-vertebral muscle relation, and cervical stability, together with shoulder girdle alignment. It includes a classification of local muscles into those providing stability or mobility, and how these are involved in patterns of hypo- and hyperactivity.

Finally there is a strong conclusion on the subject of history-taking based on clinical reasoning. This considers the fundamentals of the process, the mistakes often seen during the process, and the types of applied reasoning used in clinical practice. This is supported by clinical examples.

This method of examination allows the

clinician to observe the nature of the patients symptoms, and to clarify the history of the symptoms. A comprehensive physical examination, including neurological, cervical ROM, neurodynamics, testing and via passive accessory movement of the cranial bones maxillofacial evaluation, respiratory patterns and finally the treatment protocol. The integration of cranial techniques in the analysis of treatment is very interesting and is an introduction to, at present, subjective techniques or philosophies. This makes the reader consider the large scale of manual therapy procedures applied daily in clinical practice that require a better way of assessing their beneficial effects on a long-term basis – by also taking into account the recovery and normalizing of function, prevention of the progression of degeneration, and not only

the treatment of pain. The chapter on clinical reasoning clarifies this need and puts clinical features in perspective with the objectivity of the applied procedure.

In summary this is an ambitious book, that attempts to gather together the arsenal of philosophies, clinical techniques and principles known, at present, in the field of specialization of craniofacial pain. An effort that must be acknowledged for gathering all these different visions and giving constant fundamental reasoning for the topics involved.

An excellent book, and example for the profession. Congratulations!

Professor Mariano Rocabado
Santiago, Chile

Preface

At the start of this millennium we have to accept that in society we are faced with growing numbers of patients with long-term head and facial problems. These patients are often difficult to treat.[1] The diagnosis '(atypical) facial pain' is being used more and more by the medical profession for persistent complaints in the head and/or neck region with no physical cause. Also, diagnoses that seem clear at first, such as cervical headache, are being questioned more by clinicians. The aetiology and the pain distribution are not always as clear as was presumed in the past, so the examiner should not use nosology to label a patient too soon.[2]

Clinicians are often confronted with the same questions: what is the cause, what is the source of the complaint, what is the best treatment strategy and how do I continue to manage this patient? It is a common experience with patients who have long-term head, neck and facial pain that maximized effort does not yield the expected results. This made me, as a manual physical therapist, decide to look beyond the traditional manual therapy approach. Clinicians like G. Maitland, P. Wells, G. Rolf, P. Davies, D. Butler, M. Rocabado and S. Kraus have inspired me. The intention of this book is to contribute to a better understanding of and an improvement in the treatment and management of the often misunderstood patient with undiagnosed and long-term neck, head and facial problems.

These craniofacial problems even occur in infants. Children frequently present with a craniofacial asymmetry and a preferential posture of the head with a stiff neck. They often start life with frequent and irregular fits of crying, retardation in growth and motor skills and inexplicable attacks of fever. They are often labelled with a diagnosis of plagiocephaly or myogenic torticollis. The question arises whether this group can be linked to children who, during their school years, struggle with chronic sinusitis, middle ear infections, disturbance in concentration, motor retardation and headaches that are often diagnosed as 'migraine'. So far, there is little scientific evidence concerning these often treatment-resistant young patients.

Patients with post-traumatic head and facial pain form another group who undergo frequent medical examination and long-term treatment. Although the way to manage these patients is being described more and more effectively by means of general guidelines from the pain sciences, some of these patients are not satisfied with their treatment, partly because their problems continue to exist.

During the treatment of patients with craniomandibular and craniofacial pain – often diagnosed as atypical facial pain, trigeminal neuralgia, migraine, craniomandibular dysfunction or cervical headaches – I noticed that non-specific cranial techniques (passive mobilization of the cranial bone structures and neurodynamical tests and treatment of cranial nerve tissue) together with an explanation of the problem to the patient can have spectacular results.

The use of cranial techniques is not new. Osteopaths and chiropractors have been convinced for a long time that passive movements of the skull can influence signs and symptoms in a patient. I strongly believe that a combination of 'hands on' and 'hands off' techniques, at the appropriate time and place, can be a useful addition to treatment and can produce clear improvements in many patients with chronic craniofacial dysfunction and pain. Along with other clinicians I am also convinced that (early) treatment of children with craniofacial dysfunction can be useful to prevent future complications. However, no conclusive longitudinal studies have been performed.

While studying the literature I quickly found that there was no standardization of manual cranial techniques, not to mention fundamental clinical proof. This persuaded me to write and edit this book with Lynn Bryden.

One of our basic objectives was to initiate the standardization of cranial manual techniques within manual therapy for various patient groups (Chapters 2 and 7).

Another important goal was to introduce the reader to the use of craniocervical-mandibular and cranial techniques with an open mind (clinical reasoning). In my view manual therapy lacks gold-standard tests, in particular for patients with long-term craniofacial problems. In addition, the paradigm of manual therapy has been changing a great deal during the last few decades; from a predominantly passive approach on an impairment level to a more holistic approach in which hands-on skills play an important part in clinical decisions affecting the continued management of the patient, with regard to the level of disability. The knowledge of actual pain biology is also a useful addition to physical and manual therapy. It guides the clinician towards a different way of assessing the complex pain patient.

All in all I am convinced that the clinical reasoning model is still the most effective approach in physical and manual therapy to ensure the selection of the proper techniques and to provide tailor-made care for each individual patient. Chapter 10 deals with this in more detail. None of the manual techniques described in this book are 'recipe techniques', they are as far as possible based on literature studies. Various clinicians and researchers, all specialists in their fields, have each been invited to write a chapter to accentuate and/or substantiate clinical use and clinical evidence.

The first chapter describes recent developments in the understanding of skull growth in all its aspects. Together with Chapters 2 and 7 this provides the reader with a survey of how, based on recent literature from various disciplines (neuro-, plastic and oral surgery, orthodontics, gnathology, ENT), interpretations can be made in manual therapy. In addition the book states that manual techniques may also have a range of effects, not least at the affective–cognitive level. For instance Chapter 11 describes the cognitive processes often present in the long-term craniofacial patient. Tips and guidelines for continuing clinical management are also given in this chapter. Chapter 8 examines the current state of pain biology and from this viewpoint describes clinical patterns which can be recognized in the craniofacial patient. I think that the explanation of these pain mechanisms provides the reader, within the clinical reasoning process, with enough scope to effectively assess manual techniques and to apply them appropriately for each patient.

The actual benefits of manual therapy for the craniofacial patient are discussed in Chapter 12, illustrated by some recent results obtained using reliable measurement instruments. The craniocervical and craniomandibular regions (Chapters 5 and 6) are also considered in a practical sense, because I feel that taking an isolated cranial approach is not in line with everyday practice. These chapters also supply the reader with the tools to integrate various techniques for a more multistructural approach. We have deliberately left out the craniomandibular techniques for which good books in several languages are available.[3–8] Therefore, Chapter 9 discusses the recent rehabilitation of the importance of the muscular balance of the craniofacial–mandibular–cervical region in more detail. Chapters 3 and 4 are clinically oriented chapters on the phenomenon in children with KISS (kinematic imbalance suboccipital sprain) and long-term ear disease.

This book has been edited by physical therapists and is aimed at open-minded clinicians and researchers within physical, manual and speech therapy, dentistry, orthodontics, psychology, osteopathy and chiropractic who are interested in patients with difficult craniocervical and craniofacial problems. It is virgin territory. I hope the reader will be inspired by this humble contribution to get '*the craniofacial on the move*', in cooperation with colleagues from a variety of disciplines.

Harry von Piekartz

References

1 Zakrewska, J. M. and Hamlyn, P. J. (1999). *Facial Pain, Epidemiology of Pain*, pp. 171–203. IASP Press.
2 Leone, M., D'Amico, Grazzi, L., Attanasio, A. and Bussone, G. (1998). Cervicogenic headache: a critical review of current diagnostic criteria. *Pain*, **78**, 1–5, 7.
3 Steenks M. H. and de Wijer, A. (1989). *Craniomandibulaire Dysfunction. De Tijdstroom*
4 Rocabado, M. and Iglash, Z. A. (1991). *Musculoskeletal Approach to Maxillofacial Pain*. J. B. Lippincott Co.
5 Friction, J. R. and Dubner, R. (1995) *Oral Facial Pain and Temporomandibular Disorders. Advances in Pain Research and Therapy*, vol 21. Raven Press.
6 Kraus, S. L. (1994). *Temporomandibular Disorders*, 2nd edn. Churchill Livingstone.
7 Pertes, R. A. and Gross, S. G. (1995). *Clinical Management of Temporomandibular Disorders and Oral Facial Pain*. Quintessence Publishing Co, Inc.
8 Palla, S. (1998). *Myoarthropathien des Kausystems und Orafazial Schmerzen*. Fotoplast AG Zurich.

Acknowledgements

During the writing of this book I came to realize, more than ever, that a tough job like this can never be completed alone. I owe a great deal of thanks to many people. First, to Geoff and Ann Maitland who presented themselves more and more as a single entity. Geoff's charisma and dynamism, together with his continuing exploration in the field of manual therapy, his open mind and the natural support of his wife Ann, laid the foundation for this book.

I would also like to extend my thanks to Peter Wells, Gisela Rolf, David Butler, Peter Westerhuis, Steven Kraus, Mariano Rocabado and Jos Dibbets. They have, directly or indirectly, contributed to the realization of this book by their exceptional expertise and their enthusiasm, which gave me the necessary inspiration.

I would like to express particular appreciation to my former anatomy teacher Geert Bekkering, Professor of Anatomy, who works as a teacher at the School of Physiotherapy at the Enschede University for Professional Education, The Netherlands. He proved to be a great help with the anatomy drawings, illustrations with a style of their own. I will never forget the evenings we spent with various anatomy books in order to visualize the functional anatomy of the craniofacial region as accurately as possible. The illustrations in this book have taken some doing. Photographer Jeffrey van der Woude and our clinical model Annet Werger know all about that. Annet had to put up with quite a few hours in the cold so the right picture could be obtained. Thank you Annet! My thanks also to the patients who spontaneously declared their willingness to pose for a picture.

I have pleasant memories of the cooperation with co-authors. Without their contributions this book would not have been complete and our aims would not have been achieved.

I would like to thank Juliet Gore for her patience with a non-native speaker of English. Her critical comments regarding usage have been a particular help. Juliet, thanks for the learning process.

I received much support from the staff of Butterworth-Heinemann: Caroline Makepeace, Zoë Youd and Heidi Allen. They were always available for consultations and prepared to listen to ideas, which contributed to speedy production. That also goes for Roosi Haarer and her colleagues from

Thieme Verlag, who simultaneously translated this book into German.

As previously stated, many have contributed to the realization of this book, but I am most grateful to my near and dear ones. Irma, for co-editing and late night discussions over a glass of good wine; at those moments things were really finalized. And finally I would like to thank Tess and Kiki most of all, for their tolerance.

HJM vP

First I must thank Harry von Piekartz for inviting me to be involved in the realization of this book, which was conceived as a result of his ideas, inspiration and determination. It has at times been a steep learning curve and I am indebted to Harry for his encouragement, patience and advice. He must take all the credit for holding the project together and keeping the lines of communication open.

I would also like to thank Peter Wells for his encouragement in taking on this project, and his advice in the early stages, and Nicola Bannerman for her help with word processing. Thanks also to all the contributors for their hard work in writing their individual chapters and for their commitment to the project.

Lastly and by no means least I must thank my family. Mark – thank you for the considerable help you gave, for your time, your sympathetic ear, and for maintaining a sense of humour ! And finally a big thank you to Benedict and Alexander.

LB

1

Skull growth in relation to mechanical stimulation

H. A. J. Oudhof

Introduction

The growth process

The shape of the skull changes throughout life from embryo into old age. Quantitative changes are the most notable, and the growth process appears to be restricted to the first 20 years of life. The major growth and development manifestations are evident during the first few years of life, yet it is wrong to reserve the concepts 'growth' and 'development' exclusively for this period. This period simply demonstrates the most 'growth manifestations' but it is essentially a stage involving a quick succession of processes that continue to take place throughout life.

The return of a 'genetic' past

It is impossible to get a clear picture of skull growth without taking into account the growth of the head. In turn, the growth of the head cannot be discussed without considering overall body growth. Furthermore, if we isolate growing humans from their biological past we neglect the science of phylogeny, and consequently the genetic

contribution to ontogeny remains unexplained. It is to phylogeny that we look for explanations through the evolutionary development processes. During the ontogenetic development of humans (and therefore of the skull as well) we recognize these processes in the shape the body components take during growth and development. All morphological characteristics during growth and development are in part fragments of ancient evolution and in part products of current function.[1]

This dualism in growth is not restricted to the final modelling. Physiological processes, including growth systems, also represent systems from the remote and recent past and in part they represent current adaptation to existing environmental circumstances. To distinguish between genetic properties and properties dictated by the actual environment is therefore meaningless: nothing in the organism develops exclusively because of internal genetic potential or exclusively as a biological response to the environment. Using the biological past (genetic information), as adequate a response as possible is always given to the prevailing environmental influences. The fact that genetic properties will not be expressed without actual environmental information[1] must also be taken into account!

A biological system, modular construction

Biological systems grow according to a fixed basic principle: modular construction. This means that each individual organism, animal or plant, does not start with a completely unique method of construction. Instead, successful system units that have proved their reliability in the past are used. Such system units are called modules in biology. Modular construction methods are not only found in larger morphological units but also within the body cell itself. Thus, mitochondria construct a modular system of their own in each body cell. Mitochondria have their own DNA and essentially split independently by fission. In the body cells these mitochondria demonstrate the successful symbiosis between the purple bacteria and the plant or animal basic cell which occurred in the distant past.[1] This 'module' is also found in all human cells.

Skull growth shows a modular construction method. This implies a complex compliance and functional adaptation ability. Bone matrices form seemingly extremely complicated tissue systems with almost inconceivable mutual growth controls.[2-5] However, by following the morphogenesis step by step, the logical and systematic way in which nature forms the skull becomes evident. The resultant concepts help the modern clinician understand the behaviour of the organism better (and thus that of the patient). For instance, the mobility of the sutures continues into old age, and can be a starting point for treatment techniques in osteopathy and manual therapy.[6-10]

Indispensable mechanical influences

Hard tissues, i.e. those that are inflexible, are the basis of morphogenesis in vertebrates.[11-15] Hard tissue is bone or cartilage. Without this bone or cartilage a form cannot consolidate. Form consolidation is indispensable for the growth and development of higher organisms and, after the development of the chorda,[16] hard (and thus consolidated) tissues become increasingly important in the functional development of form.

In nature, form and function cannot be separated.[16,17] Living organisms express their functional behaviour by their current shape. In turn, expressions of functional behaviour result in a specific form.

The relative inflexibility in comparison to other more or less flexible tissues is accompanied by mechanical tensions in and around the hard tissues in the growing organism as their rigid nature prevents the total reformation of an organism. So, consolidation of form always produces mechanical tensions in an organism.

Functional changes in shape appear in quick succession during growth and development.[14] From their first appearance in the evolution of the skull the hard tissues respond to special demands: for instance, they remain able to reform while maintaining shape stability.[12] Because of this, bone tissue is extremely sensitive to mechanical stresses. The more flexible cartilage does have a reasonable ability to regenerate, but is nevertheless inferior to bone in this respect. The stiffer the hard tissue in an organism, the more it depends on its ability to regenerate for its existence. This seeming discrepancy, stability of form but dependence on mechanical stresses for this form, should always be taken into account when considering bone tissue. The skeleton is not a supporting metal construction and as such does not comply with physical strain/stress laws. Bone is never molecularly stable nor molecularly uniform. Yesterday's bone is not the same as today's bone, and the reader may even replace 'yesterday' with a few minutes or seconds. These reactive properties are at the basis of all biological systems. It would be outside the scope of this chapter to discuss all the properties and behaviour of open dissipative systems, in which all biological systems are included. For any interested reader this subject is covered in more depth in the work of Klima.[18]

For the purposes of this chapter it is sufficient to realize that biological hard tissues like cartilage and bone are very adaptive and because of this they can only maintain their shapes within a functional balance of mechanical stress. Mechanical stresses are, therefore, necessary for the existence of biological hard tissues like bone and cartilage. Loss of mechanical stress is a direct assault on the skeleton's functioning. We should realize that many experiments designed to study bone tissues have been performed in laboratory conditions, without any (normal) mechanical stresses. Much of our present knowledge about bone tissue has been gathered under 'pathological' conditions, and is therefore physiologically obsolete. Statements often heard in the clinic such as: 'this joint is overused', or, even worse: 'this joint is worn', stem directly from a static view that has no functional basis. Physiologically speaking, there is no such thing as worn or overused tissue, hopefully these clinical 'concepts' will wear away quickly!

A clinically manifest malfunction comes with a shape adapted to this function, for shape and function are inseparable. Extreme care should be taken if one wants to change the shape of the bone by means of surgery because there is a great risk of an iatrogenic malfunction. Playing with nature's building blocks has its consequences. The shape of hard tissues always has a long history, dictated by genetic and environmental information. Bone is the most tangible end product of a growing phase. By following all the growing phases step by step and simultaneously paying attention to the succession of functional developments, we will add to our knowledge of the mature situation.

The bone matrix

The bone matrix consists of all tissues in which bone develops, and includes:

1. Cartilage, the chondral matrix
2. (Subcutaneous) connective tissue, the dermal matrix
3. Existing bone tissue, the secondary matrix

Periosteal and endosteal structures, sutures and periodontia (both gomphoses), together with synovial joints, make up the secondary structures of the bone matrix. Bone matrix has a special ability to resist pressure and deformation. This ability provides the body with support and protection. Gomphoses play an important part during the enlargement of a bone matrix. These very specific joints accomplish unique, flexible connections between bones in the bone matrix. Unlike synovial joints, gomphoses pass on the external forces exerted on the bone matrix as an internal load. We will return to this very specific function of gomphoses in more detail later. Apart from the internal potential for growth, synovial joints offer the bone matrix a motion function. This motion function is obviously more explicit in the synovial joints than in gomphoses. Yet it is

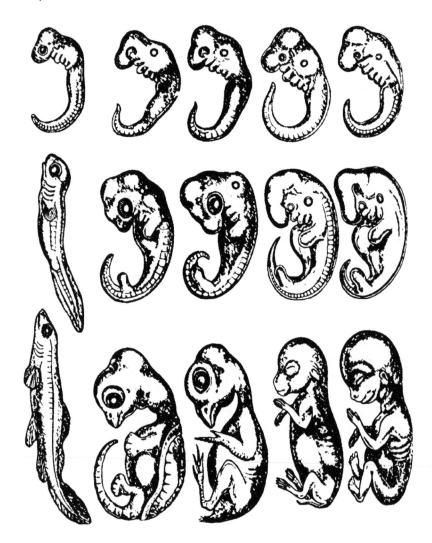

Figure 1.1 Phylogeny can be recognized in ontogeny: the embryos of fish, turtle, chicken, rabbit or man differ only slightly in this early stage[24]

a mistake to consider matrix parts, connected by means of a gomphosis, as a mechanical unity.[19] Throughout life, sutures and periodontia remain movable connections that are part of the musculoskeletal system, just like the synovial connections.

During growth, the bone matrix consolidates the shape of the head. The bone matrix changes its stress durability continually, while simultaneously enlarging itself. This has two important consequences for the processing of stress by the matrix. First, the physical properties of the matrix change. This affects remodelling of the matrix due to external mechanical stimulation.[13] Secondly, the matrix enlargement produces a larger area for mechanical stimulation. Larger matrices absorb more mechanical stimulation than smaller ones. Together, structure and size make up the tissue status of the bone matrix. The tissue status determines the transfer of mechanical stimulation by the tissue. Cartilage structures are much more elastic than bone structures.[20] Joints in a bone matrix are capable of translating mechanical loads into positional changes of a matrix part. In addition, they spread the mechanical stimulation over the bone matrix.[21] A gomphosis is particularly specialized in spreading mechanical loads over the bone matrix. This will be dealt with in the discussion of sutural and periodontal growth. So far it suffices to know that not only the size, but also the composition of the bone matrix is subject to changes during the growth and development of the skull.

The first skull growth

The development of the skull, the origin of hard tissues in the head, takes place at a time when the embryo already has a distinct shape. This shape is by no means species specific. At this stage there is very little difference in the shape of the embryo of various animal species (Figure 1.1),[1,22–24] yet the division into three primary germ layers, ectoderm, mesoderm and endoderm, has taken place in all embryos and a heart is beating. Furthermore, all the important fusion processes in the facial part of the embryo have been completed and, in the human embryo, there is a separation between the nose and the oral cavity and the face is basically formed.

From this we conclude that, in this development phase, such a non-species specific shape is the optimal answer of nature. We should also realize that in nature, successful designs are forever being repeated.[24] In biology, such successful designs are seen as modules; modules that are continually being modified to the actual demands, but in fact show strong similarities. During the development process a successful design is never completely abandoned, the modules will only differ in details and mutual relationships.

At an embryonic age of 33 days, the heart beat and the consequences of the expansive growth of the brain are by far the most important strain factors on the embryonic tissue. Because the first blood vessels are being developed in the direction of the head, this mechanical load primarily affects the head part of the embryo.[25] At this time the first hard tissues of the skull are being formed. A cartilage bone matrix is developing caudally from the brain and this cartilage will eventually develop into the nasal septum. At about the same time the first dermal bone matrices of the calvaria and the facial skull are being formed.[17] From this moment on, the shapes of the various embryos differ. Human embryos show an expansive growth of brain tissue.[26] This growth acceleration is necessary to achieve 200 billion neurons by the end of pregnancy. In the lower animal species this brain growth is less explicit.[23] The calvaria and skull base consolidate the developed shape. Because of the large difference in brain size, which varies from species to species, the shape of the hard tissues that consolidate the shape of the brain also varies. The brain too has a modular building method,[24] and the differences in shape of the basic brainstems are considerably less extensive than the differences in shape that occur between the various manifestations of the neocortex. It goes without saying that this is visible in the structure of the neurocranium. In the various animal species there are, therefore, far more similarities in the construction of the skull base than of the vault.

So far the first major conclusion is that with the introduction of hard tissues, the individual, recognizable shapes become manifest. Also, hard tissues divide the head into compartments (the neurocranium and the facial skull) that, with their structures, resist space-occupying growth processes (the brain) and stabilize the shape (Figure 1.2).[15,27]

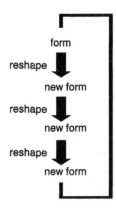

Figure 1.2 The growth process is basically the continuous development of a new form from the existing one

Growth of the skull components

Looking at skull growth, there are some remarkable details:

1. not all skull parts grow at the same pace[28,29]
2. growth originates in several centres, the growth centres[9,30]
3. non-bone parts, soft tissues, are strongly correlated with skull growth[2,17,31]
4. not all growth centres are manifest at the same time[22]
5. matrix building processes and matrix resorption processes often occur simultaneously.[32]

Many of these striking details are recognizable in the proportional variations that can be seen in the growing skull. A child is not a shrunken adult (Figure 1.3).[26] Each age

has its own proportions. During growth not only the proportions of the skull parts vary, but also the overall proportions in all parts of the skeleton. The differences in anatomical proportions can always be traced back to changes in function, occurring during growth. The brain growth function dominates the shape of the neurocranium before and during the first period after birth. This function therefore dominates the shape of the child. It is only after birth that the increasingly important breathing, sucking and swallowing functions clearly effect alterations in the anatomical shape of the facial skull. During growth the bone matrices produce an optimal form for the head, as a result of the prevalent stress in that period. Apart from the differences in shape already mentioned, the structure of the bone matrix also changes markedly.

Not all bone matrices handle stress in the same way. A chondral matrix processes the same stress in a completely different way from a dermal matrix; this is an expression of the difference in status between a chondral matrix and a dermal matrix. We will now follow the growth of the cranium and the role of the various matrices in this growth. Looking at the growth of the neurocranium and nasopharynx and the development of the teeth will give us a clear picture of the various growth mechanisms of the cranium.

The growth of the neurocranium

The neurocranium includes a chondral matrix, situated caudally to the brain, the skull base, and the various dermal matrices of the cranial roof, divided by sutures.[27,33,34] The role of the chondral matrix will be clearer if we follow it through phylogeny (Figure 1.4). In the shark the chondral matrix is a sutureless

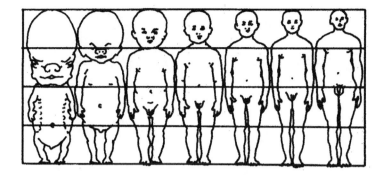

Figure 1.3 During growth enormous differences occur in the proportions of the human organism[26]

box around the brain;[26] in man part of this matrix has been reduced to a local bone matrix between the facial and the neural cranium. This large morphological difference has its origin in the inability of a chondral matrix to follow the rapid growth of the brain. Moreover, human brain growth requires a much more flexible covering than a chondral matrix is able to offer. Human brain cannot develop against a pressure larger than the systolic blood pressure.[35] Dermal matrices, divided by sutures, offer the necessary flexibility. Higher animal species, with larger brain volumes, cover their brains with dermal bone matrices. However, the tested chondral module is maintained for the boundary of the basal brainstem, albeit with some adaptations as to formation.

The large differences between the chondral and the dermal matrix in morphological processing of mechanical stimuli are clearly demonstrated by the experiments performed by Prahl.[30] She injected pregnant rats with kaolin, which largely blocks liquor absorption in fetuses, resulting in fetal hydrocephalus. In these experiments the shape of the dermatocranium changed enormously, while the shape of the chondrocranium remained unaltered. The conclusion is that the chondral matrix has

enormous (extra) buffering qualities for dealing with external mechanical stimulation, without consequences for incarnation. This leaves the shape of the skull base unaffected, even with the pathological, extravagant increase of brain volume induced by the experiment. The chondrocranium is also a mechanical buffer for 'ordinary' brain growth. The development of the dermatocranium shows a far more stress-dependent way of growth. In Prahl's experiments the dermatocranium acted like the shell of the neurocranium, forced into a balloon-like shape. The dermatocranium showed almost complete incarnation.

How does the formation of a dermal bone matrix develop?

At various places between the outermost membrane of the brain (the dura mater) and the skin, dermal bone matrices develop.[36] Various dermal matrices fuse, but not on the presumptive suture locations. Popa suggested that stress is minimal at such locations in the dermal matrices.[15] Troitzky[34] emphasized the phenomenon of the bone-fusion barrier at this location,[34] while Markens[33,37] discovered that the tissue status in these regions differs considerably from that in the fusing bone matrices. The

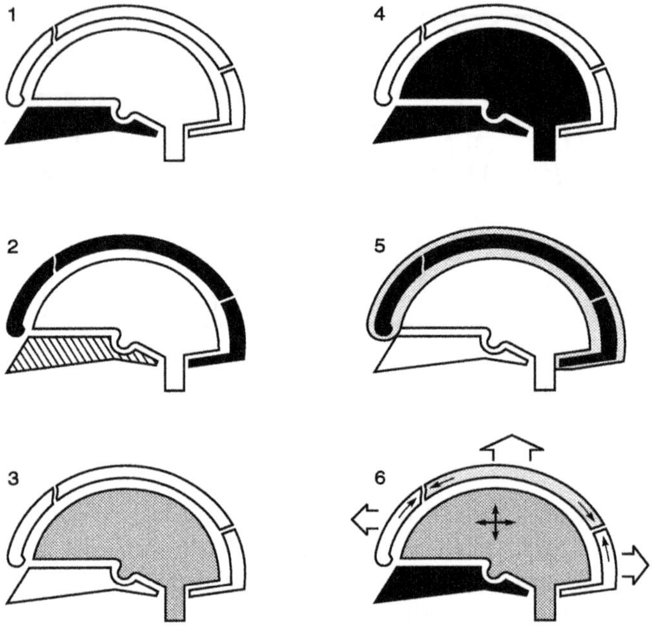

(a)

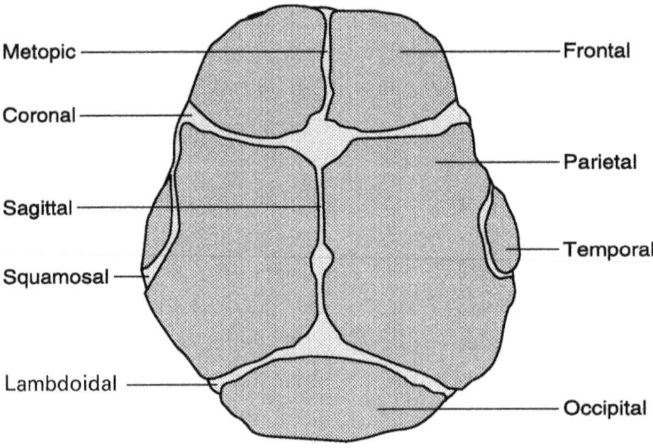

Metopic ——————————————————— Frontal

Coronal ————————————————————— Parietal

Sagittal —————————————————————

——————————————————— Temporal

Squamosal —————————————————

Lambdoidal —————————————————

——————————————————— Occipital

(b) Sutures   Bones

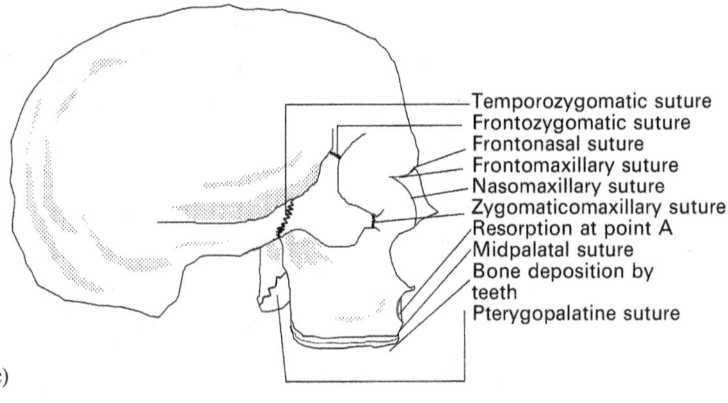

Temporozygomatic suture
Frontozygomatic suture
Frontonasal suture
Frontomaxillary suture
Nasomaxillary suture
Zygomaticomaxillary suture
Resorption at point A
Midpalatal suture
Bone deposition by
teeth
Pterygopalatine suture

(c)

Figure 1.4 (a) The neurocranium increases through various growth centres: (1) the synchondroses in the skull base (2) the sutures in the cranium. The growing brain (3) is a mechanical entity with a stable skull base (4). The sutures in the cranium allow movement of the dura mater (5). (6) The brain growth is buffered by the skull base and makes the cranium reform at the sutures. **(b)** The position of the sutures and the bones in the calvaria. **(c)** The position of the facial sutures

sutures' most important morphological function is their ability to force a separation in the growing bone matrix. Because bone–matrix fusion is prevented in the suture locations, the periostea in the sutures become separated and consequently a highly specific intrasutural fibre structure develops, induced by stress.[6,7,9,10,27] This periosteal separation stops bone growth in the suture, as periosteum is the actual border for growth! The arrangement of the intrasutural fibres guarantees a constant intrasutural fissure of approximately 250 μm, and has a function similar to that of spokes in a wheel. The spokes maintain the distance between the rim and the hub and the fibres in a suture maintain the size of the sutural fissure (Figure 1.5).

After the development of the sutural joints, the mechanical load on the dermal bone matrices, caused by brain growth, is transformed into pressure loads on the matrix. These pressure loads are established by the constant fluctuations between the systolic and the diastolic intracranial blood pressure interacting with the intracranial volume increases. This is explained below.

The vascular flow through the brain shows a constant pressure variation between systole and diastole, as does the liquor pressure. Also the absolute brain volume increases during brain growth. In addition to the rhythmical pressure fluctuations (vascular flow and liquor flow), there is a constant pressure (brain growth) exerted on the neurocranium. At its sutures, the growing vault of the skull experiences a continuously varying load.[6] This variation in load maintains the intrasutural fibre structure. The average load size (due to the constant pressure increase from the growing brain) exerts a mechanical pressure on the bone matrix through the dura mater and the sutural periostea.

Through the blood vessels in the matrix, this pressure load has its effect on the bone matrix. This also needs some further explanation.

Sutures are very special joint systems. The joint ligaments run outside and inside the joint fissure. It is well known that joint ligaments run into the bone matrix and have a sound contact with this matrix. So far, there is no essential difference between a stiff synovial joint and a suture. The suture is special in that it creates a hydraulic continuity with the medulla of the bone matrix. This continuity is created by numerous vascular connections between the suture tissue and the medullary bone tissue. These vessels transfer the internal sutural pressure directly to the medullary bone, while, conversely, all pressure fluctuations in the medullary bone itself are transferred to the suture tissue. External loads on the bone matrix lead to tensions in the bone matrix. In the sutures, these tensions are transformed into sutural movements. Consequently, these sutural movements cause pressure fluctuations in the sutural vessels. The sutural vessels pass these pressure fluctuations on to the medullary bone. During growth the results of this process are perceptible as a thickening of the cranial bone alongside the sutures. This thickening has its origin in the pressure increases within the medullary cavity around the sutures. Thus, sutures make up the stress transducers in the calvaria (Figure 1.6).

The matrix growth at the suture rims and along the dura mater increases the internal skull volume, which causes a decrease in the mean intracranial pressure. By new fission of the brain tissue, a new mean pressure increase is created. Repetitions of this process are responsible for the constantly renewed mechanical pressure on the bone matrix.

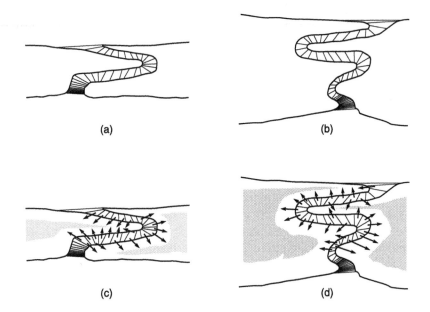

Figure 1.5 The fibre connections in a suture (a gomphosis) have a similar function to the spokes of a wheel (see Figure 1.10). They stabilize the sutural fissure, so that pressure increases within the suture can be transported to the medullary tissue in the calvaria bones. **(a)** A suture consisting of a single overlap; **(b)** a suture consisting of a plural overlap; **(c)** and **(d)** vascular connections between suture and medullary bone provide the transduction of mechanical load (see text and Figure 1.6)

The absence of blood vessels in the chondral matrix, and its elastic structure, make the skull base less susceptible to external mechanical stimulation. Furthermore, the growth rate of the brainstem is far less than that of the neocortex. The phylogenetically younger dermal matrix, which is well vascularized and basically inelastic, is the perfect mechanical closure for the skull. This structure reacts adequately to rapid volume increases of the brain and is therefore not a mechanical barrier to brain growth. In the case of the slowly growing brain of the shark, it is not important for the calvaria to be mechanically flexible; for higher animals with a continually increasing brain volume, a flexible cranial roofing is necessary.

To summarize, the neurocranium includes the skull base, the structure of which is only indirectly affected by the increases in brain volume, and the calvaria, which transforms all tensions due to brain growth directly in its morphological development. In phylogeny, the complete developmental history of a race or group of animals, this is demonstrated by the fact that the shape of the skull base undergoes far smaller changes than the shape of the vault.

The neurocranium has growth centres in its sutures and in synchondroses. Alongside the sutures, bone is created to enlarge the calvaria. Synchondroses are places where the skull base is not (yet) ossifying. The rate of fission of the cartilage cells in the synchondrosis determines the growth of the skull base. If ossification is faster than cartilage growth, the synchondrosis is closed and interstitial growth of the skull base is stopped. Because sutures do not ossify, adaptations in shape between the bones of the neurocranium remain possible throughout life. Interstitially, the neurocranium remains an active growth centre.

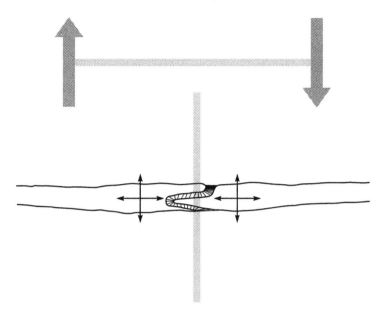

Figure 1.6 The stress transducing system of the suture (see text) transduces all tensions on the suture into strain in the bone

Outside the sutures and synchondroses, the shape of the skull bones is being constantly altered subperiosteally. Both resorption and apposition processes take place here.

The growth of the nose, and nasopharynx

The skull base experiences little stress by remodelling loads due to brain growth and, therefore, offers opportunities for the development of a nasopharynx. The ventilation, sucking and swallowing functions only start after birth and at that time a large part of the brain has been formed. Next to the chondral matrix of the nasal septum the maxillary and nasal dermal matrices grow symmetrically. The joints between these matrices are the facial and maxillary sutures. The mechanical load (from ventilation) causes an increase in these matrices and by means of the sutures the matrix parts can move away from one

another. This moving away occurs due to selective bone increases along the facial sutures.

A specific growth activity is induced by the development of the so-called pneumatic sinuses. These sinuses (the nasal cavities) are connected with the nasopharynx. Each inspiration or expiration causes a change in the mechanical pressure in the various sinuses. During growth a considerable enlargement of these cavities occurs. These enlarging cavities exert an increasing mechanical stress on the nasal skeleton. The chondral growth of the nasal septum consolidates this growth in a ventral direction, while the facial sutures are also affected by this growth process and by the consolidation of the nasal septum. In this growth process, the nasal septum acts as a bar to secure an open window. By consolidating the ventral replacement of the surrounding tissues of the nasopharynx, the cartilage in the nose acts as a stress transducer in a specific direction. The morphology of the sutures also transforms this stress into a mechanical stress on the dermal bone matrix. The growth of the nasal septum and the growth along the facial sutures is the expression of the changes in the ventilation function. The development of the nasal cavities not only contributes to an improved buffer function for the respirated air, but is also a mechanical load on the growing facial skull.

The growth of the processus alveolaris

The investing layer, the sacculus dentis, induces a dermal matrix around the dental germ layers, thereby developing a dental crypt.[38] These crypts are connected by the blood vessels (Figure 1.7a). The volume increase due to the growth of a dental germ layer increases the crypt. Such resorptive processes change the physical structure of the bone matrix. The 'growing' crypts load the bone matrix via the endosteal membrane. The mouth functions, sucking and swallowing, load the periosteal membrane of the matrix. Together these processes increase the alveolar bone volume (Figure 1.7b). Once more, the maxillary suture acts here as a stress transducer in the matrix. After perforation of the matrix, the eruption (which is completely due to the endosteal crypt membrane),[39] the endosteal crypt membrane and the periosteal membrane fuse.[9] After the opening of the dental crypts a connection (junction) appears between former endosteum, now called periosteum of the crypt, and the existing periosteum of the jaw (Figure 1.8).

Initially, only fibres form between the oral part of the periosteum and the erupting tooth, but after clinical load of the teeth the entire alveolar space, the periodontium,

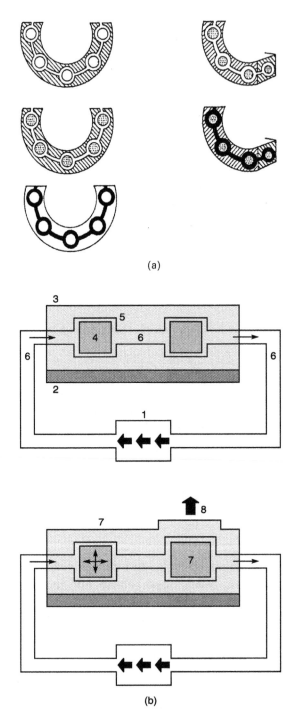

(a)

(b)

Figure 1.7 (a) The dental crypts in the alveolar bone are hydraulically connected by the vascular system. **(b)** 1 heart function; 2 mandibular bone; 3 alveolar process; 4 developing tooth; 5 dental crypt; 6 connection vessel; 7 growing tooth; 8 growth of the alveolar process

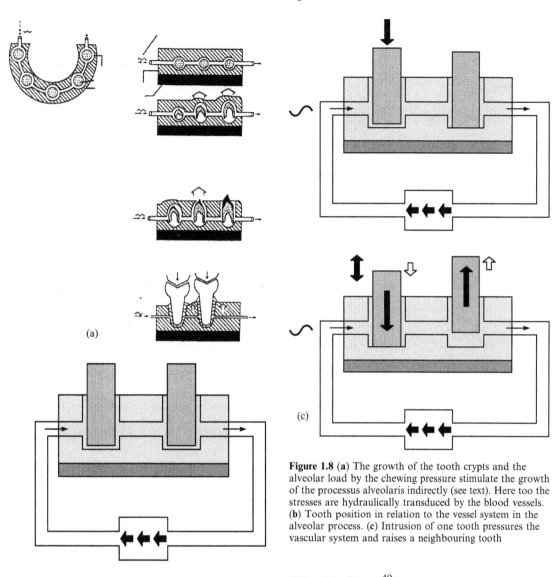

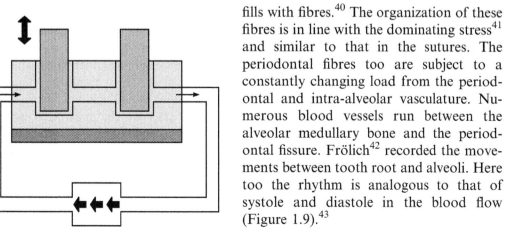

Figure 1.8 (**a**) The growth of the tooth crypts and the alveolar load by the chewing pressure stimulate the growth of the processus alveolaris indirectly (see text). Here too the stresses are hydraulically transduced by the blood vessels. (**b**) Tooth position in relation to the vessel system in the alveolar process. (**c**) Intrusion of one tooth pressures the vascular system and raises a neighbouring tooth

fills with fibres.[40] The organization of these fibres is in line with the dominating stress[41] and similar to that in the sutures. The periodontal fibres too are subject to a constantly changing load from the periodontal and intra-alveolar vasculature. Numerous blood vessels run between the alveolar medullary bone and the periodontal fissure. Frölich[42] recorded the movements between tooth root and alveoli. Here too the rhythm is analogous to that of systole and diastole in the blood flow (Figure 1.9).[43]

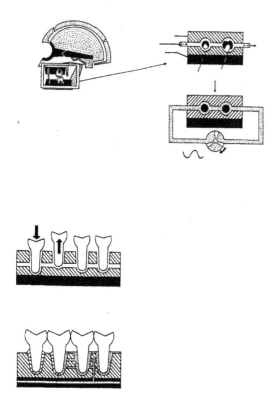

Figure 1.9 Vessel and fibre connections spread the occlusion and articulation forces over the entire processus alveolaris. The vascular flow restores the intrusion of the dental root

A special mechanical load is created by mastication. During mastication, the teeth are forced into the matrix.[27] The collective vessel connections, from periodontium to medullary bone, spread this force. The average pressure of the vascular pulse in the medullary bone is the physiological counterpressure for the chew load.[27] Chewing causes an apical movement of all elements of on average 1 mm per day, so all teeth are forced 1 mm into the jaw! During the night, the elements return to their initial positions. This highlights the load on the matrix by mastication. The influence of the mechanical stimulation on the growth of this dermal matrix will be discussed further in the section on growth regulation.

In children remarkable changes occur in the position of the deciduous teeth. As the crypt growth of the permanent teeth in the jaw proceeds, the processus alveolaris increases. This leads to spacing of the initially closed milk teeth: free spaces develop between the deciduous teeth. The germ layers of the permanent teeth are situated orally to the milk teeth, so the growing crypts increase the dental arch.

In summary, we may note that there is a great similarity in the mechanical load transmission from the teeth to the alveolar bone, and the mechanical load transmission among the bone parts bordering a suture. In both anatomical structures gomphoses develop; periodontium and suture. Basically, there is no physiological difference between sutures and periodontia; during growth both structures act as stress transducers (Figure 1.10).

The growth of the mandible

None of the chondral matrices that create the mandible in lower animal species are present in the formation of the human jaw. However, the chondral cartilage of Meckel is the first support of the complete dermal mandibular matrix,[20] which develops as two paired bars where the inferior alveolar nerve crosses Meckel's cartilage. In humans, the formation of the mandible is due to the formation of a dermal bone matrix. Meckel's cartilage controls the shape of the fusion of the two mandibular matrices in the mental symphysis.

This part of the matrix, roughly from canine to canine, has a particularly stable morphometry. The morphometry of the angle and the ramus develops under the influence of a large mechanical load, without supporting cartilage regeneration (Figure 1.11).

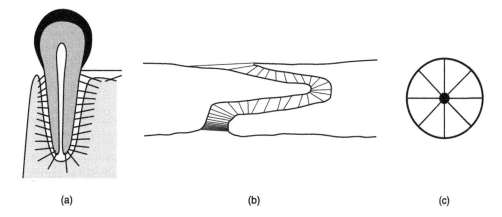

Figure 1.10 All gomphoses are basically the same and regarding mechanical function, can be compared to the spokes in a wheel (see text). **(a)** the dental gomphosis (periodontium); **(b)** the sutural gomphosis (suture); **(c)**: a wheel with spokes

The development of a secondary cartilage nucleus in this dermal bone matrix (the head of the mandible) has been ascribed to the fetal load from the skull. This secondary cartilage nucleus remains covered with matrix periosteum throughout its genesis. The temporomandibular joint is the only synovial joint in the body which is not covered by cartilage but by periosteum.

As the mastication function starts, the mandibular caput and base experience a direct mechanical load through the attached mastication muscles. The processing of these large forces is seen in the very compact matrix structure and in the chondral part of it in the caput. The fact that this chondral caput matrix is maintained throughout life highlights the necessity for durability of this part of the bone matrix.

Immediately after birth the mandible is positioned far more distally than in the adult skull. The angle is initially much bigger and the ramus can hardly be distinguished. During sucking and swallowing, the muscles bring the mandible into a more ventral position. This increases the space in the temporomandibular joint. This

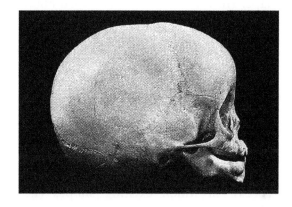

Figure 1.11 The skull of a young child shows the growth of the tooth within the alveolar bone

growth load stimulates the growth of the head of the mandible. This secondary cartilage disc is thus occurring secondary to the functional joint load. The growth keeps the joint space (despite the load) small. If a distal position of the mandible still exists (malocclusion) in adolescence, a functional activator can stimulate the growth of the head of the mandible. Such a regulation appliance stimulates the mastication muscles, which bring the jaw into a more ventral position.

Growth regulation

All living organisms, different as they may be, have two basic aspects: incarnation (the shape) and information (the function). Initially, the shapes of many embryos show great similarities. However, during development the mutual differences increase. In functional behaviour big differences develop between species, but before these functional differences are expressed, a strong resemblance in shape can be observed. Functional behaviour is, therefore, somehow associated with the development of shape, while specific functional behaviour is not possible in the absence of the necessary shape. How does an organism learn about its specific shape and what is the course of such developmental processes?

It is evident that the DNA composition of the gene plays a part in this process, but gene structure and quantity are of minor importance: a simple potato has a much more complicated DNA structure than man and the DNA of two fruit flies, identical in shape, may differ greatly.

Thus growth control is a multicausal process, in which existing shapes (i.e. current incarnations) learn to adopt subsequent shapes. External factors and functional processes (information) influence this 'learning process'. The tissue status, the receptive factor, ensures that a fish embryo grows into a fish and not into a chicken. The tissue status of a fish is only receptive to the incarnating functional stimulation that leads to the adult fish shape. Without functional stimulation, these genetic properties do not lead to growth. Each incarnation state is a perfect reaction to the current functional stimulation. During the growth phase of the organism the functional stimulation results in a reaction of the tissue status and thus growth (incarnation changes).

Returning to the growth control of the head: here too, a series of successive incarnations can be discerned. First is the development of the brain with the development of the skull base and the calvaria as a direct consequence. Here too, each new incarnation is capable of learning to grow further. When the first hard (i.e. inflexible) structures like cartilage and bone have developed in the head, this results immediately in the manifestation of new properties from the gene. Genetic information is nothing but a 'biologically solidified' past, and therefore any ontogeny is a repetition of phylogeny.

The choice of the primary nature of the bone matrix, bone or cartilage, has also been determined in a genetically distant past. Orientation depends partly on the current local functional processes and in part on the gene in the cell. Two examples from the ontogeny illustrate this.

Example 1
The area caudal to the brainstem experiences a compressing stress, on the one hand from the blood flow, which at that point in time is almost exclusively cranial in direction,[25] and on the other hand from the strongly expanding growth of the cortex. As in all embryonic areas with compressing stress, the bone matrix of first choice is cartilage.

Example 2
The area between dermal ectoderm and dura mater, the future calvaria, experiences strain load due to the growth of the neocortex. In line with the embryonic scenario, the bone matrix here is plexiform bone.

The choice of the bone matrix controls the design (the subsequent incarnation) and is, at the same time, crucial for the function (the subsequent information). Therefore, the hard tissues indirectly control the growth of the head in the successive growth phases. To put it another way: from a mechanical point of view, the hard tissue parts are the functional instruments that enable further growth. Unfortunately, this aspect is often not recognized. This has led to an unnecessarily complicated growth theory, with too many causal factors. Van Limborgh[17,44] arranged the growth systems by means of an extensive system of genetic, epigenetic and internal and external environmental factors that were divided into general and local factors. Of course, a growth theory like that explains everything, but it is questionable whether it increases clinical understanding of growth control. Furthermore, an open-minded reader may misinterpret this otherwise excellent growth theory because Van Limborgh offers the possibility of considering genetic growth factors as separate controlling influences, distinct from the grown entity. This is in contradiction to reality. The theory advanced here on possible growth control is less complicated and is a direct answer to the observations that any aware clinician can make. In this respect, it is important to realize that shape and function are linked inseparably and together make up the instrument that allows the genetic information laid down in each cell to develop.

Growth control is, therefore, only a series of developments, elaborating logically on an existing shape (incarnation). Mechanical stimulation, stemming from the initial functional processes, induces specific (embedded in the gene) morphology. A determining factor for the ideal development of this complicated combined action of shape and function is the result which is achieved in each growth phase. For it is only as a result of existing growth that the organism receives a signal (genetically embedded) for subsequent meaningful development.

Disturbances of this unique growth pattern can be seen in pathological and experimental growth results. If, for instance, a fusion process in the facial skull does not occur, as in the case of harelip, there will be a maximum adaptation but the final result is always a larger morphological defect than just a failing fusion process. The greater the disorder in the fusion processes, the greater the clinical consequences for the patient. Closing of a facial cleft cannot undo the growth disorder. In addition to the present facial cleft the adjacent skull parts are always stunted, which leads to a shortage of tissue. This shortage of tissue is the direct consequence of the inability of the organism to build on a failure in a previous growth phase. Each surgical correction of the facial cleft during growth will increase the resulting deformity to such an extent that repeated surgery will be necessary. For an optimal course of growth, a late surgical correction after growth has been completed is always the best by far. The social necessity for early surgical intervention is disregarded here.

Growth regulation has no functional priorities. The function itself regulates its influence on growth. For example, if the ventilation function is disturbed, for instance because of a restricted nasal passage during growth, less pneumatization develops in the nasal cavities. A high palate and a narrowing of the maxilla are the clinical results. Obviously, there is no such thing as a genetic morphology! All organisms have the ability to make the most of their genetically embedded growth control. However, if within the series of growth processes a morphological development fails, the growth control of the next morphological developments will always be disturbed. Thus, genetic control is dependent on the result of the previous control. This can also be regarded as a negative consequence of modular construction methods, which are typical for biological life. On the one hand, modular construction methods guarantee a solid and tested progression of successful evolutionary creations. On the other hand, this makes ontogeny dependent on successfully achieved growth phases, for the perfection of a module is the necessary starting point for a further successful morphogenesis.

Morphogenesis after the 'adult' growth result

Clinical studies into growth and development seem to be reserved for paediatrics. However, a sound understanding of growth and shape development of our musculoskeletal system is absolutely essential for adequate treatment of pathogenesis. The human body is not a machine that provides labour or products which can be stopped then restarted for the next task. On the basis of external stimulation, every body will adapt as much as possible to its (changing) circumstances. The extent of these adaptations is embedded in the genes. The duration of the pathogenesis is, therefore, likely to be very important for the consequences of this 'adaptation process'. To be able to estimate when a specific clinical function leads to the development of pathogenesis, we need to know the total functional relations in the organism. This requires a more than perfect knowledge and is, therefore, impossible.

Discussion

As far as the skull is concerned, the knowledge gained from monitoring growth and development demonstrates that in addition to the temporomandibular joints, the skull has many flexible connections, i.e. sutures and periodontia. From these 'joints' neural information flows continually. If one of these joints is disturbed, there will also be a disturbance in the total reflex framework, which may result in dysfunction and pain. Unfortunately, this is understood by only a small number of clinicians. Too often we are guided by our allegedly perfect knowledge of the musculoskeletal system. The clinician should keep in mind the behaviour of the skull and give more consideration to the fact that it is a dynamic joint complex (see also Chapter 2). This may be a basis for the development of signs and symptoms. Clinicians should influence the potential skull growth and its function, based on mechanical stimulation through the stress transducing principle, both in the young and in the old. Patients who do not react to our therapy are regarded as psychotic or, even worse, as malingerers. In his study 'Efficiency in occlusal function' Guzay[45] tries to convince us of the relation between the vertebral musculoskeletal system and the functional jaw. Much still needs to be added to our knowledge of the functioning of the sutural and periodontal musculoskeletal system. With this chapter I hope to have made a positive contribution to the discussion of the importance of the flexibility of the sutural joints. They are of crucial importance during growth, but of no less importance as parts of the cranial musculoskeletal system during function after the growth phase. They can be a cause of dysfunction and pain throughout the individual. Therefore, the clinician has to develop manual skills to examine and treat, as proposed in Chapters 2, 4 and 7.

References

1 Slack, J. M. W. (1983). *From Egg to Embryo*. Cambridge University Press.
2 Moss, M. L. and Salentijn, L. (1969). The capsular matrix. *Am. J. Orthod.*, **56**, 474–490.
3 Moss, M. L. (1972). Twenty years of functional cranial analysis. *Am. J. Orthod.*, **61**, 479–485.
4 Moss, M. L. (1958). Rotations of the cranial components in the growing rat and their experimental alteration. *Acta Anat.*, **32**, 65–86.
5 Moss, M. L. (1967). The primary role of the functional matrices in facial growth in the rat. *Am. J. Orthod.*, **55**, 566.
6 Oudhof, H, A. J. and van Doorenmaalen, W. J. (1983). Skull morphogenesis and growth: hemodynamic influence. *Acta Anat.*, **117**, 181–186.
7 Oudhof, H. A. J. (1986). Functional structure of the suture. *Nova Acta Leopoldina*, **262**, 459–464.
8 Oudhof, H. A. J. and Markens, I. S. (1982). Transplantation of the interfrontal suture in the wistar rat. *Acta Anat.*, **113**, 39–46.
9 Oudhof, H. A. J. (1978). *De betekenis van de suturae cranii in de groei van het calvarium*. Thesis, Utrecht.74
10 Oudhof, H. A. J. (1982). Sutural growth. *Acta Anat.*, **112**, 58–68.
11 Amprino, R. (1967). Bone histophysiology. *Guy's Hosp. Rep.*, **116**, 51–69.
12 Enlow, D. H. (1982). *Handbook of Facial Growth*. Saunders.
13 Enlow, D. H. (1968). Wolffs law and factor of architectonic circumstance. *Am. J. Orthod.*, **54**, 083–821.
14 Van de Klaauw, J. C. (1952). Cerebral skull and facial skull. A contribution to the knowledge of the architecture of the skull, based on literature. *Arch. Neerl. Zool.*, **9**, 369–560.
15 Popa, G. I. (1936). Mechanostruktur und Mechanofunktion der Dura mater des Menschen. *Morph. Jb.*, **78**, 85–187.
16 Sicher, H. (1952). *Oral Anatomy*. Mosby.
17 Van Limborgh, J. (1970). A new view on the control of the morphogenesis of the skull. *Acta Morph. Neerl. Scand.*, **8**, 143-161.
18 Klima, H. (1988). *Stimulation by Laserlight in Dissipative Biological Systems*. Lecture, Dallas.
19 Van der Bijl, G. (1986). *Het Individuele Functiemodel in de Manuele Therapie*. De Tijdstroom Lochum.
20 Schumacher, G. H. *et al.* (1986). Craniogenesis and craniofacial growth. *D. Ak. Natuurf.* Leopoldina.
21 Melcher, A. H. and Bowen, W. H. (1969). *Biology of the Periodontium*. Academic Press.
22 Sheldrake, R. (1988). *The Presence of the Past*. Times Books.
23 Van de Velde, J. P. *et al.* (1987). *De Ontwikkeling van het Kaakstelsel Ontogenie en Fylogenie*. Samson Stafleu.
24 Vroon, P. (1989). *Tranen van de Krokodil*. Ambo/Baarn.
25 Bruins, C. L. D. Ch. (1973). *De Arteriële Pool van het Hart*. Thesis, Leiden.
26 Shaw, J. H. *et al.* (1978). *Textbook of Oral Biology*. Saunders.
27 Oudhof, G. (1975). *Development and Growth of the Cranium*. Thesis.
28 Goose, D. H. and Appleton, J. (1982). *Human Dentofacial Growth*. Pergamon Press.
29 Massler, M. and Schour, I. (1951). The growth pattern of the cranial vault in the albino rat as measured by vital staining with Alzarin red 'S'. *Anat Rec.*, **110**, 83–101.
30 Prahl, B. (1968). *Sutural Growth. Investigation on the Growth Mechanism of the Coronal Suture and its Relation to the Cranial Growth in the Rat*. Thesis, Nijmegen.
31 Moyers, R. E. (1988). *Handbook of Orthodontics*. Yearbook Medical Publications Inc.
32 Van de Velde, J. P. (1985). *Bone Turnover and its Regulation*. Thesis, Amsterdam.
33 Markens, I. S. (1975). Embryonic development of the coronal suture in man and rat. *Acta Anat.*, **93**, 257–273.
34 Troitzky, W. L. (1932). Zur Frage der Formbildung des Schädeldaches. (Experimentele Untersuchung der Schädeldachnähte und der damit verbundenen Erscheinungen). *Z. Morph. Anthrop.*, **30**, 504.
35 Coulombre, A. J. and Coulombre, J. L. (1958). The role of the mechanical factors in the brain morphogenesis. *Anat. Rec.*, **130**, 289–290.
36 Jasper, H. H. J. and Marlet, S. (1974). Over de beenvorming in de dura mater bij dieren en mensen. *Arts en Wereld*, **7**, 5–19.
37 Markens, I. S. (1974). *De Embryonale Ontwikkeling van de Sutura Coronaria*. Thesis, Utrecht.
38 Osborn, J. W. and ten Cate, A. R. (1984). *Advanced Dental Histology*. John Wright & Sons.
39 Cahill, R *et al.* (1980). Tooth eruption: evidence for the dental follicle. *J. Oral Path.*, **9**, 189–200.
40 Bernich, S. (1960). Organisation of the periodontal membrane in rats. *Arch. Oral Biol.*, **2**, 57–63.
41 Herring, S. W. (1972). Sutures – a tool in functional cranial analysis. *Acta Anat.*, **83**, 222-247.
42 Von Frohlich, E. (1964). Die Bedeutung der Periphuren Durchblutungen des Parodontiums fur die Enstekung und therapie der Zahnbetterkrankungen. *Deut. Zahnarzt Z.*, **19**, 153–164.
43 Risinger, K. *et al.* (1996). The rhythms of human premolar eruption: a study using continuous observation. *JADA*, **127**, 100–128.
44 Van Limborgh, J. (1972). The role of genetic and local environmental factors in the control of postnatal craniofacial morphogenesis. *Acta Morph. Neerl. Scand.*, **10**, 37–47.
45 Guzay, C. M. (1991). Efficiency in occlusal function. *Basal Facts*, **7**.

Further reading

Azuma, M. (1970). Study on histological changes of the periodontal membrane incident to experimental tooth movement. *Bull. Tokyo Med. Dent. Univ.*, **17**, 149–178.

Baer, M. J. (1954). Patterns of growth of the skull as revealed by vital staining. *Hum. Biol.*, **26**, 80–126.

Bassett, C. A. L. (1962). Current concepts of bone formation. *J. Bone Jt. Surg.*, **44A**, 1217.

Bevelander, G. (1975). The fine structure of the human peridental ligament. *Anat. Rec.*, **162**, 312–326.

Bien, S. M. (1966). Fluid dynamic mechanisms, which regulate tooth movement. *Adv. Oral Biol.*, **2**, 173–201.

Bien, S. M. (1967). Difficulties and failures in tooth movement. Biophysical reponses to mechanotherapy. *EOS Rep. Congress Bern*, **53**, 55–62.

Bjork, A. A. (1964). Sutural growth of the upper face studied by the implant method. *Trans. Eur. Orthod. Soc.*, **40**, 48–64.

Boger, C. C. and Neptine, C. M. (1962). Patterns of blood supply to teeth and adjacent tissues. *J. Dent. Res.*, **41**, 158–171.

Borkland, G. A., Herley, J. D. and Irving, I. T. (1958). A histological study of the regeneration of completely disrupted periodontal ligament in the rat. *Arch. Oral Biol.*, **21**, 349–354.

Bosten, J. M. and Keeman, R. M. (1967). The formation of Sharpey's fibers in the hamster under non functional conditions. *Arch. Oral. Biol.*, **12**, 1331–1336

Bundgaard, M., Melsen, B. and Terp, S. (1986). Changes during and following total maxillary osteotomy (le fort 1 procedure): encephalometric study. *Eur. J. Orthod.*, **8**, 21–29.

Carels, C. and Van de Linden, F. P. G. M. (1987). Concepts on functional appliance's mode of action. *Am. J. Orthod.*, **92**, 162–168.

Chandler, H. (1971). *Textbook of Neuranatomy.* **XXVI**, 417–431.

Crennley, B. (1964). Collagen formation in normal and stressed periodontium. *Periodontics*, **2**, 53–61.

Eastoe, J. E. (1968). Collagen and tissue architecture. *Dent. Pract.*, **18**, 267–273.

Epker, B. N. and Frost, H. M. (1965). Correlation of bone resorption and formation with physical behavior of loaded bone. *J. Dent. Res.*, **44**, 33–41.

Giblin, N. and Alley, A. (1944). Studies in skull growth. Coronal suture fixation. *Anat. Rec.*, **88**, 143–153.

Girgis, F. G. and Pritchard, J. J. (1958). Effects of skull damage on the development of sutural patterns in the rat. *J. Anat.*, **92**, 39.

Girgis, F. G. and Pritchard, J. J. (1958). Experimental production of cartilage during the repair of fractures of the skull vault in rats. *J. Bone Jt Surg.*, **40B**, 274.

Griffin, C. I. (1972). Organisation and vasculature of human periodontal ligament mechanoreceptors. *Arch. Oral Biol.*, **17**, 713–921.

Ham, W. A. (1969). *Histology.* Lippincott.

Jackson, D. S. (1957). The formation and breakdown of connective tissue. *Connective Tissue.* S Tunbridge. CdRE: 62–76.

Justus, R. A. (1970). Mechanical hypothesis for bone remodeling induced by mechanical stress. *Calc. Tiss. Res.*, **5**, 222–235.

Kahlberg, K. (1974). Influence of periosteum on healing of tibial defects in the rat. *Odont. Rev.*, **25**, 157–164.

Khouw, F. E. (1970). Changes in vasculature of the periodontium associated with tooth movement in the rhesus monkey and dog. *Arch. Oral Biol.*, **15**, 1125-1132.

Körber, K. H. (1970). Periodontal pulsation. *J. Periodont.*, **41**, 382.

Kvam, E., Øsbøll, B. and Slagvold, O. (1973). Growth in width of the frontal bones after fusion of the metopic suture. *Acta Odont. Scand.*, **33**, 227–232.

Lacroix, P. (1948). Le mode de croissance du perioste. *Arch. Biol. Paris*, **59**, 379–391.

Linden-Aronson, S., Woodside, D. G. and Lindstrom, A. (1986). Mandibular growth direction following adenoidectomy. *Am. J. Orthod.*, **89**, 273-283.

Loaneli, C. (1987). *Permanent Maxillary Crypts in Man. A Study of Postnatal Development.* Thesis, Groningen.

Markens, I. S. (1970). The presence of alkaline phosphatase in coronal suture of the rat. *Acta Anat.*, **102**, 319–323.

Markens, I. S. and Oudhof, H. A. J. (1976). The occurrence and function of oxytalan fibers. *Netherl. Dent. J.*, **83**, 6-18.

Markens, I. S. and Oudhof, H. A. J. (1979). A study on the occurrence of alkaline phosphatase in the sutura interfrontalis of Wistar rats. *Acta Anat.*, **104**, 431–438.

Markens, I. S. and Oudhof, H. A. J. (1980). Morphological changes in coronal suture after replantation. *Acta Anat.*, **107**, 289–296.

Markens, I. S. and Taverne, A. A. R. (1978). Development of cartilage in transplanted future coronal sutures. *Acta Anat.*, **100**, 428–434.

Melcher, A. H. (1967). Remodelling of the periodontal ligament during eruption of the rat. *Arch. Oral Biol.*, **12**, 1649–1651.

Nanda, R. and Hickory, W. (1984). Zygomaticomaxillary suture adaptations to anteriorly directed forces in rhesus monkeys. *Angle Orthod.*, **54**, 199–210.

O'Brien, C. (1958). Eruptive mechanism and movement in the first molar of the rat. *J. Dental Res.*, **37**, 467–484.

Persson, M. (1973). Structure and growth of facial sutures. *Odont. Rev.*, **24**, 26.

Pritchard, J. J., Scott, J. H. and Girgis, F. G. (1956). The structure and development of cranial and facial sutures. *J. Anat.*, **90**, 73.

Quintarelli, G. (1959). The normal vascular architecture of the mandible periodontal membrane and gingiva in dogs. *Alabama Dent. Rev.*, **7**, 13–24.

Romulo, L. (1974). Histochemistry of ossification *Internat. Rev. Cyt.*, **II**, 283–306.

Rych, P. (1972). Ultrastructural cellular reactions in pressure zones of the ratmolar periodontium incident to orthodontic tooth movement. *Acta Odont. Scand.*, **30**, 575-593.

Schumacher, G. H. (1962). Anatomie und Fysiologie de Paradontium. *Deutsche Stomatol.*, **12**, 305.

Stockli, P. W. *et al.* (1987). Myofunktionelle Therapie. *Fortschr. der Kieferorthop.*, **48**, 460–463.

Storey, E. (1973). Tissue response to the movement of bones. *Am. J. Orthod.*, **64**, 229–247.

Storey, E. (1973). The nature of tooth movement. *Am. J. Orthod.*, **63**, 292-314.

Storey, E. (1972). Growth and remodelling of bones. *Am. J. Orthod.*, **2**, 142–165.

Strong, R. M. (1926). The order, time and rate of ossification of the albino rat skeleton. *Am. J. Anat.*, **36**, 313–352.

Stutzmann, J. and Petrovic, A. (1986). Ist der Bionator ein Orthopadisches und/oder ein Orthodontisches Gerat. Eine experimentelle klinische Studie. *Fortschr. Kieferorthop.*, **47**, 254–280.

Tarvonen, P. L. and Koski, K. (1987). Cranialfacial skeleton of 7-year-old-children with enlarged adenoid. *Am. J. Orthod.*, **91**, 300–304.

Van Beest, H. (1977). *Morfologie en Groei-activiteit van Faciale Suturen*. Thesis, Nijmegen.

Van de Linden, F. P. G. M. (1986). *Facial Growth and Facial Orthopedics*. Quintessence.

Van Doorenmaalen, W. J. (1986). Environmental factors in sutural growth. *Nova Acta Leopoldina*, **262**, 447–449.

Van Doorenmaalen, W. J. and Oudhof, H. A. J. (1981). Functional structure of the sutura cranii. *Verh. Anat. ges.*, **75**, 243.

Wagemans, P. A. H. M. *et al.* (1986). The postnatal development of frontonasal suture. *J. Dent. Res.*, **65**, 558.

Wagemans, P. A. H. M., van de Velde, J. P. *et al.* (1988). Sutures and forces: a review. *Am. J. Orthod.*, **94**, 129–141.

Wedl, C. Über Gefasskrauel im Zahnpereost. *Virchow's Arch.*, **85**, 175.

Weinmann, J. P. and Sicher, H. (1955). *Bone and Bones*. Mosby.

Young, R. G. (1962). Autoradiographic studies on postnatal growth of the skull in young rats injected with tritiated glycine. *Anat. Rec.*, **143**, 1.

2

Features of cranial tissue as a basis for clinical pattern recognition, examination and treatment

H. J. M. von Piekartz

Introduction. What lies above the atlanto-axial joint?

Most clinicians with a manual therapy background are trained in the fundamental examination and treatment of the cervical spine. For example there are standardized tests to screen for vertebral artery insufficiency[1] and reliability, and validity studies of intervertebral spinal movements have been undertaken.[2] But what about the structures above the atlanto-axial joint (excluding the temporomandibular joint)? Cranial tissue is still neglected by manual therapists in clinical situations as a subject for research. If we are open-minded and try to recognize clinical patterns that are probably related to the craniofacial region; perhaps we can better understand patients with long-term problems, for example: migraine, atypical facial pain, hemifacial spasm, tinnitus, trigeminal neuralgia, chronic sinusitis, pain after facial pareses, motor retardation and headache in children. With reference to recent literature and personal experience, differing terminology and methods of examination of the cranium are discussed in this chapter.

Terminology and definitions

The skull bones

Different terminology has been used in the literature to describe the same tissues. Clinicians who predominantly use passive movements in examination, treatment and assessment are helped by a classification which has clinical relevance, but is also understood by other professions. Therefore, the following terminology and definitions from the literature may be helpful.

Cranium: the skull without its mandible.
Neurocranium: the cranium without the facial bones.
Viscerocranium: the facial skeleton.
Calvaria: skullcap formed by frontal, occipital and parietal bones.
Skull base: temporal, sphenoid and occipital bones (Figure 2.1).[3,4]

From a clinical viewpoint these definitions are helpful. Personal clinical experi-

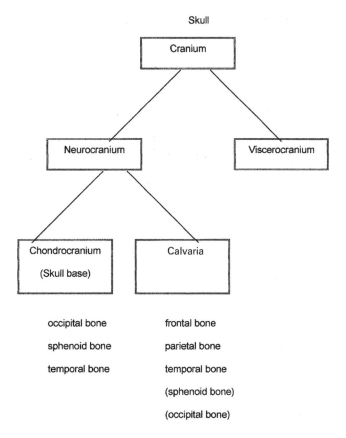

Figure 2.1 Anatomical classification of the cranium (adapted from Bourekas and Lanzieri, 1994[3])

ence suggests that passive movements of the neurocranial bones will cause different reactions depending on the area of the cranium that is influenced.

For example:

- The qualities of pain in the neurocranium are generally duller and greater in area. The facial skeleton has a more localized and sharper quality of pain.
- Facial bone mobilization after trauma generally responds faster than neurocranial bone mobilization in the same situation.
- Associated symptoms such as vertigo, dysphagia and dysarthria are easily reproduced or more easily reduced

with techniques on the neurocranial bones than on the facial skeleton.

Dynamic features of the cranium

Little is known about cranial bone motion. The commonly held belief that the cranial bones fuse in early life has been shown to be false.[5] Histological studies have supported the idea that the articulating surfaces of the cranial bones allow a small degree of movement.[6,7] Orthodontic and dental journals have published more articles relating to the field of cranial adaptation, changes and movement of the

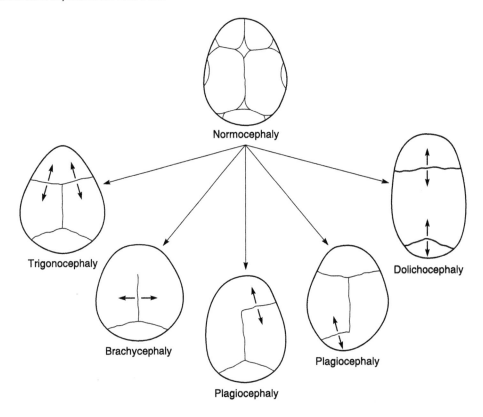

Figure 2.2 Types of craniosynosthosis. Trigonocephaly: malformation characterized by a triangular configuration of the cranium mostly in the frontal region. Brachycephaly: premature closure of the sutures between both parietal bones (sagittal sutures). Plagiocephaly: an asymmetric craniostenosis due to premature closure of the lambdoid and coronal sutures on one side, which is expressed in an asymmetrical face and neurocranium. Dolichocephaly: premature closure of coronal and lambdoid suture, which is expressed in an disproportionately long head (Adapted from Xu, Shephard and Xu[44])

cranium, in the past ten years than in the entire history of this field. Studies of skull growth measured by cephalometry have made enormous progress.[8–16] Owing to these new developments it is now known that the process of ossification starts in the mid-twenties, that the cranial sutures may remain open throughout life and that some motion and flexibility last into old age. It is now accepted that the cranium is not a rigid sphere of solid bone which ossifies in early life, rather it adapts to and changes with its environment independently.[17–22] Clinical evidence of this is seen in plastic and reconstructive surgery after premature craniosynostosis (closing of the sutures) (Figure 2.2). Corrections of persisting cranial deformities can still be made at 12 years of age.[23–30]

The nature of cranial movement (cranial dynamics)

The nature of the movements between the cranial bones still remains unclear. However, there is recognition among many clinicians (osteopaths, chiropractors, manual therapists, orthodontists and dentists) and researchers that the cranium has some mobility.[31–34]

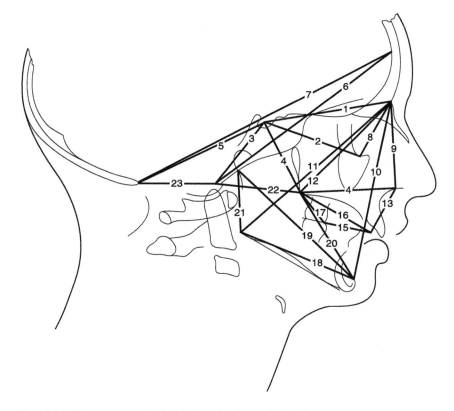

Figure 2.3 Different mathematical models predict the cranial facial growth in children, which can help the orthodontist in making clinical decisions. The numbers in the figure correspond with the main landmarks used during cephalometry (Adapted from de Bruin, 1993[16])

An overview of the different hypotheses on cranial bone movements (cranial dynamics) found in the literature follows.

Continuous, predictable and rhythmic motion

This type of cranial movement is widely regarded as the fundamental principle underlying cranial pathomechanics and is described by Sutherland[35] as one of the fundamental theories of osteopathy.[32,36,37]

Spontaneous, unpredictable motion

Cranial bones may move independently from each other. There is no consistent pattern of motion. Upledger and Vredevoogd maintain that the pressure of the vascular and cerebrospinal fluid circulations influence this motion of the bones.[32,36,38]

Movement by transduction of forces

Stresses and pressures are transduced through the skull and build up forces so that growth is stimulated in the whole craniofacial mandibular and cervical complex. The sutures play an important role in this stress-transducer mechanism.[39–42] This principle is well-known in orthodontic, dental and paediatric plastic surgical literature and is used in these fields. For example, in long-term cochlear implantation of auditory protheses in children it is known that the skull adapts without significant deformity.[43,44] The masticatory system (for example muscle tone and direction of forces),[34,45] the position of the mandible (condyle),[46,47] the teeth,[48–50] and the craniocervical junction[51–53] all influence cranial growth and form. The reverse also occurs. Patients with ocular torticollis (torticollis caused by abnormal eye position, strabismus) often develop facial asymmetry. A reduction in this facial asymmetry is made possible quite easily using strabismus surgery.[54,55] Orthodontists use mathematical models (cephalometry) to analyse the growth and change in forces using a specific splint therapy so that the dysfunction of the masticatory system and the craniofacial complex adapts in a favourable way (Figure 2.3).[16,56,57] Other external forces, for example cosmetic deformities of the orbit due to wearing glasses or a prolonged single sleep position (prone or supine), can promote deformation of the skull in young children.[58,59] (For more information see Chapter 1.)

In summary, it can be hypothesized that the cranial bones move owing to external forces, with the sutures playing an important role.[32] The nature of the movement and the effect upon the sutures of different forces related to the position and growth of the cranial bones is still unknown.[32,52,53] In other words, the dose–response relationship between the applied forces and the resulting effects on the biological tissue of the suture, followed by cranial bone changes, is still an open question.[60] Different therapeutic strategies such as cranial surgery, eye correction at an early age and manual therapy give empirical results, however, future investigations and studies of sutural growth and its regulation of cranial bone movements could lead to a better understanding of these clinical effects.

The sutures as a potential source of symptoms

Most previous studies on sutures have concentrated on the relationship between external forces and suture morphology,[31,37,60–69] and the biochemical responses during changes of cranial bone forces *in vitro* in animals and humans.[63,70–75] The question remains, can sutures be a source of nociceptive input and can this present with typical clinical patterns? Even within well-known organizations such as the International Association of the Study of Pain (IASP) or classifications of craniofacial pain or headache such as the Bell classification, there is no description of 'suture pain' or 'suture dysfunction'.[76]

Neuroanatomical, neurobiological and neurochemical studies of the sutures related to pain or other symptoms which may give clinicians a basis to explain unfamiliar or new clinical patterns are rare.[77,78] However, well-known classic studies that may help are those of Retzlaff and Mitchel,[36] and Bourekas and Lanzien.[3] They investigated cranial sutures using electronmicroscopy and revealed a high level of vascularization and innervation in the connective tissue and sutural ligaments.

Yen and Suga[71] and Meikle *et al.*[73] discovered differently innervated collagen types intrasuturally using electrophoresis. This collagen tissue was widely and abundantly present, and changed in response to short-term and long-term force application.[70] The function and type of nerve fibres which accompany these collagenous tissues have not been established.[70,71]

When sutures have Aδ and C fibres, abnormal forces on the sutures may cause neurobiological and mechanical changes which change the vascular system in the cranial region and which may, in turn, cause pathophysiological changes in the suture.[61] It can be hypothesized that passive movement of the cranium could possibly relieve forces within the sutures, which would be followed by changes in the local tissue and thus a reduction in the symptoms caused by these articulations, if indeed they are innervated.

Can the sutures be seen as a part of a joint complex?

One group of scientists, including traditional anatomists and clinicians, and orthopaedic surgeons, regards the skull as a rigid osseous structure with immovable sutures. This theory is predominantly based on the study of cadavers.[4,69,79,80] The other group, which includes orthodontists, cranial morphologists and those who are involved with manual therapy (for example manipulative physiotherapists, osteopaths and chiropractors), believes that the suture is a functional articulation that adapts constantly relative to its environment, even into old age.[31,75,81–86] In *Gray's Anatomy*, the suture has been described as a *solid* non-synovial joint with interosseous connective tissue (fibrous *joint*).[4] Linking the words 'solid' and 'joint' seems contradictory. The variation in the terminology used to describe the contact of two cranial bones pervades the literature on the subject. 'Fibrous' or 'solid connections' and 'articulations' or 'joints' are used in the same context and in the same literature, which can be confusing.[69,73,87–91]

Sutures:
- are structures between the bones which are recognized by membranous ossification and made of dense fibrous connective tissue and are pliable and flexible (Bourekas – a radiologist).[3]
- are solid non-synovial joints with interosseous connective tissue (William and Warwick – anatomists).[4]
- form a strong (band of) union between adjacent bones while permitting slight movements (Pritchard – anatomist).[92]
- are bony connections, which have autonomous growth capacity, and which can be influenced by local external forces (Wagemans – orthodontist).[31]

From a clinical perspective a joint can be defined in a more 'open-minded' way, for example 'functional unit' may be appropriate. A good example of this is Maitland's definition:[93] 'Any non-contractile tissue which moves or is moved independently from other tissue during any active or passive movement'. It may be concluded that the suture has the potential to be a joint-like structure, which can in turn be responsible for dysfunction, pain and other symptoms. Passive movements can be useful tools with which to examine and treat the cranial bone tissue. However, the clinician has to be aware that during the application of passive movement to the cranium it is not only the tissues in the region of the individual suture (joint) that are being examined, as in the examination of a peripheral joint – rather that compression and decompression forces are being transmitted through the cranial and perhaps intracranial tissues.[94–103]

Which structures can be influenced by passive movements?

The anatomy of the craniofacial region is enormously complex and includes many different structures (bones, nerves, blood vessels etc.).[104] As a clinician it is important to reflect on which structures one can

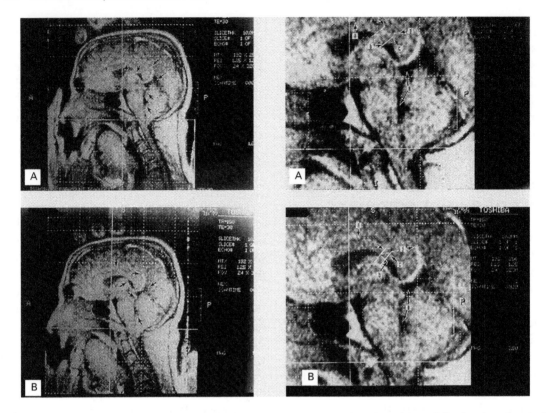

Figure 2.4 Mid-sagittal MRI scan of an adult human brain, before (A) and after (B) the cranial mobilization. Note how brain tissue has moved (black arrows in picture B on the left side), particularly the corpus callosum (a), lateral ventricle (b) the fornix column and the fourth ventricle (e) (picture B on the right side). (From Pick, 1994), A preliminary single case magnetic resonance imaging investigation into maxillary frontal-parietal manipulation and its short-term effect upon the intracranial structures of an adult human brain. *J. Manipul. Physiol. Ther.*, **17**, 168–173 by kind permission of Lippincott Williams & Wilkins[125])

influence with 'hands on' examination and treatment. The main structures are briefly discussed below.

Cranial bones, sutures and nerves.

Please refer to the section on cerebrospinal fluid following, and also to Chapters 1 and 7, which describe the behaviour of these structures in detail.

Dural attachments

The meninges have a firm attachment to the inside of the atlas and the occiput, and also to the connective tissue within the cranial sutures.[74,75] Butler (1991) has already described the nervous system as an electrical, chemical and mechanical continuum.[78]

A strong correlation has been suggested between (the influence of) the condition of the dura, suture morphology and the cerebrospinal circulation.[105–112] Abnormal conditions of the dura influence the growth, the shape of the cranium and its environment.[113–117] Abnormal short-term or long-term forces change the mechanical and physiological condition of the dura.[118–121] The effect of extracranial pressure on intracranial membranes, brain and dura mater has been demonstrated.[122–123] Pick,[125] for example, undertook a single case study using a magnetic resonance imaging investigation into passive movements of the maxillary frontal-parietal region and their short-term effects upon the intracranial structures of an adult human brain. Positional changes were seen in the corpus callosum (fornix column) and the lateral vesicle. This study supports the hypothesis that cranial passive movements influence the brain (Figure 2.4). Other studies on humans suggest that passive movements of the different cranial bones transfer effects to the dural meningeal system so that the environment of the brain can be altered.[119–121]

Intracranial vascularization

Important functions of the vascular system of the cranium are as follows:

- the cranial bones form a solid wall for the brain which bathes in a pool of blood; it is known that a change in skull pressure of intracranial and external origin can compromise or change the blood flow of intracranial blood vessels.[111,126,128]
- cranial vault bones are active in blood cell formation.[76,89,129]
- the rich innervation of the intracranial blood vessels by the sympathetic nervous system. The brain utilizes 20% of the total oxygen uptake of the body and needs a good blood supply. One factor that restricts blood flow to the brain is cerebrovascular resistance.[32] During various experiments it has been observed that there is a close relationship between the vascular innervation of the cranial bones and the central regulation system – hypophysis, trigeminal nucleus and periaqua-

ductal grey (PAG). No one has yet identified clear pathways from the sutures to specific areas of the nervous system.[130–133]

In the clinic I have observed that passive movements applied to the patient's cranium can change physical reactions, which are possibly based in altered autonomic reactions. For example, the feeling of a warm head with reduction of the 'pumping' headache, together with flushing, slowly increasing vertigo and sweating during or after the application is not unusual. It is true to say that in the clinic we observe these clinical patterns and believe that they are due to a vascular reaction, but clinical evidence of and fundamental research into this are still lacking.[60]

Cerebrospinal fluid (CSF)

The cranium provides an ideal container for the CSF. CSF circulation is necessary for the transport of substances such as neurotransmitters, nutrients, and waste products required to maintain the homeostasis of the central nervous system.[4,134–136]

The CSF and associated intracranial dynamics, such as the nature of the CSF circulation, the driving forces of the CSF and the major routes for the absorption of the CSF, are altered in pathological situations such as hydrocephalus, Parkinson's disease, meningitis and cranial neuropathy.[135,137–140] Clinicians suggest that something similar occurs in minor pathologies – for example, post-traumatic headache, craniomandibular dysfunctions and atypical facial pain – but this has not been proven. When one applies manual techniques to the facial region, one may sometimes see unexpected changes in the patient's signs and symptoms, perhaps related to the CSF. Some unexpected

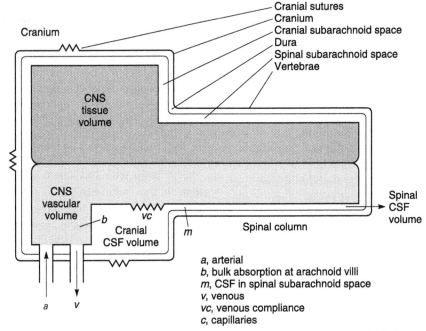

Figure 2.5 This model accounts for the dynamic and steady-state volume–pressure buffering characteristics of the intact cranium and spinal cord. The total cranial compliance arises in part from the system's ability to distribute its internal volumes of blood (arterial (*a*) and venous (*v*)) and CSF into the systematic venous circulation (*b*) and/or CSF into the spinal subarachnoid space (*m*). The cranial bone mobility (but also the intracranial fluid movement) contributes to the total cranial compliance. This depends on the suture compliance and the increase of intracranial volume (CNS tissue volume and CNS vascular volume) (adapted from Heisey, S. R. and Adams, T., 1993[142])

patient reactions after application of passive movement on the cranium were:

- 'My sciatic pain changed a few hours after that pressure on my skull.'
- 'The low back pain suddenly stopped after the treatment.'
- 'My depressed feelings and the headaches have decreased. I feel much fitter than over the last 2 months.'
- 'The burning eye pain was severe for a long time after the treatment.'

A possible hypothesis could be that the CSF moves *and* that biochemical changes occur during and after cranial intervention. Adams and Heisey[141,142] showed the importance of cranial bone mobility in anaesthetized cats, using a newly developed instrument for quantification of cranial bone movement, by measurement of CSF

movements. When the intracranial volume (ICV) increases the cranium adapts (using the phenomenon described above), which can be called cranial compliance. The total cranial compliance depends on the mobility of intracranial fluid and movement of the cranial bones at their sutures, when there is an increase in ICV (Figure 2.5). Even with small increases in ICV, cranial bone mobility plays an important role. This suggests that in minor pathological changes the CSF dynamics may also occur, and that the movement of cranial bones during examination or treatment may change the CSF dynamics.

The brain

Studies have shown that frontal and lateral impact injuries to the brain mass affect the dura and the cranial membranes.[143–144] Fewer studies have investigated the influence of passive movements on the brain mass. Pick showed the short-term effect of passive movements on an adult human brain in a preliminary single case study, which is described earlier (Figure 2.4).[125] Margulies *et al.*,[144] Adams *et al*[141] and Heisey and Adams[142] described the importance of the role of the sutural system in total cranial compliance. By increasing the intracranial volume, the important role played by the brain in movements of the cranial bones at their sutures has been demonstrated.[32,37,141,145] Conversely it can be hypothesized that changing pressure on the cranium influences intracranial pressure and, therefore, influences the movement and forces in the brain. Osteopaths have believed for a long time in the powerful effects of cranial techniques on the brain and dura. They describe the brain as a motile organ with inherent rhythmic movements, and are strongly convinced that head position and dural tension also influence the brain motility.[38,146,147] Studies show that on movement from the neutral position to maximal flexion of the head, there is a strong increase in tension of the dura and the intracranial membranes, and the brainstem lengthens by about 1 cm.[148,149] Cinematography of the brain after laminectomy shows shape changes of the brain and a characteristic lateral translation.[74,89] The intracranial volume (ICV) and pressure could also be influenced and can have consequences for examination and treatment by cranial dynamics.[138]

Cranial nervous tissue

Within the cranium there are numerous sites where nerves may be impinged upon by soft tissue at bony ridges or foraminal openings. There are many vulnerable points and potential mechanical interface (tissue which contacts the peripheral nervous system) problems for the cranial nerves, which may in due course reflect as mechanical and/or physiological changes in the nervous system. This may lead to a cranial peripheral neuropathy.[104,150,151] Passive movements may reduce (or increase) pressure in intra- or extracranial structures by changing the pathodynamics of these nerves. For detailed information see Chapter 7.

The muscles

Masticatory and neck muscles cross the cranial articulations and can influence the osseous relationships and intra-articular stress patterns of the cranial vault.[152–156] Studies have shown that resection of cranial muscle during growth on mammals revealed changes in craniofacial growth due to muscle balance.[151,157–161] In humans there are also hypotheses on neuromuscular (im)balance and craniofacial morphology. For example, with long-term bruxism there may be a significant correlation between the large diameter of the (masseter) muscle and the asymmetry of the face.[155,157] Further, with congenital torticollis, the sternocleidomastoid muscle pulls more at the dorsolateral side of the cranium and changes the skeletal balance, which can in turn be expressed as cranial asymmetry and morphological changes of the first cervical vertebra (Figure 2.6).[162–164] Knowledge of the quality, behaviour and mechanisms of cranial, cervical and jaw muscle pain has improved during the last decade.[162] However, there appear to be no direct studies concerning the contribution of pain or symptom distribution from the cranium in such situations. Clinically it may often be noted that cranial muscle tone

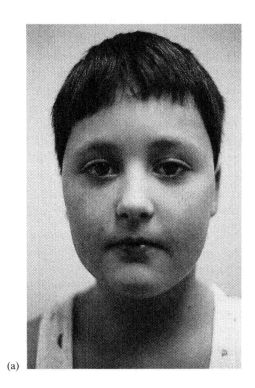

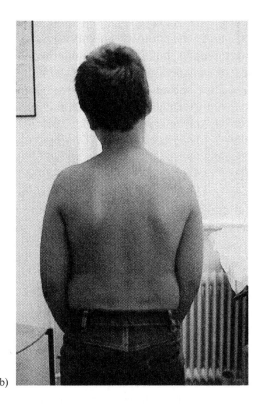

(a) (b)

Figure 2.6 (a) A 9-year-old male patient with the diagnosis of congenital muscular torticollis, with the main complaints of unilateral headache (right side) and disturbance of concentration. Note the asymmetry in the face (orbits, ears, frontal region). **(b)** The same patient with an asymmetrical position (side flexion of the neck towards the left elevation, left shoulder, elevated scapula)

decreases alongside the relief of symptoms in this region following treatment with passive movements, and this suggests a strong functional relationship between these structures. (For more information about this subject see Chapter 9.)

'Hands on' skills. A basis for assessment and management strategies

The terms 'hands on' and 'hands off' have been clearly described clinically by McIndoe.[165] As a physiotherapist and psychologist she emphasized the need for both strategies, especially for patients in a chronic pain state. As a strategy Hands on is mainly used to identify the sources of

the symptoms and to classify the pain mechanisms, but can also have a role in monitoring reactivity, as a form of communication and for education, rather than a quick fix.[65,78] A decision needs to be taken on whether other strategies should be used, such as other manual techniques, treatment with equipment or other 'hands off' management. Hands off in the right framework can lead to skills for self-help and self-treatment.[166] The disadvantages of hands on are that it can lead to nocebo[167] and can discourage active participation. Passive movement of the cranial region may be a basic hands on tool for further clinical management of patients with a variety of clinical presentations (see also Chapter 7).

Examples of examination and treatment by passive movements of cranial tissue

The only types of passive movements applicable to the cranium are accessory movements (movements which cannot be performed actively by the patient but only passively by another person).[93] The movement direction of accessory movements is defined by the direction in which the clinician performs the accessory movement, for example an antero-posterior movement of the zygoma or longitudinal movement of the temporal bone. An advantage of testing movements in differing directions is that clinical decisions can remain open as to which possible structure(s) influence the cranial dysfunction and pain. Multiple structures, and also multiple pathobiological mechanisms, may influence the signs and symptoms of any particular patient.[93,168]

Dependent upon the clinical presentation of the patient's problems, passive movement to different regions of the cranium is indicated. As a result of my clinical experience with manual techniques the strategy shown in Table 2.1 is suggested.

Table 2.1

Neurocranium	General techniques	Occipital-frontal region
		Occipital region
		Frontal region
		Temporal region
		Parietal region
	Specific techniques	
Viscerocranium	General techniques	Orbit
		Zygoma
		Maxilla
	Specific techniques	

When the symptoms of the patient are thought to relate to the craniofacial region in most cases neurocranial techniques are proposed, because they have more influence in changing stress or effecting movement of larger regions of the cranium. Therefore, it is often useful to apply techniques in different regions as described above. Which region one starts with can depend, for example, on the pain area, history and observation. When a patient complains of symptoms in the temporomandibular region, primary examination of the temporal region is indicated.

When from the history and from observation it is clear that the patient has a plagiocephaly, occipital-frontal examination makes sense in most cases. General techniques are in my opinion useful:

- to gain an impression of severity, irritability and the pain state from which the patient suffers.
- to give information about which region has (relevant) dysfunction related to the patient's symptoms and to give an indication of whether to examine that region with more specific techniques.
- to allow the patient to become familiar with cranial techniques in general.

When the clinician feels that the responses to passive movements in one or more region(s) are abnormal, they can decide to examine or treat this region with more specific accessory movements of that bone or its neighbouring bones. The following are some techniques which are commonly used together. They are:

- general compression technique of the occipital-frontal region.
- transverse movement of the sphenoid-occipital region.
- rotation of the maxilla around the sagittal axis.

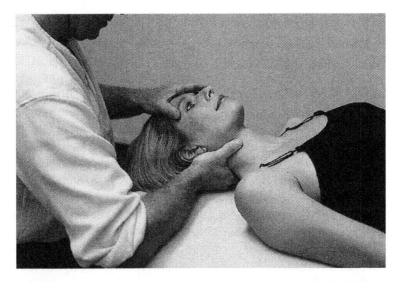

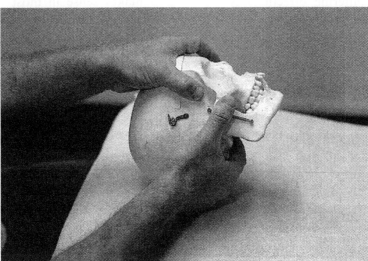

Figure 2.7 General compression technique of the occipital-frontal region

General compression technique of the occipital-frontal region

Starting position and method

The patient lies supine; you sit to the right of the patient with your right hand resting on the plinth. Hold the patient's occipital bone with the tips of your fingers on the left side. Place your left hand on the frontal bone keeping both elbows flexed and maintaining contact with your trunk (Figure 2.7). Apply increasing pressure with your left hand posteriorly while at the same time moving the right hand anteriorly in the opposite direction. By doing this you are increasing pressure on the cranium. Grasp with the whole volar side of both hands so that the pressure is evenly distributed.

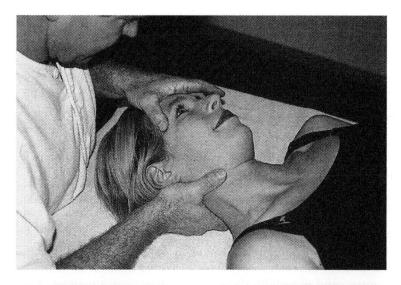

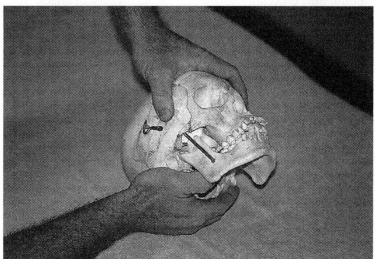

Figure 2.8 Transverse movements of the sphenoid bone in the occipital-sphenoid region

The same starting position can be used to create a decompression technique. Begin with your hands in the same position, make an anterior movement avoiding squeezing your thumb and fingers together, then make a posterior movement with your right hand.

The occipital-frontal compression is one of the most general movements because it influences many cranial tissues between the occipital and frontal bones. It also gives you an idea of the amount of force you need to apply relative to the condition of the patient. An advantage is that when using this technique you can easily modify the movement by an angulation to release or increase the patient's symptoms – for example, a post-whiplash patient with moderately irritable symptoms such as dizziness and dull headache which are reproduced by general compression but decreased by an angulation laterally towards the hand that cups the occipital bone. In cases where angulation changes the patient's symptoms, it is useful to examine the occipital region (the occipital bone and their neighbouring bones) in more detail, e.g. the occipital-sphenoid region (see below).

Transverse movement of the occipital-sphenoid region

Starting position and method

This technique is a common examination and treatment technique used when one has assessed that the general accessory movements of the cranium, and especially those in the occipital-sphenoid region, significantly change the symptoms of the patient.

Have the patient lying supine and comfortable and sit or stand at his head. Cup his occipital bone in your right hand, your elbow resting on the plinth. Hold the greater wings of the sphenoid bone between the tips of your thumb and index finger of your left hand (Figure 2.8). Steady your left forearm against your trunk during movement of the sphenoid bone to prevent extraneous movement.

Once again, it is important that it is your body and not your hands that create the movement. Apart from anchoring your forearm against your trunk, concentration on your thumb, index and middle fingers will help you to do this. Watch that the distance between the two fingers is always the same, ensuring that you avoid any increase in tone in your hand muscles. Ask the patient to inform you of any increase in localized pressure from your fingers.

Comment

The occipital-sphenoid joint is often one of the first regions to be examined. Some reasons for this might be:

- the relatively long duration of suture mobility, which can be a source of dysfunction and pain.[169] Researchers have varying opinions about the age at which union of the sutures occurs relative to the other cranial bones.
- the sphenoid bone and its foramina have the largest share of craniofacial growth, which can be a predisposition for neuropathies (see also Chapter 7).[170]
- because general signs and symptoms can be traced to deformation or dysfunction in this region, and this has consequences for neighbouring bones and foramina. The jugular foramen, which is formed by the temporal and occipital bone at the base of the skull, is a case in point. The jugular vein drains blood from the cranial vault, where cranial nerves IX, X and XI pass through the same foramina. Hence symptoms related to intracranial fluid congestion can be explored.[171] Clinicians are convinced of the significance of symptoms such as gag reflex problems, taste abnormality at the back of the tongue, problems with speech and swallowing, vagal symptoms like cranial arrhythmia, digestive disturbances and abnormal tone in the sternocleidomastoid and trapezius muscles.[32,169]

Rotation of the maxilla around the sagittal axis

This is a general intraoral technique of the facial region (viscerocranium). The aim of this technique is to establish whether the signs and symptoms are predominantly provoked from the maxillary region rather than the orbits or zygoma. When you find abnormal responses such as extreme stiff-

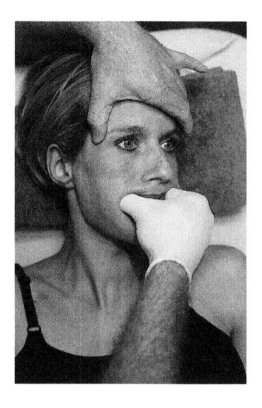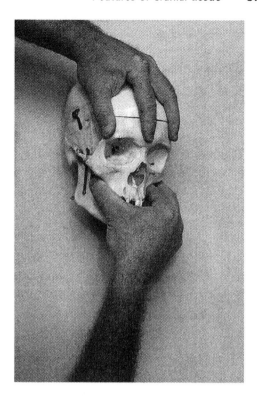

Figure 2.9 General rotations of the maxilla around the sagittal axis

ness on left and right rotation or reproduction of the patient's symptoms, this gives an indication that you should explore this region further with other accessory movements or neighbouring bones.

Starting position and method

The patient lies supine and is comfortable and relaxed. The plinth is at the height of your iliac crest. A small towel against the contralateral side of the head can be useful, particularly during rotation and transverse movements. The web space of your left thumb and left index finger span the frontal bone and stay on the right lateral border of the frontal bone or are contacting both greater wings of the sphenoid. This depends

on which is the main joint to be examined, the maxillofrontal or maxillosphenoid joint. Your right index finger is placed left and right intrabuccally on the maxilla above the teeth and beneath the zygomatic process. Contact the couch softly with the trunk and fix the medial side of the right elbow against your trunk so that you can bend over the patient (Figure 2.9).

During the movement make a slow trunk movement in the direction of the mobilization and prevent right forearm and hand movement. The distance between your right thumb and right index fingers stays the same without increasing local pressure on the bones. When the maxilla is too small on the lateral side, the longitudinal movement to caudal can be better accomplished using a unilateral technique.

During clinical observation I believe that

signs and symptoms related to asymmetry of the cranium, malocclusions, tempero-mandibular joint dysfunctions, neuropathic pain from the maxillary nerve and maxillary sinusitis indicate the need for assessment and, if necessary, further treatment of this region.

The reader will have realized that only a few examination and treatment techniques have been described but that doses have not been prescribed (force and duration of the application) or given their place in the overall management. These two factors, can be related to the:

- age of the patient: at around 30 morphological changes of connective tissue, constitution of blood vessels and innervation in and around the sutures occur.[92,172]
- region of the cranium: different regions seems to have different patterns of suture changes with age.[31,173]
- pathology: pathology can provide clues as to whether you will be able to make adjustments to the region and the intensity of passive movements. For example, a child with a moderate headache which may be related to craniosynosthosis needs long-term local techniques in the region of the craniosynosthosis.
- clinical patterns: recognition of clinical patterns can influence the treatment techniques together with the doses you choose. For example, a whiplash patient with an increase in tone of the right upper trapezius and sterno-cleidomastoid muscles fits with the hypothesis of a (minor) accessory nerve problem. Examination of the occipital region is proposed because the accessory nerve runs through the jugular foramen, which is formed by part of the occipital bone.[104]

- pain state: the pain mechanism behind the patient's symptoms can influence the way you apply cranial tissue techniques. For example, a patient with a nociceptive pain pattern is probably helped more by local manual techniques of the cranium with a progressive increase of duration and force to make the local tissue healthier, in contrast to a patient with secondary allodynia and hyperalgesia where the central nervous system is dominantly involved. These techniques will probably be more general, employing mild to minimal force without aggravating the symptoms, and also used for other purposes such as explanation as part of further management.[174]

Below is a clinical example where dominant cranial dysfunctions were strongly related to the patient's symptoms.

A clinical example

An 8-year-old boy with a 2-year diagnosis from his paediatrician of 'muscular torti-collis' complains of a dull headache, dominantly in the vertex region, which began 3 years ago with a progressive nature. This occurs two or three times a week for several hours, especially in the evening. He has difficulties with concentration and his teacher has recognized dyslexic behaviour, but no intellectual deficit. During inspection and palpation a right small orbit, small not prominent right zygomatic bone, and prominent left frontal region were observed (Figure 2.10a). He has an antalgic head posture to the right and increased muscle tone in the right cervical spine region (trapezius, semispinalis and levator scapulae muscles) which is painful to local pressure. Elevation and protraction

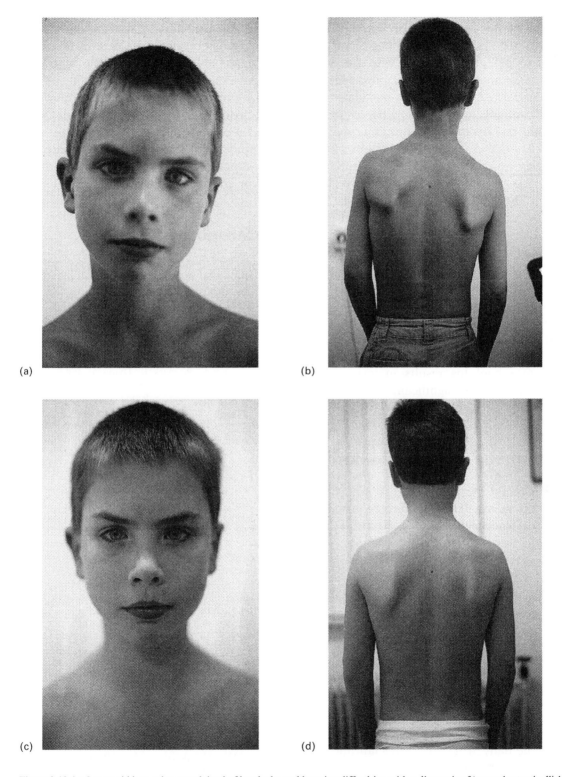

Figure 2.10 An 8-year old boy, who complained of headache and learning difficulties, with a diagnosis of 'muscular torticollis', (a) and (b) before and (c) and (d) after craniofacial management.

of this right scapula was also noted (Figure 2.10b). The right coronal suture was not easy to palpate compared with the other side. Examination of the occipital-sphenoidal region reproduced his headache and clear stiffness could be palpated in the frontal and occipital regions. The hypothesis was that a minor frontal right plagiocephaly was contributing to his symptoms. After six treatments over 2 months consisting of mobilization of cranial tissue and minor upper cervical spine mobilization together with muscle balancing exercises, the asymmetry in his face was less (Figure 2.10c). A more active posture was noted with a less antalgic head posture, and the increased muscle tone and palpation pain of the muscles had gone (Figure 2.10d). His parents noted that he complained less about headache, laughed more than before and at school his results in writing and mathematics were significantly improved as reported by his schoolteacher.

Summary and conclusion

- Cranial bone motion is still under discussion. There is some biomechanical evidence that the cranium adapts to forces and that the human adult sutures are still open in older age.[35,41,60]
- Clinically it is observed that dysfunction of the cranium is expressed in specific clinical patterns and that passive movement of the cranium can change these signs and symptoms dramatically in both younger patients and adults.
- Passive accessory movements of the cranium can easily be integrated into the daily work of a clinician and can be an important part of treatment and management, where clinical evidence

of the individual patient is essential.[77]

- Clinicians should be careful to scrutinize the literature about the behaviour of cranial dynamics. The clinical reasoning approach is, at this moment, probably still the best strategy to follow. More research, probably with an experimental design, is needed to support the effectiveness of treatment of cranial tissues.[49,69,141,175]

References

1 Grant, R. (1996). Vertebral artery testing – the Australian Physiotherapy Association Protocol after 6 years. *Man. Ther.*, **1**, 149–153.
2 Jull, G., Bogduk, N. and Marsland, A. (1988). The accuracy of manual diagnosis for cervical zygapophysial joint pain syndromes. *Med. J. Aust.*, **148**, 233–236.
3 Bourekas, E.C. and Lanzieri, C.F. (1994). The calvarium. *Sem. Ultrasound, CT, MRI*, **15**, 424–453.
4 William, P. L., Warwick, R., Dyson, M. and Bannister, L. H. (1989). *Gray's Anatomy*. Churchill Livingstone.
5 Bernardy, M., Donauer, E. and Neuenfeldt, D. (1994). Premature craniosynostosis. A retrospective analysis of a series of 52 cases. *Acta Neurochir. (Wien)*, **128**, 88–100.
6 Brandt, I. (1986). Developmental biology, prenatal growth. In: *Human Growth* (F. Falkner, J. M. Tanner, eds), p. 168. Plenum.
7 Von Karolyi, L. (1971). *Anthropometrie*. Fischer UTB.
8 Brodie, A. G. (1941). On the growth pattern of the human head. From the third month to the eighth year of life. *Am. J. Anat.*, **68**, 209–262.
9 Low, W. D. (1970). The cross-sectional, longitudinal and mixed longitudinal methods in the study of human growth. *Z. Morphol. Anthropol.*, **62**, 249–258.
10 Pearl, M., Finkelstein, J. and Berman, M. R. (1972). Temporary widening of cranial sutures during recovery from failure to thrive. A not-uncommon clinical phenomenon. *Clin. Pediatr.*, **11**, 427–430.
11 Eiben, O. (1977). Changes in body measurements and proportion of children, based on Kormend growth study. *Acta Med. Auxol.*, **9**, 38–39.
12 Komenda, S. and Klements, J. (1978). *Proportion of Body Dimensions in Children and Youth*. SPN.
13 Farkas, Gy. L. and Nyilas, K. (1988). Head measurement parameters in 23 338 3 to 18 year old Hungarian children. *Acta Biol. Szeged.*, **34**, 139–153.
14 Prokopec, M., Zlámalová, H., Lipková, V. and Grunt, J. (1991). Comparison of basic body dimensions of Czech and Slovak children and youths. *Cs. Pediat.*, **46**, 205–213.

15 Hajnis, K. and Petrásek, R. (1993). Cranial and thoracic circumference as criteria of body development. *Z. Morphol. Anthropol.*, **79**, 343–353.

16 De Bruin (1993). *A Mathematical Model Applied to Craniofacial Growth*. Thesis, Rijksuniversiteit Groningen.

17 Wolff, J. (1892). *Das Gesetz der Transformation der Kochen*. A.H. Hirschwald, Berlin.

18 Perrie, S. M., Huggler, A., Russenberger, M. *et al.* (1969). The reaction of cortical bone to compression. *Acta Orthop. Scand. Suppl.*, **125**, 19–29.

19 Duterloo, H. S. and Enlow, D. H. (1970). A comparative study of cranial growth in Homo and Macaca. *Am. J. Anat.*, **127**, 357–368.

20 (a) Hassler, C. R., Rybicki, E. F., Simonen, F. A. and Weis, E. B. (1974). Measurements of healing at an osteotomy in a rabbit calvarium: the influence of applied compressive stress on collagen synthesis and calcification. *J. Biomech.*, **7**, 545–550. (b) Hassler, C. R., Rybicki, E. F., Cummings, K. D. and Clark, L. C. (1980). Quantification of bone stresses during remodeling. *J. Biomech.*, **13**, 185–190.

21 Schock, C. C., Noyes, F. R., Crouch, M. M. and Mathews, C. H. E. (1975). The effects of immobility on long bone remodelling in the Rhesus monkey. *Henry Ford Hosp. Med. J.*, **23**, 107–115.

22 Todd, J. T., Mark, L. S., Shaw, R. E. and Pittenger, J. B. (1980). The perception of human growth. *Sci. Am.*, **242**, 132–134.

23 Gellad, F., Haney, P., Sun, J. *et al.* (1985). Imaging modalities of craniosynostosis with surgical and pathological correlation. *Pediatr. Radiol.*, **15**, 285–290.

24 Jane, J. and Persing, J. (1986). Neurosurgical treatment of craniosynostosis. In: *Craniosynostosis Diagnosis, Evaluation, and Management* (M. Cohen Jr, ed.) pp. 249–320. Raven.

25 Delashaw, J. B., Persing, J. A., Broaddus, W. C. and Jane, J. A. (1989). Cranial vault growth in craniosynostosis. *J. Neurosurg.*, **70**, 159–165.

26 Goodrich, J. (1991). Craniofacial reconstruction for craniosynostosis. In: *Plastic Techniques in Neurosurgery* (J. Goodrich, K. Post and R. Argamaso, eds.) pp. 75–108. Thieme.

27 Fatah, M. F. T., Ermis, I., Poole, M. D. and Shun-Shin, G. A. (1992). Prevention of cranial reossification after surgical craniectomy. *J. Cranifac. Surg.*, **3**, 170–172.

28 Roddi, R., Vaandrager, J. M., Gilbert, P.M. and van der Meulen, J. C. (1993). Reshaping of the skull in the early surgical correction of scaphocephaly. *J. Craniomaxillofac. Surg.*, **21**, 226–233.

29 Drake, D. B., Persing, J. A., Berman, D. E. and Ogle, R. C. (1993). Calvarial deformity regeneration following subtotal craniectomy for craniosynostosis: a case report and theoretical implications. *J. Craniofac. Surg.*, **4**, 85–90.

30 Blake, D. P. (1994). The use of synthetics in cranioplasty: a clinical review. *Mil. Med.*, **159**, 466–469.

31 Wagemans, P. A. H. M., van de Velde, J.-P. and Kuijpers-Jagtman, A. M. (1988). Sutures and forces: a review. *Am. J. Orthod. Dentofac. Arthop.*, **94**, 129–141.

32 Ebner, J. A. (1994). An overview of cranial manipulation. In: *Chiropractic Approach to Head Pain* (D. D. Curl, ed.), pp. 338–348. Williams and Wilkins.

33 Van Vuuren, C. (1991). A review of the literature on the prevalence of Class III malocclusion and the mandibular prognathic growth hypotheses. *Aust. Orthod. J.*, **12**, 23–28.

34 Kiliaridis, S., Johansson, A., Haralson, T. *et al.* (1995). Craniofacial morphology, occlusal traits, and bite force in persons with advanced occlusal tooth wear. *Am. J. Orthod. Dentofacial Arthop.*, **107**, 286–292.

35 Sutherland, W. G. (1939). *The Cranial Bowl*. Free Press Co.

36 Retzlaff, E. and Mitchell, F. (1987). *The Cranium and its Sutures*. Springer-Verlag

37 Retzlaff, E. W., Michael, D. K. and Roppel, R. M. (1975). Cranial bone mobility. *J. Am. Osteopath. Assoc.*, **74**, 138–146.

38 Upledger, J. E. and Vredevoogd, J. D. (1988). *Craniosacral Therapy*. Eastland Press.

39 Dullemeijer, P. (1972). Methodology in craniofacial biology. *Acta Morph. Neerl. Scand.*, **10**, 9–23.

40 Oudhof, H. A. J. (1982). Sutural growth. *Acta Anat.*, **112**, 58–68.

41 Jaslow, C. R. (1990). Mechanical properties of cranial sutures. *J. Biomech.*, **23**, 313–321.

42 Buchman, S. R., Bartlett, S. P., Wornom, I. L. III and Whitaker, L. A. (1994). The role of pressure on regulation of craniofacial bone growth. *J. Craniofac. Surg.*, **5**, 2–10.

43 Eby, T. L. and Nadol, J. B. (1986). Postnatal growth of the human temporal bone: implications for cochlear implants in children. *Ann. Otol. Rhinol. Laryngol.*, **95**, 356–364.

44 Xu, J., Shepherd, R. K., Xu, S. A. *et al.* (1993). Pediatric cochlear implantation. Radiologic observations of skull growth. *Arch. Otolaryngol. Head Neck Surg.*, **119**, 525–534.

45 Osborn, J. W. (1993). Orientation of the masseter muscle and the curve of Spee in relation to crushing forces on the molar teeth of primates. *Am. J. Phys. Anthropol.*, **92**, 99–106.

46 Owen, A. H. (1987). Orthodontic/orthopedic therapy for craniomandibular pain dysfunction part A. Anterior disk displacement, review of literature. *J. Craniomandib. Pract.*, **5**, 357.

47 Ayoub, A. F. and Mostafa, Y. A. (1992). Aberrant mandibular growth: theoretical implications. *Am. J. Dentofacial Orthop.*, **101**, 255–265.

48 Rocabado, M. (1983). Biomechanical relationship of the cranial, cervical and hyoid regions. *Phys. Ther.*, **1**, 62–68

49 Rocabado, M. and Tapia, V. (1987). Radiographic study of the craniocervical relation in patients under

orthopaedic treatment and the incidence of related symptoms. *J. Craniomandib. Pract.*, **5**, 36–46.

50 Christensen, L. R., Kjaer, I. and Graem, N. (1993). Comparison of human dental and craniofacial maturation on prenatal profile radiographs. *Eur. J. Orthod.*, **15**, 149–154.

51 Poole, M. D. and Briggs, M. (1990). The cranio-facio-cervical scoliosis complex. *Br. J. Plast. Surg.*, **43**, 670–675.

52 Biedermann, H. (1995). The manual therapy of newborn infants and young children. *Vopr. Kurortol. Fizioter. Lech Fiz. Kult.*, **4**, 48–49.

53 Sinsel, N. K., Opdebeeck, H., Lesaffre, E. *et al.* (1995). Maxillofacial growth after neck burn injury at a young age: an experimental study in the rabbit. *Plast. Reconstr. Surg.*, **96**, 1588–1599.

54 Goodman, C. R., Chabner, E. and Guyton, D. L. (1995). Should early strabismus surgery be performed for ocular torticollis to prevent facial asymmetry? *J. Pediatr. Ophthalmol. Strabismus*, **32**, 162–166.

55 Chang, P. Y., Tan, C. K., Huang, Y. F. *et al.* (1996). Torticollis: a long-term follow-up study. *Acta Paediatr. Sin.*, **37**, 173–177.

56 Yen, E. H., Pollit, D. J., Whyte, W. A. and Suga, D. M. (1990). Continous stressing of mouse interparietal suture fibroblasts in vitro. *J. Dent. Res.*, **69**, 26–30.

57 Willinger, R., Taleb, L. and Kopp, C. M. (1995). Modal and temporal analysis of head mathematical models. *J. Neurotrauma*, **12**, 743–754.

58 Mittelviefhaus, H. (1994). Optical improvement of deforming facial asymmetry with eyeglasses. *Klin. Monatsbl. Augenheilkd.*, **204**, 241–243.

59 Huang, C. S., Cheng, H. C., Lin, W. Y. *et al.* (1995). Skull morphology affected by different sleep positions in infancy. *Cleft Palate Craniofac. J.*, **32**, 413–419.

60 Rogers, J. S. and Witt, P. (1997). The controversy of cranial bone motion. *JOSPT*, **26**, 95-102.

61 Basset, C. A. L. (1971). Biophysical principles affecting bone structure. In: *The Biochemistry and Physiology of Bone* (G. H. Bourne, ed.), pp. 1–76. Academic Press.

62 Basset, C. A. L. (1972). A biophysical approach to craniofacial morphogenesis. *Acta Morphol. Neerl. Scand.*, **10**, 71–86.

63 Cutler, B. S., Hassig, F. H. and Turpin, D. L. (1972). Dentofacial changes produced during and after use of a modified Milwaukee brace on Macaca Mulatta. *Am. J. Orthod.*, **61**, 115–137.

64 Droschl, H. and Graber, T. M. (1975). The effect of heavy orthopedic forces on the sutures of the facial bones. *Angle. Orthod.*, **45**, 26–33.

65 Enlow, D. H. (1982). *Handbook of Facial Growth*. WB Saunders Company.

66 Furtwängler, J. A., Hall, S. H. and Koskinen-Moffett, L. K. (1985). Sutural morphogenesis in the mouse calvaria: the role of apoptosis. *Acta Anat. (Basel)*, **124**, 74–80.

67 Hinrichsen, G. J. and Storey, E. (1968). The effect of force on bone and bones. *Angle. Orthod.*, **38**, 155–165.

68 Johanson, V. A. and Hall, S. H. (1982). Morphogenesis of the mouse coronal suture. *Acta Anat. (Basel)*, **114**, 58–67.

69 Persson, M. (1973). *Structure and Growth of Facial Sutures*. Thesis, Odontol. Revy., 24.

70 Yen, E. H. K., Suga D. M. and Chiang, S. (1980). Identification of collagen type synthesized in interparietal suture during orthopedic stress. *J. Dent. Res.*, **59**(SI), 903.

71 Yen, E. H. K. and Suga D. M. (1981). Collagen and noncollagenous protein synthesis in adult cranial suture in vitro. *J. Dent. Res.*, **60**(SI), 579.

72 Yen, E. H. K. and Suga D. M. (1982). Immunohistochemical localization of type I and type III collagen in calvarial suture. *J. Dent. Res.*, **61**(SI), 183.

73 Meikle, M. C., Heath, J. K., Hembry, R. M. and Reynolds, J. J. (1982). Rabbit cranial suture fibroblasts under tension express a different collagen phenotype. *Arch. Oral Biol.*, **27**, 609–613.

74 Hall, S. H. and Decker, J. D. (1986). Proteoglycan distribution during initial mineralization of intramembraous bone. *J. Dent. Res.*, **65**(SI), 349–355.

75 Johnson, P. M. and Hall, S. H. (1986). Purification of 2 distinct proteins which react with antiosteonectin antibody. *J. Dent. Res.*, **65**(SI), 279–286.

76 Merskey, H. and Bogduk, N. (1994). *Classification of Chronic Pain*. IASP Press.

77 Jones, M., Jensen, G. and Rothstein, J. (1995). Clinical reasoning in physiotherapy. In: *Clinical Reasoning in the Health Profession* (J. Higgs and M. Jones, eds), pp. 72–87. Butterworth-Heinemann.

78 Butler, D. S. and Gifford. L. S. (1999). *The Dynamic Nervous System*. Workbook, NOI-Press

79 Lohman, A. H. M. (1977). *Vorm en Beweging. Leerboek van het Bewegingsapparaat van de Mens*. Bohn, Scheltema & Holkema.

80 Sabotta, J. and Becher, H. (1972). *Atlas der Anatomie des Menschen*. Urban & Schwarzenberg.

81 Van Limborgh, J. (1972). The role of genetic and local environmental factors in the control of postnatal craniofacial morphogenesis. *Acta Morphol. Neerl. Scand.*, **10**, 37–47.

82 Brandt, H. C., Shapiro, P. A. and Kokich, V. G. (1979). Experimental and postexperimental effects of posteriorly directed extraoral traction in adult Macaca fascicularis. *Am. J. Orthod.*, **75**, 301–317.

83 Jackson, G. W., Kokich, V. G. and Shapiro, P. A. (1979). Experimental and postexperimental response to anteriorly directed extraoral force in young Macaca nemestrina. *Am. J. Orthod.*, **75**, 318–333.

84 Engdahl, E., Ritsilä, V. and Uddströmer, L. (1978). Growth potential of cranial suture bone/autograft. II. An experimental microscopic investigation in young rabbits. *Scand. J. Plast. Reconstr. Surg.*, **12**, 125–129.

85 Scott, J. H. (1962). The growth of the craniofacial skeleton. *Ir. J. Med. Sci.*, **488**, 276–286.

86 Moss, M. L. (1972). Twenty years of functional cranial analysis. *Am. J. Orthod.*, **61**, 479–485.

87 Taveras, J. M. (1988). Anatomy and examination of the skull. In: *Radiology: Diagnosis-Imaging-Intervention* (J. M. Taveras and J. T Ferrucci, eds), pp. 1–9. Lippincott.

88 Gooding, G. A. (1971). Size and shape. In: *Radiology of the Skull and Brain: The Skull*, vol 1 (T. H. Newton and D. G. Potts, eds), pp. 141–153. Mosby.

89 Hahn, F. J., Chu, W. K. and Cheung, J. Y. (1984). CT measurements of cranial growth: normal subjects. *Am. J. Neuroradiol.*, **5**, 155–157.

90 Reynolds, J. (1987). The skull and spine. *Semin. Roentgenol.*, **23**, 168–175.

91 Madeline, L. A. and Elster, A. D. (1995). Suture closure in the human chondrocranium: CT assessment. *Radiology*, **196**, 747–756.

92 Pritchard, J. J., Scott, J. H. and Girgis, F. G. (1956). The structure and development of cranial and facial sutures. *J. Anat.*, **90**, 73–90.

93 Maitland, G. D. (1986). *Vertebral Manipulation*, 5th edn. Butterworths.

94 Van der Klaauw, C. J. (1946). Cerebral skull and facial growth. *Arch. Neerl. Zool.*, **7**, 16.

95 Van de Linden, F. P. G. M. (1968). Bone dynamics in the cranial skeleton. *Folia Med. Neerl.*, **11**, 150–155.

96 Christmann, C., Knop, H., Köhler, G. *et al.* (1977). Zum Stossmechanismus am kindlichem Hirnschädel. *Verh. Anat. Ges.*, **71**, 1309; Christmann, C., Möller, M. and Pawletta, A. (1977). Dezelerations-und Akzelerationstraumen des menschlichen Schädels. *Anat. Anz.*, **142**, 314.

97 Hoyer, H.-E. and Zech, M. (1980). Die Verformund des menschlichen Schädels beim Stoss. *Unfallheilkunde*, **83**, 30–34.

98 Richtsmeier, J. T. and Cheverud, J. M. (1986). Finite element scaling analysis of normal growth of the human craniofacial complex. *J. Craniofac. Genet. Dev. Biol.*, **6**, 289.

99 Richtsmeier, J. T. and Lele, S. (1993). Quantitative analysis of growth: Models and theoretical considerations. *Biol. Rev.*, **68**, 381.

100 Hildebolt, C. F., Vannier, M. W. and Knapp, R. H. (1990). Validation study of skull three-dimensional computerized tomography measurements. *Am. J. Phys. Anthropol.*, **82**, 283.

101 Carter, D. R., Wong, M. and Orr, T. E. (1991). Musculoskeletal ontogeny, phylogeny and functional adaptation. *J. Biomech.*, **24**, 3.

102 Kowalski, C. J. (1993). Data analysis in craniofacial biology with special emphasis on longitudinal studies. *Cleft Palate Craniofac. J.*, **30**, 111–120.

103 Ohman, J. C. and Richtsmeier, J. T. (1994). Perspectives on craniofacial growth. *Clin. Plast. Surg.*, **21**, 489–499.

104 Patten, J. (1995). *Neurological Differential Diagnosis*, 2nd edn. Springer-Verlag.

105 Moss, M. L. (1975). Functional anatomy of cranial synostosis. *Child's Brain*, **1**, 22–33.

106 O'Rahilly, R. and Müller, F. (1986). The meninges in human development. *J. Neuropathol. Exp. Neurol.*, **45**, 588–608.

107 Opperman, L. A., Passarelli, R. W., Morgan, E. P. *et al.* (1995). Cranial sutures require tissue interactions with dura mater to resist osseous obliteration in vitro. *J. Bone Miner Res.*, **10**, 1978–1987.

108 Andres, K. H. (1967). Über die Feinstruktur der Arachnoidea und Dura mater von Mammalia. *Z. Zellforch.*, **79**, 272–295.

109 Rogers, L. C. and Payne, E. E. (1961). The dura mater at the cranio-vertebral junction. *J. Anat.*, **95**, 586–588.

110 Beasley, A. B. and Kuhlenbeck, H. (1966). Some observations on the layers of dura mater at the cranio-vertebral transition in the human newborn. *Anat. Rec.*, **154**, 315.

111 Markowski, I. (1931). Über die Entwicklung der Falx cerebri und das Tentorium cerebelli des Menschen mit Berücksichtigung ihrer venösen sinus. *Ztschr.f. d. ges. Anat.*, **159**, 33–58.

112 McLone, D. G. (1980). The subarachnoid space: A review. *Child Brain*, **6**, 113–130.

113 Moss, M. L. and Young, R. W. (1960). A functional approach to craniology. *Am. J. Phys. Anthropol.*, **18**, 281–292.

114 Dias, M. S. and Leland Albright, A. (1989). Management of hydrocephalus complicating childhood posterior fossa tumors. *Pediatr. Neurosci.*, **15**, 283–290.

115 Hentschel, F. (1990). Das rezividierende chronische Subduralhämatom Pachumeningeosis haemorrhagica interna. *Zent. Bl. Neurochir.*, **51**, 119–123.

116 Murai, H., Kira, J., Kobayashi, T. *et al.* (1992). Hypertrophic cranial pachymeningitis due to Aspergillus flavus. *Clin. Neurol. Neurosurg.*, **94**, 247–250.

117 Haines, D. E. and Harkey, H. L. (1993). The 'subdural' space: a new look at an outdated concept. *Neurosurg.*, **32**, 111–120.

118 Bakay, L. Jr (1941). Die Innervation der Pia mater, der Plexus choriodei und der Hirngerfässe. *Arch. Psychiatr. Nervenkr.*, **113**, 412–416.

119 Courville, C. B. (1965). Contrecoup injuries of the brain in infancy. *Arch. Surg.*, **90**, 157–165.

120 Merchant, R. E. (1984). Pacchionian bodies. In: *Illustrated Encyclopedia of Human Histology* (R. V. Kristic, ed.). Springer.

121 Földes, V., Mojzes, L. and Antal, A. (1987). Vitale Reaktionen in Pacchioni-Granulationen. *Z. Rechtsmed.*, **98**, 165–173.

122 Kostopoulos, D. C. and Keramidas, G. (1992). Changes in elongation of falx cerebri during craniosacral therapy techniques applied on the skull of an embalmed cadaver. *J. Craniomandib. Pract.*, **10**, 9–12.

123 Kragt, G., Ten Bosch, J. J. and Borsboom, P. C. F. (1985). Measurement of bone displacement in a macerated human skull induced by orthodontic forces: a holographic study. *J. Biomech.*, **12**, 905–910.

124 Wood, J. (1971). Dynamic response of human cranial bones. *J. Biomech.*, **4**, 1–12.

125 Pick, M. G. (1994). A preliminary single case magnetic resonance imaging investigation into maxillary frontal-parietal manipulation and its short-term effect upon the intercranial structures of an adult human brain. *J. Manipulative Physiol. Ther.*, **17**, 168–173.

126 Bleistein, J. and Jerusalem, F. (1984). Konservative therapie der subduralen Hämatoms. *Aktuell Neurol.*, **11**, 121–123.

127 Laumer, R. (1986). Das chronische subdruale Hämatom unter dem Bild der zerebrovaskulären Insuffizient. *Nervenheilkunde*, **5**, 238–240.

128 Pichert, G. and Henn, V. (1987). Konservative Therapie chronische subduralhämatome. *Schwiez Med. Wochensch.*, **117**, 1856–1862.

129 Cohn, S. H., Vaswasi, A. *et al.* (1976). Effect of aging of bone mass in adult women. *Am. J. Physiolog.*, **230**, 143–148.

130 Mayberg, M. R., Zervas, N. T. and Moskowitz, M.A. (1984). Trigeminal projections to supratentorial pial and dural blodd vessels in cats. Demonstrated by horseradish peroxidase histochemistry. *J. Comp. Neurol.* **223**, 46–56.

131 Markowitz, S., Saito, K. and Moskowitz, M. A. (1988). Neurogenically mediated plasma extravasation in the dura mater: effect of ergot alkaloids. A possible mechanism of action in vascular headache. *Cephalagia*, **8**, 83–91.

132 Herskovitz, M. S., Hallas, B. H. and Singh, I. J. (1993). Study of sympathetic innervation of cranial bones by axonal transport of horseradish peroxidase in the rat: preliminary findings. *Acta Anat.*, **147**, 178–183.

133 Wright, A. (1995). Hypoalgesia post-manipulative therapy: a review of a potential neurophysiological mechanism. *Man. Ther.*, **1**, 11–16.

134 Greitz, D. (1993). Cerebrospinal fluid circulation and associated intracranial dynamics. A radiologic investigation using MR imaging and radionuclide cisternography. *Acta Radio. Suppl.*, **386**, 1–23.

135 Tulen, J. H., Man in 't Veld, A. J., Dzoljic, M. R. *et al.* (1991). Sleeping with and without norepinephrine: effects of metoclopramide and D,L-threo-3,4-dihydoxyphenylserine on sleep in dopamine bea-hydroxylase deficiency. *Sleep*, **14**, 32–38.

136 Feinberg, D. A. (1992). Modern concepts of brain motion and cerebrospinal fluid flow. *Radiology.*, **185**, 630–632.

137 Newman, N. J. (1992). Multiple cranial neuropathies: presenting signs of systematic lymphoma. *Surv. Ophthalmol.*, **37**, 125–129.

138 Letson, G. W., Gellin, B. G., Bulkow, L.R. *et al.* (1992). Severity and frequency of sequelae of bacterial meningitis in Alaska native infants. Correlation with a scoring system for severity of sequelae. *Am. J. Dis. Child.*, **146**, 560–566.

139 Ledin, T., Bynke, O. and Odkvist, L. M. (1995). Influence of cerebrospinal fluid tapping on dynamic equilibrium in suspected hydrocephalus. *Acta Otolaryngol. Suppl.*, **520** 2, 317–319.

140 Ondarza, R., Velasco, F., Velasco, M. *et al.* (1994). Neurotransmitter levels in cerebrospinal fluid in relation to severity of symptoms and response to medical therapy in Parkinsons's disease. Stereotact. *Funct. Neurosurg.*, **62**, 90–97.

141 Adams, T., Heisey, R. S., Smith, M. C. and Briner, B. J. (1992). Parietal bone mobility in the anesthetized cat. *J. Am. Osteopath. Assoc.*, **92**, 599–622.

142 Heisey, S. R. and Adams, T. (1993). Role of cranial bone mobility in cranial compliance. *Neurosurgery*, **33**, 869–877.

143 Ruan, J. S., Khalil, T. and King, A. I. (1991). Human head dynamic response to side impact by finite element modeling. *J. Biomech. Eng.*, **113**, 276–283.

144 Margulies, S. S., Thibault, L. E. and Gennarelli, T. A. (1990). Physical model simulations of brain injury in the primate. *J. Biomech.*, **23**, 823–836.

145 Wealthall, S. R. and Smallwood, R. (1974). Methods of measuring intracranial pressure via the fontanelle without puncture. *J. Neurol. Neurosurg. Psych.*, **37**, 88–96.

146 Cottam, C. (1984). *Cranial Manipulations Roots References*. Coraco.

147 Greenman, P. E. (1970). Roentgen findings in the craniosacral mechanism. *J. Am. Osteopath. Assoc.*, **70**, 1–12.

148 Breig, A. (1976). *Adverse Mechanical Tension in the Central Nervous System*. Almqvist & Wiksell International.

149 Doursonian, L., Alfonso, J. M., Iba-Zizen, M. T. *et al.* (1989). Dynamics of the junction between the medulla and the cervical spinal cord: an in vivo study in the sagittal plane by magnetic resonance imaging. *Surg. Radiol. Anat.*, **11**, 313–322.

150 Moller, A. R. (1991). The cranial nerve vascular compression syndrome. *Rev. Treat. Acta Neurochir.*, **113**, 18–23.

151 Dyck, P. J. and Thomos, P. K. (1993). *Peripheral Neuropathy.* Vol 2. 3rd edn. W. B. Saunders.

152 McNamara, J. A. Jr (1972). Neuromuscular and skeletal adaptations to altered oral facial function monograph #1. *Cranial Facial Growth Series*, Ann Arbor. Centre for Human Growth and Development, The University of Michigan.

153 McNamara, J. A. Jr and Arbor, A. (1973). Neuromuscular and skeletal adaptations to altered function in the orofacial region. *Am. J. Orthod.*, **64**, 578–606.

154 Grant, P. G. (1972). *Biomechanical Analysis of the Masticatory Muscles of the Rhesus Macaque (Macacca malluta)*. Thesis, University of California.

155 Enlow, D. H. (1986). *The Human Face*. Harper & Row.

156 Trainor, P. G., McLachlan, K. R. and McCall, W. D. (1995). Modelling of forces in the human masticatory system with optimization of the angulations of the joint loads. *J. Biomech.*, **28**, 829–843.

157 Washburn, S. L. (1947). The relation of the temporal muscle to the form of the skull. *Anat. Rec.*, **99**, 239–248.

158 Avis, V. (1959). The relation of the temporal muscle to the form of the coronoid process. *Am. J. Phys. Antrop.*, **3**, 210–220.

159 Schumacher, G. H. and Dokládal, M. (1968). Über unterschiedliche Sekundärveränderungen am Schädel als Folge von Kaumuskelsektionen. *Acta Anat.*, **69**, 378–392.

160 Rönning, O. and Kylämarkula, S. (1979). Reaction of transplanted neurocentral synchrondrosis to different conditions of mechanical stress. A methodological study on the rat. *J. Anat.*, **128**, 789–801.

161 Kylämarkula, S. (1988). Growth changes in the skull and upper cervical skeleton after partial detachment of neck muscles. An experimental study in the rat. *J. Anat.*, **159**, 197–205.

162 Knutson, F. (1961). Growth and differentiation of the postnatal vertebra. *Acta Radiol.*, **55**, 401–408.

163 Christensen, L. V. (1967). Facial pain from the masticatory system induced by experimental bruxism. A preliminary report. *Tandae gebladet*, **74**, 175–182.

164 Stohler, C. S., Zhang, X. and Ashton-Miller, J. A. (1992). An experimental model of jaw muscle pain in man. In: *Biological Mechanisms of Tooth Movement and Craniofacial Adaptation* (Z. Davidovitch, ed.), pp. 503–511. The Ohio State University College of Dentistry, Columbus.

165 McIndoe, R. (1995). Moving out of pain. Hands-on or hands-off. In: *Moving Out of Pain* (M. Shacklock, ed.), pp. 153–160. Butterworth-Heinemann.

166 McIndoe, R. (1994). A behavioural approach to the managment of chronic pain. A self management perspective. *Austr. Fam. Physician*, **23**, 2284–2292.

167 Wall, P. D. (1994). The placebo and the placebo response. In: *Textbook of Pain* (P. D. Wall and R. Melzack, eds), pp. 1297–1308. Churchill Livingstone.

168 Butler, D. S. (1999). Integrating pain awareness into physiotherapy–wise action for the future. In: *Topical Issues in Pain* (L. Gifford, ed.), pp. 1–23. NOI Press.

169 Upledger, J. E. (1988). Dysfunctions of the craniosacral dural membrane system: diagnosis and treatment. In: *Craniosacral Therapy* (J. E. Upledger and J. D. Vredevoogd, eds), pp. 60–87. Eastland Press.

170 Williams, P. L., Warwick, R., Dyson, M. and Bannister, L. H. (1989). *Gray's Anatomy*. Churchill Livingstone.

171 Martins, A. N., Wiley, J. K. and Myers, P. W. (1972). Dynamics of the cerebrospinal fluid and the spinal dura mater. *J. Neurol., Neurosurg, Psych.*, **35**, 468–473.

172 De Cock, J. (1988). *Manuele Therapie Etio- en Osteopatie in de Cranial Regio*. Private publisher.

173 Cobb, W. M. (1955). The age incidence of suture closure. *Am. J. Antropol.*, **13**, 394.

174 Wittink, H. and Michel, T. H. (1997). *Chronic Pain Management for Physical Therapists*. Butterworth-Heinemann.

175 Worth, D. R. (1995). Movements of the head and neck. In: *Grieve's Modern Manual Therapy*, 2nd edn (J. D Boyling and N. Palastnaga, eds), pp. 53–66. Churchill Livingstone.

3

Primary and secondary cranial asymmetry in KISS children

H. Biedermann

Introduction

We all 'know' what symmetry is but we would be hard put to give a precise or concise definition. Mathematical definitions of symmetry do not sit well with living things. Strictly speaking nobody is symmetrical, but symmetry is nevertheless perceived as ideal in art and nature,[1] and might even convey evolutionary advantages to its bearer.[2,3] This point of view has not remained unchallenged.[4] A comprehensive treatment of symmetry and its evolutionary role can be found in Møller and Swaddle.[5*] Blickhorn[6] reviewed a recent publication by Furlow[7] '...fluctuating asymmetry could account for almost all heritable sources of variability in IQ'. This is but one hint of the importance of symmetry as a marker or cause of other more fundamental problems. The impairment of senso-motor development in KISS children seems to point to the same conclusions.

Complete symmetry is empty, dead.[8] Had there not been a little asymmetry right after the Big Bang we, and all the universe around us, would not be here. The analysis of the structural principles behind this initial 'symmetry problem' fertilized research in scientific areas as far apart as nuclear physics and ethology.[9] A person or object needs a certain amount of symmetry to be considered beautiful, but the addition of a little bit of asymmetry can really make us like what we see.[4] Strong asymmetry on the other hand is seen as 'sick'.[10] Between these two extremes the ideal has to be found by intuition or trial and error.

For structures connected to sensory input symmetry is more than an embellishment: most of the information has to be related to a three-dimensional analysis of its origin and here symmetry of the supporting structure simplifies processing. Strong asymmetry necessitates a higher level of 'input-correction' and is therefore of evolutionary disadvantage.

The KISS syndrome

The term KISS refers to *k*inematic

---

*French-speaking readers can find a summary in: *Anders Pape Møller La Nature Préfère la Symetrie. LA RECHERCHE 304 DÉCEMBRE 1997* (Møller teaches in Paris). Some of the material is accessible via < www.oup.co.uk/MS-asymmetry >

imbalances due to suboccipital strain. These can be regarded as one of the main reasons for asymmetry in posture and consequently asymmetry of the osseous structures of the cranium and the spine. In 20 years of treatment of small children and newborn babies for a variety of problems we saw more than 5000 children under the age of 2 years. Based on these cases we realized that the suboccipital region – between the occiput and C3 (the craniocervical area) – plays a very important role in the sensomotor development, exceeding the symptoms seen at that time and reaching far into adolescence and even adulthood. Cranial asymmetry, functional asymmetries and asymmetrical neurological patterns all contribute to this diagnosis.

The term KISS syndrome is used to bring together a seemingly non-coherent group of symptoms and ailments found in newborn and small children, its dominant feature being the torticollis, often combined with an asymmetry of the head (Table 3.1).

Table 3.1 Spontaneous complaints reported by the parents[1] (n = 263)

Complaint	Percentage
Torticollis	89.3
Reduced range of head movements	84.7
Cervical hypersensitivity	76.0
Cranial asymmetry	40.1
Opisthotonos	27.9
Restlessness	23.7
Forced sleeping posture	14.5
Unable to control head movements	9.5
Uses one arm much less	7.6

All statistical material presented here is based on a catamnestic study of 263 babies treated between July 1994 and June 1995. Of the total of 554 babies seen in our consultation these were the ones we could still locate directly by a phone call or via the doctors and/or physiotherapists who sent them initially

Cranial asymmetry and the phenomena observed in association with it are beginning to receive more attention. Understanding the importance of a symmetric sensomotor development during the first year allows us to analyse some problems which appear much later in a new context. Seen from this perspective, cranial asymmetry of small children can be an early warning sign, indicating an imbalance in sensomotor development which may eventually lead to both morphological and neurofunctional disorders.[7] One does not need to treat asymmetry in babies as such. However, timely treatment to achieve a symmetrical posture and morphology goes a long way to prevent both current problems and later complications. Having traced back a lot of schoolchildren's problems to initial asymmetries of posture,[11] one can attribute much more importance to them than their unremarkable symptomatology initially suggests. Asymmetry in posture and cranial configuration are a symptom, a sign calling our attention to the underlying condition that might be triggering it (Figure 3.1). By focusing on this prime mover we can successfully treat functional and morphological asymmetry as well.

As is often seen in the history of medical knowledge, our frame of reference changes over time. In 1727 Nicolas Andry, who coined the word 'orthopaedics', had already mentioned the treatment of torticollis as one important field of this new discipline. In going back to the roots we understand that good posture in children was at the forefront of orthopaedic diagnostics and treatment. Ortho-Paedics – 'rightening the young' – has such an importance for Andry that he used this concept as the definition of the medical procedures he published in his book. This fundamental underpinning of the new discipline was lost in later centuries, and Andry's eminently functional approach had to make way for the mechanistic paradigms which have dominated orthopaedics in the last decades.

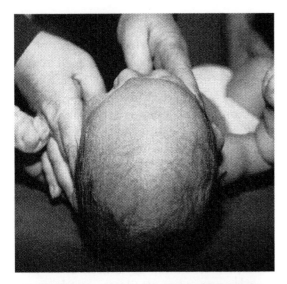

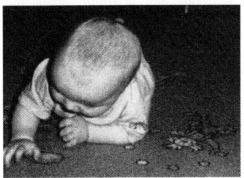

Figure 3.1 Two KISS babies with their cranial asymmetries. Both pictures were taken by the parents and are reproduced here with their kind permission. They show in both cases a right-convex KISS situation with the accompanying cranial scoliosis, microsomy of the left side of the face, flattening of the right occipital region and a seemingly asymmetrical positioning of the ears. All these morphological asymmetries need many months to subside. The important sign at the control 3 weeks after the initial treatment is the free movement of the cervical spine

Asymmetry in newborn babies remained a well-known problem, although one which was often thought to disappear spontaneously if left alone long enough. For a long time it was linked to malfunction of the sternocleidomastoid muscle. 'The etiology of congenital muscular torticollis remains a mystery despite intensive investigation' is a commonly held view, see Davids *et al.*[12] most authors still put the blame on birth trauma of the sternocleidomastoid muscle.[13,14] The symptom was thought to be the cause. At least in the early phases, the shortened and thick sternocleidomastoid muscle is so prominent that it is a 'natural' culprit. This chapter argues that it is a co-victim of the underlying trauma to the articular structures of the cervical spine and as such it is not a good starting point for therapy or analysis. It is far better used as an indicator of the improvement brought about by other therapeutic measures.

There is a controversy about how to react to a fixed or asymmetric posture in newborn babies. Some consider this a 'physiological scoliosis' and think it wears off without treatment.[15,16] More recent papers stress the importance of asymmetries in perception and posture for the development of more severe consequences later on.[17] Buchmann remarked, 'The existence of an asymmetrical range of tilt in the suboccipital region of a child is no big deal. Only if additional signs accompany this, an immediate treatment might be necessary'.[18] Asymmetry is frequently found in testing newborns[19,20] and its clinical significance has to be carefully examined. Seifert published data of unselected groups of newborn babies where she found that more than 10% of all newborns show signs of asymmetry of the functioning of the upper cervical spine.[21]

Nobody advocates a treatment schedule where all these initially asymmetrical babies have to be treated routinely, but these babies should be re-examined later on and treated if the functional deficit has not subsided spontaneously after 4–6 weeks. We would propose to take a large margin, especially as manual therapy is a low-risk procedure, quite uncomplicated and does not need to be repeated more than once or twice.

Keessen *et al.* showed that the accuracy of the proprioception of the upper limb is reduced in cases with idiopathic scoliosis and spinal asymmetry.[17] As we know that the proprioception of the arms depends heavily on a functioning suboccipital region,[22] functional deficits in this region should be corrected as soon as possible.

During 15 years of experience with children suffering from postural asymmetries we were able to show that the most efficient treatment of these cases can be a single treatment of a very mild passive impulse (thrust technique) to the upper cervical spine. Almost all symptoms that led to the presentation of the babies in our office subsided during 3 weeks after the intervention (Table 3.2).

Table 3.2 Improvement after single treatment for KISS-related problems. Answers of parents interviewed 6–18 months after treatment (216 answers of 263 interviews)

Time after treatment	No.
0–24 hours	102
1–7 days	34
8–14 days	25
15–21 days	33
22–28 days	22

While almost half of the cases reported an improvement soon after craniocervical manual therapy, a smaller group needed some reaction time and the effects of the therapy appeared only 2–3 weeks later (no other treatment applied during the first 3 weeks).

A short summary of the biomechanics of birth

'Head stabilization ... is a complex process involving the interaction of reflexes elicited by vestibular, visual and proprioceptive signals'.[23] Most of the afferent proprioceptive signals originate from the craniocervical junction. Any obstacle impeding these afferential signals will have many more extensive consequences in a nervous system

in formation, which depends on appropriate stimuli to organize itself.[24,25] 'Most of the cerebral development lies still in the future for the newborns';[26] this development 'begins at the head.'[27] Head stabilization and an adequate supply of sensory input from the craniocervical junction are essential for the ripening of the central nervous system.

These delicate structures undergo considerable stress during delivery, as the evolution of bipedal gait necessitated a radical restructuring of the human pelvis. The initially straight birth canal had to be bent to fit the new anatomical situation. Our ancestors in Central Africa had a pelvis construction much better adapted to upright gait.[28] The increased cranial circumference of the modern newborn makes the situation even worse. The birth canal is one of the most dangerous obstacles we ever have to traverse.[29] Wischnik showed in experimental studies of the biomechanics of delivery[30,31] that during delivery the head is rotated about 90° and pressed against the trunk by the contractions of the uterine muscles. A majority of newborns suffer from microtrauma of brainstem tissues in the periventricular areas.[32] The injury of the intracranial and subcranial structures is thus the rule, not the exception. The ability of most newborns to overcome and repair these lesions shows the enormous capacity of the not yet fully developed brain to cope. Now that we understand that complete brain development – which lasts at least until the fifth year – depends on consistent sensory inputs, the importance of imbalances for the efficient repair of cerebral lesions becomes evident.

This area is beyond the scope of this chapter, but it opens fascinating opportunities for the improvement of the therapy schedule for cerebral palsy and similar neuropaediatric problems.

The trauma of the suboccipital structures inhibits the functioning of the proprioceptive feedback-loops. The motor development, though pre-programmed, cannot develop normally. These systems are fault-tolerant and able to overcome considerable difficulties and restricted working conditions. But the price for this is a reduced capacity to absorb additional stress later on. Children who undergo this kind of trauma may show only minor symptoms in the first months of their lives, e.g. a temporary fixation of the head in one position, and may 'recover' spontaneously. Later on, at the age of 5 or 6 years, they suffer from headaches, postural problems or diffuse symptoms like sleeping disorders, being unable to concentrate, etc. Quite a large number of those children suffering from one of these 'three-letter-word' syndromes such as MCD (minimal cerebral damage), POS (psycho-organic syndrome), ADD (attention deficit disorder) and the like, have a functional disorder of the upper cervical spine as one of their problems.

In our practice we learned to look for symptoms of functional lesions of the upper cervical spine in the newborn-phase of children who came to us at school age with postural or behavioural problems. Their successful manual therapy suggested functional disorders of the cervical spine were the main cause of their disorders and we looked back into their developmental history to find the starting point of their ailments. As a rule we found signs of KISS-related problems in these cases, e.g. a fixed posture during the first months, sleeping problems, and many more.

The incentive to define the KISS syndrome was purely practical. Having found an efficient and low-risk way of treating the asymmetries of small children we had to redefine some pathogenetic concepts. If the shortened sternocleidomastoid muscle lengthens spontaneously after a manipulation of the upper cervical spine it cannot be burdened with the responsibility of causing a torticollis. The shortened muscle is only a symptom, albeit quite a prominent one.

Two typical developmental patterns need to be analysed when examining babies with asymmetry problems. In the first group the cranial and postural asymmetry is clearly visible from day one. Immediately after delivery the posture of the head and neck as well as the configuration of the cranial bones is asymmetrical. The gynaecologist or the midwife can show this to the parents.

In the second group, the baby appears symmetrical after birth. Beyond the 'normal' distortions of the cranial structures nothing obvious is seen. The asymmetrical posture is observed only 4–8 weeks later and develops gradually, together with other KISS symptoms.

There is no need to treat every newborn who shows signs of cranial asymmetry; quite frequently this asymmetry subsides spontaneously in the first 3–6 weeks. Over-zealous therapy is more often than not unnecessarily irritating. Most of the initially asymmetrical babies are able to straighten themselves out if given enough time. Having said this, we must emphasize that these initially asymmetric babies should be screened after 5–7 weeks and treated at that time if symptoms persist.

Head control is accomplished between the second and third months. Only then can you meaningfully examine the babies in order to check and treat for cranial and postural asymmetries. If such symptoms are found, the distinction between the two patterns outlined above helps to give insight into the probable cause of the asymmetry. At a later stage in the child's development the two patterns which we have identified become less important as a tool for analysing the cause of the asymmetries.

The treatment of cranial asymmetry is not only achieved by pushing or pulling the cranium into a more or less symmetrical form. Since the ancient Egyptians applied head bandages to their newborns to give them a 'beautiful' head, it has been well known how malleable a structure the newborn's head is. It does not serve any useful purpose to 'rectify' the cranial asymmetry itself. Once the functional deficits behind it are treated the asymmetry diminishes gradually. Whatever asymmetry is still there afterwards interferes only inasmuch as it blocks normal functioning of sensory input and proprioception. To treat plagiocephaly with redression helmets[33,34] is to confuse the symptom with the cause, similar to the myotomy of the sternocleidomastoid muscle still advocated by many clinicians. But the effects of a functional asymmetry on the morphology of the skull or the muscle cannot simply be reversed by eradicating these secondary signs. Once this is accepted the treatment schedules become much more efficient, and simplified, too. Another more functional approach is to facilitate the delicate movements of the different osseous partners, i.e. craniomobilization therapy, which is presented in Chapters 2 and 4.

The clinical picture of the KISS syndrome

It is next to impossible to identify the exact reason why an individual baby has KISS-related problems. Sometimes we find massive asymmetries in babies with a completely empty anamnesis. In other cases the children had everything going against them: oblique intrauterine positioning, a long and difficult birth using extraction aids in the last phase and marked cranial deformation immediately after birth. But 6–10 weeks later some of these children are without any KISS-type symptoms and are straight as an arrow. It is, therefore, exceedingly difficult to define the origin and outcome in any one individual child. However, after examining 100 or more children a picture emerges.

The risk groups we found in our statistics were:[35,36]

- long labour
- extraction with vacuum etc.
- twins or triplets
- prenatal positional anomalies.

Any combination of these factors is possible. An obliquely positioned fetus has more difficulties in adapting to the contortions of the birth canal and long labour often results in the use of extraction aids, etc.

The common denominator is the mechanical stress exerted on the most vulnerable structures, i.e. the cerebral tissues and the craniocervical area with its high density of sensory and transport structures.

What we have found in these cases can be put into four categories:

1 asymmetry in posture
2 asymmetry in movement
3 asymmetry in morphology
4 'asymmetry' in behaviour, i.e. non-appropriate reactions to external stimuli.

This categorization, as with any attempt to impose order on a clinical picture, should be viewed with some caution. As a closer examination of the symptoms shows, they are so common that their significance for the diagnosis of a KISS case can only be taken for granted if they occur in combination. The asymmetry – functional or morphological – is the leading sign. The presence or absence of a cranial (i.e.

morphological) asymmetry determines the need for manual therapy. Physiotherapy without direct treatment of the cranio-cervical junction has proved to be insufficient.

The main symptoms and signs found in the newborns and small children (up to 24 months old) referred to us for treatment were:

- tilt posture of head and spine, torticollis
- opisthotonos, often with a KISS spot, i.e. an asymmetrical abrasion of the hair of the occipital part
- uniform sleeping posture; difficulties in finding convenient sleeping position
- sleeping disorders; the baby often woke up crying during the night
- asymmetric motor patterns and posture of trunk and extremities: the arm at the concave side is less frequently used
- in cases with prominent retroflexion of the head the arms are often held in an fixed extroverted position: 'chicken-wings'
- extreme sensitivity of the neck to palpation, tearing the hair, especially on one side
- cranial scoliosis or plagiocephaly, combined with a flattened occipital region
- unilateral microsomy, i.e. swelling of one side of the facial soft tissues
- blockages of the iliosacral joints, asymmetries of the gluteus muscles
- asymmetric development and range of movement of the hips, especially of the concave side
- 'three-months-colic', often combined with
- cry babies, i.e. constant crying and visible discomfort without apparent infection etc.

- fever of unknown origin, loss of appetite and other symptoms.

We have to be careful not to over-emphasize the importance of the torticollis and/or C-scoliosis in the discussion of the KISS syndrome. It is like a self-fulfilling diagnosis to regard these signs as the most important. Most children are referred for manual therapy primarily because this kind of asymmetrical posture is apparent. To put these two specific conditions at the top of the list is a circular argument: as we have noted they are the most prominent features, but not necessarily the most important causal agents. We saw that other less specific symptoms often precede the asymmetry and certainly the morphological changes of the skull.

For many decades the treatment of these babies consisted of putting them into braces, gypsum casts while sleeping or leather bandages to 'redress' their asymmetrical spinal posture. A latecomer to this kind of mechanical treatment schedule is the 'corrective helmet'.[33]

The outcome of the treatment of babies coming with *all* the symptoms mentioned above shows that whereas postural or cranial asymmetry may be the most visible problem – and the problem most easily connected to a malfunction of the upper cervical spine – the other ailments are as effectively treated by manipulation. One example is the 'cry-babies': once we can exclude the 'usual suspects', i.e. respiratory or gastrointestinal infections, manipulation of the occipitocervical region is singularly effective.

Form follows function

Immediately after birth babies regularly show signs of the forces exerted on the cranial structures. As a rule the resulting configuration of the head allows clinicians to analyse the delivery mode, i.e. how the head was positioned while passing through the birth canal. Frequently an asymmetric cranial configuration is combined with the remnants of a haematoma.

These morphological signs of the birth trauma disappear during the first weeks. At this stage we can distinguish between those cranial asymmetries caused by the deformation of the osseous structures of the skull during passage through the birth canal and the asymmetries induced by an asymmetrical posture. In our view the second group is by far the larger. Apart from the very few cases of primary unilateral microsomy (we see less than 1% in the babies treated), a cranial asymmetry starts as a postural asymmetry. The functional deficit, if left alone long enough, leads to the morphological change. Two types of asymmetry are discernible:

Primary asymmetry: facial and cranial scoliosis in the sagittal *and* frontal plane. The primary asymmetry can be seen immediately after delivery and is easily distinguishable from cranial misalignment as it includes a scoliotic posture of the cervical spine or the whole body. Needless to say, it is impossible to draw a sharp line between this and secondary asymmetry. The newborn babies who display this kind of fixed and asymmetrical posture tend to have been in an oblique position during the last weeks of pregnancy or at least did not move much during this time.

Secondary asymmetry: unilateral flattening of the occiput due to forced retroflexion. The secondary asymmetry gradually develops after birth and is, therefore, only remarked on after some time, usually 6–8 weeks after birth.

The primary asymmetry group is the smaller of the two; in our case histories

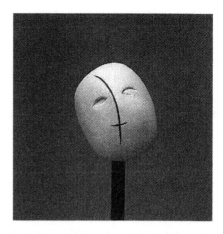

Figure 3.2 This clay doll shows the typical signs of cranial asymmetry found in KISS babies. A left-convex case is shown. The symptoms of these children are a left-convex posture of the trunk, retardation of hip development on the right, less spontaneous movements of the right arm and leg, inability to roll over to the right and to look to the right as well as refusal to bend the head to the left. The morphological signs on the head are a less developed cheek on the right, a 'smaller' eye on the right, a c-shaped and left-convex facial midline (i.e. microsomy of the right half of the face) and a flattening of the left side of the occiput

the percentage varies between 20% and 30%. A much larger group of newborns consists of those who are straight at birth. Only after 6–10 weeks do these babies develop a more asymmetrical posture. Initially the parents may try to counteract this posture preference by putting toys or other stimuli on the less used side. In some cases this simple manoeuvre does the trick. In others the babies will not react when their preferred toy is put at the 'wrong' side, or they will try to reach it and cry out in frustration when they cannot. In these babies an internal obstacle keeps them from using the 'wrong' side. Interestingly enough, the more subtle signs of KISS syndrome often precede the clinical development of the asymmetry itself. Before a tilted head or a C-scoliosis is seen the babies cause concern because they cry incessantly, are restless and irritable and do not want to get into bed. The mothers of these children spend hours carrying them around and singing them to sleep. 'I have to make sure she is fast asleep in my arms before I can try to put her to bed' is a remark they frequently make. This chain of events makes it probable that the starting point of the whole problem is a painful neck. As newborn babies cannot react specifically to an irritant, they display the well-known signs of dysphoria. A 3-month-old baby who cries may not necessarily do so because of neck pain – there are many other reasons for it – but this is at least one sound reason we should take into consideration.

The origin of the baby's discomfort is not necessarily obvious to the onlooking parent, paediatrician or child physiotherapist. One of the less pleasant ways to 'explain the problem away' is to blame over-attentive mothers. Nobody doubts that overattention can provoke such reactions in a 3- or 4-year-old, but in the first months of their life the little ones simply do not have the means to analyse this maternal attitude, let alone the capacity to react to it. As is often the case in the analysis of the first months, we mistakenly extrapolate from what we presume to be correct in older children or adults into this early developmental stage, forgetting that a symptom displayed at 9 years and the same symptom displayed at 6 months do not necessarily have the same cause.

When we began treating small children we did not draw a sharp line between different types of asymmetry; anything not symmetrical was considered to be of the same kind. It was only after having seen a number of cases that we were able to distinguish between two types of asymmetry; one primarily located in the frontal plane, i.e. scoliotic posture, the other in the sagittal plane, i.e. hyperextension or ophistotonic posture.

These two types of asymmetry can occur separately or together. The most common type combines a markedly scoliotic posture with a retroflexion component. Again this does not necessarily mean that this represents the majority of treatable cases, only the most easily perceptible and thus diagnosable clinical picture.

We have seen an interesting development in the contact between ourselves and paediatricians. The initial group of babies sent to us represented a fairly 'typical' collection of little patients with a 'classical' C-scoliosis. After having seen the effects of treatment on these children, colleagues are more aware of the other signs connected to the KISS syndrome but less obviously cervicogenic at first sight, such as cry-babies, sleeping disorders or frequent vomiting. Babies are then referred to us based on the less 'obvious' symptoms. It is less the screening for asymmetries than for the secondary symptomatology which becomes the dominant feature in our collaboration. Colleagues send babies with 'colic', cry-babies or children who have problems swallowing; they are also a bit asymmetrical, but this asymmetry is not such as to force the mother to go to the paediatrician or to make the latter think about referring the baby for manual treatment. We have to be alert to the range of problems originating from the malfunctioning of the cervical spine and the abnormal form of the cranium before we can recognize the possible benefits of therapeutic intervention. The postural asymmetry and its morphological repercussions attract our attention to the cervical symptomatology.

A window of opportunity

The acquisition of any skill requires a learning period and a predisposition to learn. The optimal point in time for a specific ability is embedded in the phylogenetically fixed development pattern. Language acquisition is the example we are frequently and painfully confronted with: whereas our children absorb another language without any effort, we grown-ups labour and toil and will never achieve the same level of effortless mastery our children achieve before puberty.

All our capacities, be they concerned with movement or perception, build on physiological and mental abilities previously learned. The earlier a basic skill's learning phase is situated in the 'normal' chain of events, the more its faulty acquisition will interfere with cognitive or motor developments later on. Head control is situated very early on in this chain of events, which is one reason why the long-term consequences of its malfunctioning are so far reaching. This is also the primary reason why we should check and treat even minor signs of asymmetry of the posture or form of the head. They may not look very impressive, but they can cause a derailment of the kinesiological development and thus necessitate much more extensive treatment in later years. Kinematic imbalances lead to behavioural and morphological asymmetries. 'Symmetric individuals appear to have quantifiable and evolutionary significant advantages over their asymmetric counterparts'.[5] We found signs of asymmetry and KISS in the newborn period of 72% of the schoolchildren we saw (and treated successfully) for headaches, postural and behavioural problems. The seeds of problems which surfaced at age 8 or 10 years could be traced back to KISS symptoms before verticalization, i.e. during the first year. This is the main reason why a vigilant attitude towards minor signs of functional asymmetry in this first stage of neuromotor development is necessary.

Even successfully treated babies continue to carry the imprint of their initial asymmetry with them. In times of exhaustion or after periods of rapid growth they will display the former asymmetrical posture again, at least temporarily. In most cases these symptoms subside spontaneously and no treatment is necessary. Only if the asymmetry persists for more than a few days should one intervene therapeutically.

Treatment

Manual therapy is by definition a craft and, therefore, dependent on the skills and attitude of the individual clinician. The etymological root of the German word 'Behandlung' (treatment) indicates how basic a principle this is, as does the narrower term 'mani-pulation', its latinized form. Where does manual therapy end, where do massage, osteopathy, chiropractic start? The answer depends on one's individual standpoint. We know how the 'normal' diagnostic examination of a patient already alters the clinical situation; you cannot draw a sharp line between test and therapy, far less limit whatever positive effect is exerted on the patient for exclusive use by one professional group. We can only give some guidelines in teaching the treatment of functional vertebrogenic disorders, nothing more. However, there are some essentials that help to maximize efficiency and minimize the amount of time necessary. By reading Andry's book written at the beginning of the eighteenth century, you will find a lot of those manual techniques which you read about in contemporary publications as the newest trick in town. Naegeli's book,[37] originally written 100 years ago, lists some of our 'modern' techniques in another context, but with comparable indications. This list can be expanded almost indefinitely. This is one reason why no 'how-to' guide is given here. The technique an individual therapist uses depends as much on his or her individual abilities as on the material framework in which they have to function. It is quite useless to tell somebody who has to work in a slum to use an X-ray of the cervical spine. So I want to limit the 'do's and don't's' to one warning. *Do not treat too often*!

Simple as this advice may sound it is extremely difficult to follow. All parties concerned want success as soon as possible, and rightly so. But it is the task of the professional to know when to expect a result from treatment, and once we know that this may take more than 2 weeks we must convey this information to the parents. Overzealous therapy is one of the main reasons for unsatisfactory results. Initially, we regularly told parents to resume other therapies immediately after manual therapy 'to make the best use of the liberation of movement provided by the soft manipulation'. We were quite astonished to see that in some cases where this was not possible (a parent was sick, the physiotherapist on holiday etc.) the results were better than normal. This led us to experiment with a therapy pause of 2–3 weeks after manipulation, and we found reproducibly better results following that rule.

Having said that, one is still pushed to show how the treatment works; just to dispel the notion that there is such a thing as a 'magic touch', let us describe the procedure.

If you want to treat a small child, take your time to win the confidence of the parents first. Remember that anxious parents transmit their fear to the child. The excitement and nervousness this causes the little patient cannot be easily overcome! One always has to consider the almost axiomatic assumption that: 'a very effective therapy has to have very impressive side-effects'. I can look back on more than 5000 newborns I have treated, most of them (80%) were treated to the satisfaction of their parents and physicians with one manipulation, without a single serious complication. But those who have just started to work in this field have to make do with less experience and must still be able to transmit confidence to the parents.

Why not stick with the 'classic' methods of physiotherapy and gradual treatment?

- Suboccipital strain is the leading factor. Without its removal the symptoms can be dealt with by physiotherapy, but the reappearance of symptoms caused by suboccipital strain can later necessitate manipulation at or after entering school.
- Removal of suboccipital strain is the fastest and most effective way to treat the symptoms of KISS; one session is sufficient in most cases (81% once, 16% twice).
- Manual therapy of the craniocervical region leads to the disappearance of problems not reported by the parents, because they did not see any connection with the vertebral spine. Later on, and especially when we made retrospective inquiries, we heard time and again 'that Lars (or Laura) sleeps (or eats) much better since the treatment', is 'another child altogether' etc.
- This therapy requires cooperation from the babies and their parents, whereas most forms of physiotherapy have to rely on the compliance of the parents.

We do not treat the cranial asymmetry itself. It is considered a symptom of an underlying problem. Treating the upper cervical spine and optimizing its function-

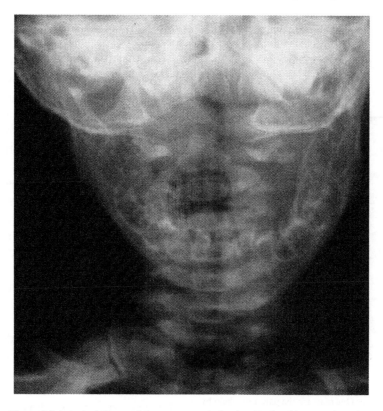

Figure 3.3 A typical X-ray of the upper cervical spine. To be able to analyse the occipitocervical (o/c) junction care has to be taken to open the baby's mouth wide enough to allow the projection of the o/c-junction between the teeth. The alignment of the head has to be scrupulously observed to avoid projection effects. This picture shows a marked lateralization of occiput–C1 and indicates a scoliotic posture of the body with a left-convexity. It is important to emphasize that the atlas moves to the convexity in babies before verticalization. Afterwards C1 is pushed into the concavity by a tilt head, due to the angle between the orientation of the joint plane C0/C1 and C1/C2[39,40]

ing re-establishes the full range of motion in the head and neck and thus induces a re-symmetry of the morphologically altered cranial bone tissue. While the functional improvement is detectable after 2–3 weeks, the diminution of the cranial asymmetry takes many months. It is important to draw the attention of the parents to the functional level of the problem, otherwise they become impatient and tend to want over-treatment.

The procedure used is basically a minimal impulse manipulation. The baby lies on the examination table in front of the therapist.

After the kinesiological and neurological examinations, the child is put on their back and we check the segments of the cervical spine. These findings are compared with the X-ray analysis. It is important to be patient; agitated children are particularly difficult to examine. Careful friction massage of the short muscles of the neck helps manual palpation. Contrary to the situation in adults, there is no 'limit of the range' for a manipulative thrust. One has to be very delicate and it helps to remember that we cannot improve the outcome by using more force. We measured the forces used in

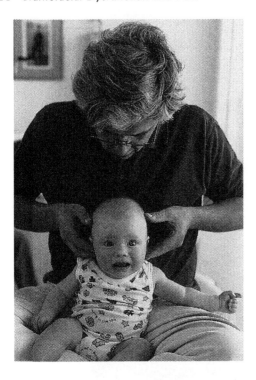

Figure 3.4 For treatment the baby is positioned on its back in front of the therapist. One may ask the parents to help by fixing the trunk and legs, but in most cases this is not necessary. The technique most commonly used is a mild transverse impulse to C1 or C2, depending on the palpatory and/or radiological analysis

the treatment of babies and adults.[38] The force used for treating babies is 15–20% of that used in adults.

In most cases the direction of the impulse is determined by the radiological findings (85%) (Figure 3.3). In the other cases the orientation of the torticollis, the palpation of segmental dysfunction or the local pain reaction helps to establish the best approach. The manipulation itself consists of a short thrust with minimal force of the proximal phalanx of the medial edge of the second finger. It is mostly lateral; in some cases the rotational component can be taken into account (Figure 3.4). If retroflexion is the main component of the fixed posture, the manipulation can be applied via the transverse process of C1 in a sagittal direction.

We believe that selection of the specific technique without functional analysis of the radiography of the cervical spine lessens the effectiveness of this treatment. As it is not that easy to get good X-rays some clinicians tend to dismiss the necessity of consulting the radiological findings. Apart from the improved treatment technique, a correct analysis also reveals morphological problems in 6–8% of cases.[41] During the first 18 months standard X-rays – an antero/posterior plate of the cervical spine including the suboccipital region – have to be of optimal quality, and no manipulation in the suboccipital region should be done without them.

The technique itself needs subtlety and long years of experience in the manual treatment of the upper cervical spine of adults and schoolchildren. In the hands of the experienced the risk is minimal; we have not yet encountered any serious complications. The forces used during the manipulation were tested with a calibrated pressure gauge; they do not exceed the force used to push a bell-button energetically. Most children cry for a moment, but stop as soon as they are in their mothers' arms. In three cases (out of 5000 infants) the children vomited after the treatment; this had no negative effect on the outcome, and there were at least as many babies vomiting already during the routine test to determine their neurological status.

Results

The main aim of any therapy should be to result in the best possible outcome with the least time and expense needed. The method proposed here fulfils these demands, but with one drawback: we have to have a little patience.

From the 263 cases (152 male, 109 female) randomly drawn from the 554 babies treated between June 1994 and June 1995, some data are published here. Two hundred and thirteen babies were treated only once, 41 twice. Only 3% were treated more often (four babies three times, and two babies each four or five times). To get a feeling for the kind of result one can expect from well-applied manual therapy, an evaluation by the paediatricians and/or physiotherapists who sent the children is needed first.

From our sample of 263 children we were able to reach 195 paediatricians for evaluation. Their replies are presented in Table 3.3. These results can be related to the different main symptoms as shown in Table 3.4.

Some details are worth mentioning:

- It does take some time for the treatment to have an effect, regardless of the symptom treated.
- In most cases no further therapy was necessary, or if so was vastly more effective. Less than half the children treated received additional physiotherapy after the minimal thrust of the craniocervical region.
- Functional changes precede the morphological improvement and here soft-tissue asymmetries (for example the cheeks in a unilateral microsomy) disappear much faster than osseous asymmetries.
- The flattened back of the head improves faster than the asymmetrical forehead; the former takes 3–5 months to be almost symmetrical, whereas the latter might take almost a year. If the babies are older than 9 months at the first treatment the parents must be warned that a functionally irrelevant asymmetry may persist.
- These results are only obtainable in babies treated before or at least at their verticalization. After the first birthday the effectiveness of the functional therapy decreases rapidly.

In some very rare cases one is tempted to use the term 'malign asymmetry' to classify those babies where a correctly applied treatment does not lead to the expected outcome, regardless of the fact that no

Table 3.3 Evaluation by the paediatricians

Very content with the effect of the treatment	40.5%	79
Content with the effect of the treatment	31.3%	61
Moderately content with treatment	2.6%	5
Not content with treatment	2.6%	5
Cannot comment	23.1%	45

The evaluation of the parents was as follows:

Very content with the effect of the treatment	62.7%	165
Content with the effect of the treatment	24.7%	65
Moderately content with treatment	9.1%	24
Not content with treatment	3.0%	8
Cannot comment		0

Table 3.4 Symptoms for referral

Symptom	(very) Good result after				Improved	No change	Total
	1 day	1 week	2 weeks	3 weeks			
Torticollis	78	28	33	19	40	25	223
Ophistotonos	10	6	5	7	12	5	45
Restless/crying	26	5	6	2	6	7	52
Fixed sleeping position	16	3	3	6	4	1	33

complicating details appear. If the expected improvement does not materialize, check for the following:

1 Was there trauma immediately before or after the manipulation?
2 Did you treat too often and/or with insufficient time between the manual treatment?
3 Did the mother continue the physiotherapy immediately after the manual therapy? (Something frequently seen if the mother is a 'professional', e.g. a physiotherapist).
4 Did you overlook a complicating neurological problem?
5 Did you overlook a morphological problem in the cervical or upper thoracic spine?

It is quite surprising how often one of these reasons emerges. To help distinguish between an adverse effect of the treatment and other factors, it is important to be very precise about the timing. Sometimes the parents come and tell us: 'After the treatment she got a lot worse'. Precise questioning reveals that the initial reaction was unspectacular or positive and only after 'some gymnastics the other day'; 'being roughed up by his elder brother'; 'stumbling over her sister's bike' etc. did things get worse.

In most cases the symptoms stop spontaneously if we leave them long enough and nobody interferes prematurely. Even the best-intentioned additional treatment is too much, and usually less is more. If the symptoms resume or have an increased intensity, do consider malignancy, even if the initial treatment improved the situation for days or weeks. At the least after the second relapse it is of paramount importance to ask for a neuropaediatric examination including MRI or comparable procedures.[41–45]

Individual and interpersonal reproducibility

As previously mentioned, we are dealing with a form of therapy which depends to a large extent on the degree of competence the individual clinician has at his or her disposal. Therefore, comparisons between different clinicians are difficult. If one therapist is able to treat a given problem, it is not necessarily true that all those who have a diploma in manual therapy or chiropractics will be able to do the same just by following the same procedure. This basic problem of interpersonal comparison is shared by most medical and paramedical activities. Think about psychotherapy or surgery, and also something as routine as massage or a hairdo – all these services rendered to others may be absolutely individually reproducible but are not necessarily of the same quality when administered by another person.

Basic as it may seem, this fundamental dilemma is rarely addressed in scientific publications. Everybody feels much more at ease with the assumption that you just have to have enough lessons and gather sufficient diplomas to be as good as anyone else. It is certainly not good marketing for our concept of KISS therapy to address this problem, but when dealing with a topic as sensitive as manual therapy in small children the issue cannot be avoided.

Epilogue

Having arrived here you might want to ask yourself (and me): well, it sounds more or less convincing, but how can I be sure that this is it? There are so many other propositions, not least in this book, and this one does sound too simple to be true. We could refer to the usage of the acronym KISS in business education, where management consultants use KISS to say 'Keep it simple, stupid!', but the final proof is the success of the treatment schedule based on the ideas outlined here. In almost 80% of the cases, one treatment only was sufficient. We do have to keep in mind that a lot of other problems mimic the same symptomatology, but if you keep the whole picture in focus you should be able to avoid these pitfalls. If and when there is reason to believe that a given clinical situation is primarily caused by a functional problem of the upper cervical spine, the therapy proposed here is simple, effective and diagnostically undemanding. If it does not succeed, nothing is lost besides 2 or 3 weeks' time. If it succeeds, mother and child are spared a lot of time- and energy-consuming treatments, and things are indeed kept simple.

References

1 Enquist, M. and Arak, A. (1994) Symmetry beauty and evolution. *Nature*, **372**, 169–172.
2 Thornhill, R. and Gangestad, S. W. (1993). Human facial beauty: averageness, symmetry and parasitic resistance. *Hum. Nat.*, **4**, 237–269.
3 Shackelford, T. K. and Larsen, R. J. (1997). Facial asymmetry as an indicator of psychological, emotional, and physiological distress. *J. Pers. Soc. Psychol.*, **72**, 456–466.
4 Swaddle, J. P. and Cuthill, I. C. (1995). Asymmetry and human facial attractiveness: symmetry may not always be beautiful. *Proc. R. Soc. Lond.*, **261**, 111–116.
5 Møller, A. P. and Swaddle, J. P. (1997). *Asymmetry, Developmental Stability and Evolution.* Oxford University Press.
6 Blickhorn, S. (1997). Symmetry as destiny – taking a balanced view on IQ. *Nature*, **387**, 849–850.
7 Furlow, F. B., Armijo-Prewitt, T., Gangestad, S. W. and Thornhill, R. (1997) Fluctuating asymmetry and psychometric intelligence. *Proc. R. Soc. Lond. B. Biol. Sci.*, **264**, 823–9.
8 Landau, T. (1989). *About Faces.* Doubleday.
9 Tarassow, L. (1993). *Symmetrie, Symmetrie! Strukturprinzipien in Natur und Technik.* Spektrum Akademischer Verlag.
10 Parson, P. A. (1990). Fluctuation asymmetry: an epigenetic measure of stress. *Biol. Rev.*, **65**, 131–145.
11 Biedermann, H. (1996). *KISS-Kinder.* Enke.
12 Davids, J. R., Wenger, D. R. and Mubrak, S. J. (1993). Congenital muscular torticollis: sequela of intrauterine or perinatal compartment syndrome. *J. Pediatr. Orthop.*, **13**, 141–147.
13 Slate, R. K., Posnick, J. C., Armstrong, D. C. and Buncic, J. R. (1993). Cervical spine subluxation associated with congenital muscular torticollis and craniofacial asymmetry. *Plast. Reconstr. Surg.*, **4**, 1187–1195.
14 Suzuki, S., Yamamuro, T. and Fujita, A. (1984). The aetiological relationship between congenital torticollis and obstetrical paralysis. *Int. Orthop.*, **8**, 75–81.
15 Bratt, H. D. and Menelaus, M. B. (1992). Benign paroxysmal torticollis of infancy. *Jt Bone J. Surg.*, **74**, 449–451.
16 Kamieth, H. (1988). Die chiropraktische Kopfgelenks-diagnostik 'unter funktionellen Gesichtspunkten' nach Palmer- Sandberg- Gutmann aus schulmedizinisch-radiologischer Sicht. *Z. Orthop.*, **126**, 108–116.
17 Keesen, W., Crow, A. and Hearn, M. (1993). Proprioceptive accuracy in idiopathic scoliosis. *Spine*, **17**, 149–155.
18 Buchmann, J., Bülow, B. and Pohlmann, B. (1992). Asymmetrien der Kopfgelenksbeweglichkeit von Kindern. *Man. Medizin*, **30**, 93–95.
19 Rönnqvist, L. (1995). A critical examination of the Moro response in newborn infants – symmetry, state relation, underlying mechanisms. *Neuropsychologia*, **33**, 713–726.
20 Groot, Ld (1993). *Posture and Motility in Preterm Infants.* Fac. Bewegingswetenschappen. Amsterdam, Vrije Universiteit, p. 155.
21 Seifert, I. (1975). Kopfgelenksblockierung bei Neugeborenen. *Rehabilitation* (Suppl.), **10**, 53–57.
22 Hassenstein, B. (1987). *Verhaltensbiologie des Kindes.* Piper.
23 Schor, R. H., Kearney, R. E. and Dieringer, N. (1988). *Reflex Stabilization of the Head, Control of Head Movement.* Oxford University Press, pp. 141–166.
24 Hassenstein, B. (1977). *Biologische Kybernetik.* Quelle & Meyer.
25 Prechtl, H. F. R. (1977). *The Neurological Examination of the Full-term Newborn Infant.* Heinemann.
26 Buchmann, J. and Bülow, B. (1983). Funktionelle Kopfgelenksstörungen bei Neugeborenen im Zusammenhang mit Lagereaktionsverhalten und Tonusasymmetrie. *Man. Med.*, **21**, 59–62.
27 Flehmig, I. (1979). *Normale Entwicklung des Säuglings und ihre Abweichungen.* Thieme.
28 Lovejoy, C. O. (1988). Evolution of human walking. *Sci. Am.*, **259**, 82–89.
29 Lierse, W. (1984). *Das Becken, V Lanz Wachsmuth: Praktische Anatomie*, Springer.
30 Wischnik, A., Nalepa, E. and Lehmann, K. J. (1993). Zur Prävention des menschlichen Geburtstraumas I.

Mitteilung: Die computergestützte Simulation des Geburtsvorganges mit Hilfe der Kernspintomographie und der Finiten-Element-Analyse. *Geburtshilfe Frauenheilkunde,* **53**, 35–41.

31 Govaert, P., Vanhaesebrouck, P. and de-Praeter, C. (1992). Traumatic neonatal intracranial bleeding and stroke. *Arch. Dis. Child,* **67**, 840–845.

32 Chagnon, S. and Blery, M. (1982). Entroses et luxations du rachis cervical chez l'enfant. *J. Rad. Med. Nucl.,* **63**, 465–470.

33 Draaisma, J. M. T. (1997). *Redressie Helm Therapie bij Plagiocephalie, Voorkeurshouding bij Zuigelingen.* Lustrum, VCNN, pp. 6–9.

34 Clarren, S. K., Smith, D. W. and Hansen, J. W. (1981). Helmet treatment for plagiocephaly and congenital muscular torticollis. *J. Pediatr.,* **1**, 92–95.

35 Biedermann, H. (1993). Das Kiss-Syndrom der Neugeborenen und Kleinkinder. *Man. Med.,* **31**, 97–107.

36 Biedermann, H. (1992). Kinematic imbalances due to suboccipital strain. *J. Man. Med.,* **6**, 151–156.

37 Naegeli, O., (1953). *Nervenleiden und Nervenschmerzen.* Haug.

38 Koch, L. E. and Girnus, U. (1998). Kraftmessung bei Anwendung der Impulstechnik in der Chirotherapie. *Man. Med.,* **36**, 21–26.

39 Jirout, J. (1990). *Röntgenologische Bewegungsdiagnostik der Halswirbelsäule.* Fischer.

40 Wackenheim, A. (1975). *Roentgen Diagnosis of the Cranio-Vertebral Region.* Springer.

41 Shafrir, Y. and Kaufman, B. A. (1992). Quadriplegia after chiropractic manipulation in an infant with congenital torticollis caused by a spinal cord astrocytoma. *J. Pediatr.,* **120**, 266–269.

42 Gutmann, G. (1987). Hirntumor Atlasverschiebung und Liquordynamik. *Man. Med.,* **25**, 60–63.

43 Visudhiphan, P., Chiemachanya, S. *et al.* (1982). Torticollis as the presenting sign in cervical spine infection and tumor. *Clin. Pediat.,* **21**, 71–76.

44 Turgut, M., Akalan, N., Bertan, V. *et al.* (1995). Acquired torticollis as the only presenting symptom in children with posterior fossa tumors. *Child. Nerv. Syst.,* **11**, 86–88.

45 Bussieres, A., Cassidy, D. and Dzus, A. (1994). Spinal cord astrocytoma presenting as torticollis and scoliosis. *JMPT,* **17**, 113–118.

4

Manual therapy movements of the craniofacial region as a therapeutic approach to children with long-term ear disease

H. E. M. Spermon-Marijnen and J. R. Spermon

Introduction

Over the years many children suffering from various complaints have been treated in our practice. The number of children who were also suffering from chronic ear disease was remarkable. Most of these children were under 10 years of age with the greatest number being between 3 and 6 years of age. The ear disease, otitis media with effusion (OME), is one of the most common diseases of childhood.[1] Because OME has frequently been associated with hearing loss, many children have been treated with ventilation tubes or other methods such as paracentesis, antibiotics, adenoidectomy or tonsillectomy.

In view of the fact that most of the treatments had a moderate effect or no effect, these children were referred to our clinic by their general clinicians based on the view, 'if it doesn't do any good, it doesn't do any harm either'. With the knowledge of manual therapy, introduced by van de Bijl,[2] 60 children were inspected and treated with passive movements of the craniofacial region over the last 6 years. Forty-nine children were treated successfully and 11 showed no change.

This remarkable result prompted some research and with the aid of the literature an important explanation has been suggested: chronic ear disease cannot be explained by the function of the middle ear alone. It seems very important to maintain the mobility of the craniofacial region in the vulnerable first years of childhood.

Treatment of the cranium by passive movements as a therapeutic approach in children with chronic ear pain can only be undertaken after studying the movements of the cranium and trying to locate the source of the symptoms.

Definition of otitis media with effusion

Otitis media with effusion is an inflammation of the middle ear in which a collection of liquid is present in the middle ear space; the tympanic membrane is intact. The duration (not the severity) of the effusion can be acute (less than 3 weeks), subacute (3 weeks to 2–3 months) or chronic (longer than 3 months). The most important distinction between this type of disease

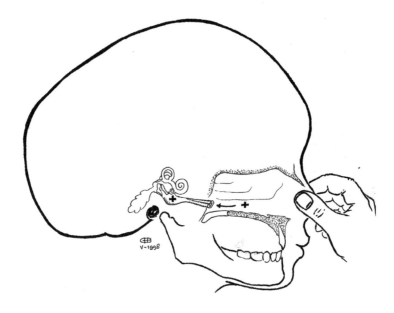

Figure 4.1 The Valsalva manoeuvre. As a result of the increased pressure in the nasopharynx the air is pushed into the middle ear, if the Eustachian tube has not been closed

and acute otitis media (acute 'suppurative' otitis media) is that the signs and symptoms of acute infection are lacking in OME (e.g. otalgia, fever), but hearing loss may be present in both conditions.

Prevalence of long-term otitis media with effusion

Otitis media with effusion is one of the most common diseases that affect young children. The presence of fluid in the middle-ear cavity usually results in a mild to moderate hearing loss. The Nijmegen Otitis Media Study (1984–1987), in which 1328 children were screened for OME serially at the ages of 2–4 years, showed that 80% of the children experienced at least one episode of OME before the age of 4 years.[1]

The literature shows that the otologic sequelae of early persistent OME vary from abnormalities of the tympanic membrane to more serious conditions such as adhesive otitis or cholesteatoma. These structural sequelae are associated with varying degrees of hearing loss. The conductive hearing loss associated with concurrent OME is considered to be responsible for adverse effects on language development as shown in the Nijmegen Otitis Media Study. It is not known whether OME has a permanent effect on language ability.

Aetiology and pathogenesis of otitis media with effusion

The aetiology and pathogenesis of OME is multifactorial; the anatomy and function of the Eustachian tube and the mastoid air cells, the age of the child and facial changes are the key components. For children with recurrent episodes of acute otitis media or otitis media with effusion, anatomical or physiological abnormality of the Eustachian tube appears to be one of the most important factors.

The Eustachian tube is part of a continuous system including the nose, nasopharynx, middle ear and the mastoid air cells. The respiratory mucosa is continuous throughout this system. Thus, signs and effects of inflammation, infection or obstruction in one area are likely to be reflected in other areas.

The anatomy of the continuous system

Anatomy of the Eustachian tube

The Eustachian tube is divided into a posterior osseous one-third and an anterior cartilaginous two-thirds. The osseous Eustachian tube (protympanum) lies completely within the petrous portion of the temporal bone and is directly continuous with the anterior wall of the superior portion of the middle ear.[3] The healthy osseous portion is open all the time, in contrast with the cartilaginous portion, which is closed at rest and opens during swallowing or during the Valsalva manoeuvre (Figure 4.1).

The cartilaginous tube is closely applied to the basal aspect of the cranium and is fitted to a sulcus tubae between the greater wing of the sphenoid bone and the petrous portion of the temporal bone. It is firmly attached at its posterior end to the osseous orifice by fibrous bands and usually extends some distance (3 mm) into the osseous portion of the tube.[2]

The tubal lumen is shaped like two cones joined at their apices. The junction of the cones is the narrowest point of the lumen and has been called the 'isthmus'. The lumen at this point is 2 mm high and 1 mm wide.[4] The lumen has a constant height, and there are only small differences be-

tween the height of the isthmus in the child and that in the adult.[5,6]

In adults the Eustachian tube lies at an angle of 45 degrees in relation to the horizontal plane, whereas in infants this inclination is only 10 degrees (Figure 4.2).[3] The tube is longer in the adult than in the infant and young child. The Eustachian tube in the infant is about half as long as in the adult; it averages about 18 mm. The cartilaginous tube represents somewhat less than two-thirds of the distance, whereas the osseous portion is relatively longer and wider in diameter than in the adult. Since the infant and young child have a shorter Eustachian tube than the adult, nasopharyngeal secretions may reflux more readily into the middle ear through the shorter tube.[7]

As a result of this the function of the tube is less efficient in young children than in adults.

Anatomy of the nasopharynx

The nasopharynx lies behind the nasal cavities and above the soft palate. On the lateral wall is a prominence, the torus tubarius, which protrudes into the nasopharynx. This prominence is formed by abundant soft tissue overlying the Eustachian tube. Anterior to this is the nasopharyngeal orifice of the tube. On the posterior wall lie the adenoids or pharyngeal tonsil, composed of abundant lymphoid tissue (Figure 4.3).

Anatomy of the middle ear

The middle ear is an irregular, laterally compressed, air-filled space lying within the petrous portion of the temporal bone between the external auditory canal and the inner ear. At birth, the cavity is of adult size (Figure 4.4).

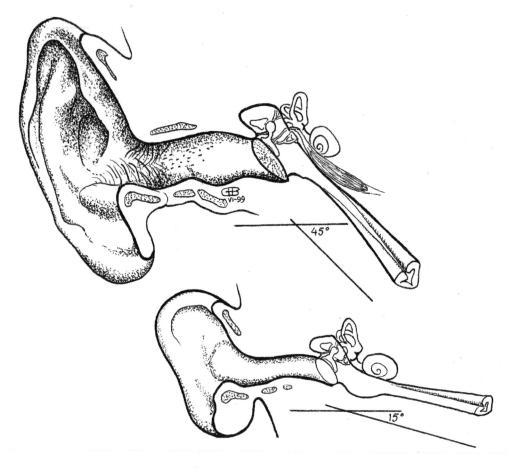

Figure 4.2 The anatomical difference between the Eustachian tubes of infants and adults

Anatomy of the tympanic membrane and the ossicles

The tympanic membrane is a thin, semi-transparent membrane that separates the middle ear from the external ear canal. It measures about 8–10 mm in diameter and is oriented downward and inward (Figure 4.4). The outer margin is thickened and forms a fibrocartilaginous ring, the tympanic annulus, which is fitted into a sulcus in the bony tympanic ring. Superiorly, where the ring is deficient, the tympanic membrane is lax and thin. This triangular region of the tympanic membrane is called the pars flaccida, or flaccid part, and communication between the external and middle ear may occur in this area. The remaining eight-ninths of the tympanic membrane is called the pars tensa. The tympanic membrane decreases in vascularity with increasing age.[8]

The ossicles bridge the middle ear cavity and provide mechanical transmission of vibrations from the tympanic membrane to the oval window and inner ear. The most lateral is the malleus, which is connected to the tympanic membrane on its internal surface. The middle ossicle is called the incus. The most medial ossicle is the stapes, which is connected to the oval window.

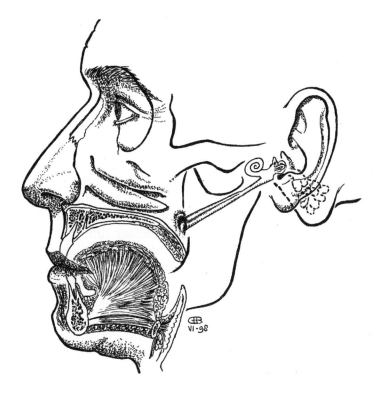

Figure 4.3 The Eustachian tube is a part of a system of continuous organs including the nose, nasopharynx, middle ear and mastoid air cells

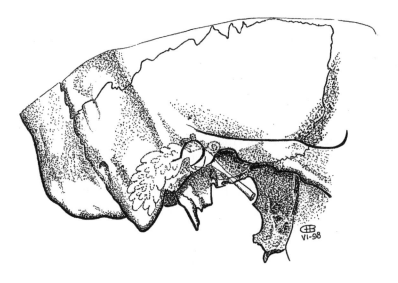

Figure 4.4 The anatomy of the external, middle and internal ear

Anatomy of the mastoid air space

Directly posterior to the cavity above the superior border of the tympanic membrane is a large air space called the mastoid antrum. The antrum serves as a communication between the middle ear and the mastoid air cells. The mastoid refers to that portion of the petrous temporal bone that lies posterior to the middle ear cavity (see Figure 4.4).

The quite small mastoid process of the infant develops into the sizable protuberance of the adult. In the newborn the mastoid process is very small with few air cells. Between the second and fifth years the number of air cells increases, with a maximum number of cells between the sixth and twelfth years. Incomplete development of pneumatization has been associated with OME.[9]

The function of the continuous system

The function of the Eustachian tube

Eustachian tube obstruction can be either functional or mechanical or both. Functional Eustachian tube obstruction results from persistent collapse of the tube. This obstruction is common in infants and younger children since the amount and stiffness of the cartilage support of the Eustachian tube is less than in older children and adults. In infants and younger children, active tubal opening is probably impaired by a lack of stiffness of the cartilage support during contraction of the tensor veli palatini muscle.[10,11] Functional obstruction may result in persistent high negative middle ear pressure. Otitis media has usually been caused by an upper respiratory tract infection. This results in congestion of the respiratory mucosa throughout the system, continuous with the Eustachian tube. Obstruction develops at the narrowest portion of the tube, the isthmus. This obstruction results in middle ear negative pressure. If ventilation occurs when there is a high negative middle ear pressure, nasopharyngeal secretions can be aspirated into the middle ear and result in an acute bacterial otitis media. If ventilation does not occur, persistent functional Eustachian tube obstruction could result in sterile otitis media with effusion. Nose blowing, crying, close-nose swallowing or ascent in an aeroplane could create high positive nasopharyngeal pressure.

Usually the Eustachian tube is closed, it opens during nose blowing, etc. and thereby permits the equalization of the middle ear pressure and atmospheric pressure. The nasal resistance (Figure 4.5) also influences Eustachian tube function (in particular the steady state pressure and the closing pressure will increase with increasing nasal resistance).[12] The nasal resistance is greater on the side of the affected ear in patients with unilateral chronic otitis media.[13] All infants with unrepaired cleft palates have otitis media as a result of functional obstruction of the Eustachian tube.[14]

Mechanical obstruction of the Eustachian tube may be intrinsic or extrinsic. Intrinsic obstruction could be the result of abnormal geometry, which compromises the lumen of the Eustachian tube. The most common factor is inflammation due to infection or allergy. Extrinsic obstruction could be the result of increased extramural pressure due to compression secondary to a tumour or adenoid mass.[15] Improved patency of the Eustachian tube was related to a reduction of extrinsic mechanical obstruction following adenoidectomy in animal model OME.[16,17]

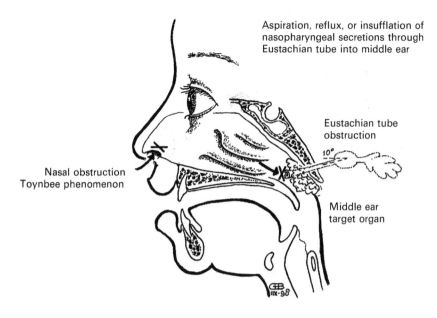

Aspiration, reflux, or insufflation of
nasopharyngeal secretions through
Eustachian tube into middle ear

Eustachian tube
obstruction

Nasal obstruction
Toynbee phenomenon

Middle ear
target organ

Figure 4.5 The relation between nasal resistance, Eustachian tube and otitis media

In conclusion, Eustachian tube function improves with advancing age, which is consistent with the decreasing incidence of otitis media from infancy to adolescence.[18]

The function of the mastoid air cell system

The role of the mastoid air cell system is probably to act like a tank of gas available to the relatively smaller middle ear cavity. In case of reduced middle ear pressure the mastoid air cells act as a reservoir of gas, resulting in higher pressure.[9]

It is generally believed that a cause and effect relationship exists between chronic middle ear inflammatory conditions and suppressed growth of the pneumatized cellulae. Continuous inflammatory changes of the epithelium of the middle ear cavity and the degree and duration of the air cavity's inflammatory condition cause the suppression of the pneumatization at the growing stage of the mastoid process. So the suppression of the growth of the cellulae is closely related to a persistent state of otitic inflammation such as OME in the early stages of growth.[19]

At the University of Turkey, research was completed into the relationship between OME and the craniofacial skeleton (CFS).[20] OME is a disease of childhood and this period is characterized by active growth of the craniofacial skeleton. The bony Eustachian tube, the portion of the tensor veli palatini (TVP) muscle and the mastoid air cells are smaller in children with OME. Enlow[11] suggests that the deviations in the growth process of the nasomaxillary complex lead to corresponding imbalances in the bony tube and vertical portion of the TVP.

However, since regional imbalances often tend to compensate for one another to provide functional equilibrium, improvement of the tubal function occurs with age.[11,20]

The age of the child

The age of the child is one of the most important factors, since most studies of the epidemiology of OME show that the disease has a peak in infancy and declines rapidly after the age of about 6 years. In addition, the structure and function of the Eustachian tube and the child's immunity are usually more mature after 6 years of age. Swarts and Rood[6] reported that there is a change in the angle between the tensor veli palatini muscle and the cartilage with development, which could be related to the efficiency of tubal dilation and the increased frequency of OME in infants and young children. As already mentioned, the length of the tube is shorter in children under the age of 7 years.[7]

Two diseases are fundamental in the development of chronic otitis media. These are mastoiditis and Eustachian tube dysfunction. Both diseases occur most frequently in younger age groups and can be differentiated. Mastoiditis occurs most frequently in infancy, while Eustachian tube dysfunction occurs between the age of 3 and 7 years. Prevention should be focused on these two diseases. Early recovery from mastoiditis, recognition of the tube dysfunction and providing ventilation of the middle ear will prevent the development of chronic otitis media.[21]

Cranial characteristics at different ages

At birth the overall length of the cranium has completed approximately 60–65% of its growth and it will increase rapidly, reaching about 90% of its full size at the age of 5 years.[22]

The growth of the brain slows after about 3 or 4 years and so will the cranium, but the facial bones continue to enlarge for many more years.

The nasal and jaw regions in particular grow much faster so that the face enlarges inferiorly. The nasal bridge becomes more prominent, the whole face expands, the frontal, maxillary and ethmoidal sinuses enlarge and the quite small mastoid process in the infant develops into the sizable protuberance of the adult.

Growth of the vault

The growth of the vault is rapid during the first year and slower up to the seventh, by which time it has reached almost adult dimensions. The shape of the vault is not directly related to cerebral growth but to genetic factors and the great range of cranial indices and shapes in racial groups supports this. Growth in breadth occurs at the sagittal, sphenofrontal, sphenotemporal and occipitomastoid sutures and petro-occipital cartilaginous joints, while growth in height occurs at the frontozygomatic and squamosal sutures, pterion and asterion.

Thickening of the vault and development of external muscular markings are related to the development of the masticatory and neck muscles. The mastoid process is a visible bulge in the second year and invaded by air cells by the sixth.

Growth of the base

This is responsible for much of the cranial lengthening, mostly at the cartilaginous joints between the sphenoid and occipital bones. It is largely independent of cerebral growth and continues at the occipitosphenoid synchondrosis until the eighteenth to twenty-fifth years, a period prolonged by continued expansion of the jaws to accommodate erupting teeth and by growth in the muscles of mastication and those of the nasopharynx. Disproportionate growth of the brain and face will have an effect on the development of the cranial base.[22]

Growth of the face

The ethmoidal and the orbital and upper nasal cavities have almost completed growth by the seventh year. Orbital and upper nasal growth is achieved by sutural accretion with deposition of bone on the facial aspects of the margins. The maxilla is carried downwards and forwards by expansion of the orbits and nasal septum and sutural growth, especially at the fontanelles and zygomaticomaxillary and pterygomaxillary sutures.

In the first year, growth in the width occurs at the symphysis menti and midpalatal, internasal and frontal sutures; but such growth is diminished or even ended when the symphysis menti and frontal suture close during the first few years, even though the midpalatal suture persists until mature years. Facial growth in this period continues to puberty and is later linked with the eruption of permanent teeth.

The height and width of the maxilla below the level of the palate are related to the eruption of the teeth and development of the supporting alveolar bone. The alveolar bone supporting the teeth best exemplifies adjustment of a skeletal element to the environment. This bone develops only to support the teeth and disappears when the teeth are removed. When a tooth is exposed to even a very gentle pressure, the alveolar bone reacts quickly with resorption on the pressure side of the tooth and apposition to the tension side. Stretching of the periodontal ligament, whose fibres are inserted into the bone and the tooth, creates the tension. Thumb sucking can interfere with dentoalveolar adjustment and will cause a malocclusion.[23]

After sutural growth, near the end of the second year, expansion of the facial skeleton is by the surface accretion on the face, alveolar process and palate, with resorption in the walls of the maxillary sinuses, the upper surface of the hard palate and the labial aspect of the alveolar process.

The facial changes with regard to otitis media with effusion

The external appearance of the baby's face does not reveal the truly striking enormity of the dental battery developing within it. The teeth are a dominant part of the infant's face as a whole, yet they are not even seen. The parent does not usually realize they are already there at all, much less suspect the massiveness of their extent. Parents do not realize that a vast magazine of unerupted teeth hidden to the eyes occupy the whole midface. After eruption of the teeth there is much more space within the maxillary sinuses, and hence the ventilation function of the sinuses will be improved (Figure 4.6).

Oudhof[24] has already indicated that particular growth activity is caused by the development of the so-called pneumatic cavities. These cavities have a particular influence on the increase of the buffer capacity of our respiratory system and they also exert a mechanical force on the growing facial part of the skeleton. In case of a disturbance in respiratory capacity, e.g. as a result of decreased nasal airflow, a decrease in pneumatic volume of the maxillary sinuses could be the result. This could lead to a disturbed mechanical force on the growing facial bone structures, causing the palate to be higher and the maxilla narrower with regard to their anatomical structure.

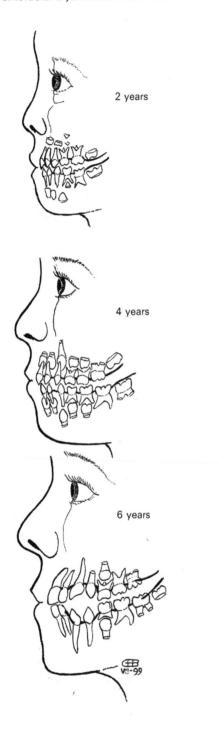

Figure 4.6 The relation between the development of the teeth and the maxillary sinus. After eruption of the permanent teeth, there is much more space within the maxillary sinus, so ventilation and drainage functions will be improved

Elevated nasal resistance, as a result of nasal mucosal swelling and adenoidal hyperplasia, has been associated with an increased incidence of mouth breathing, which may lead to alterations in facial morphology.[12] It is thought that prolonged oral respiration during critical growth periods in children initiates a sequence of events that commonly result in dental and skeletal changes. In the chronic mouth breather, excessive molar tooth eruption is almost a constant feature, causing a clockwise rotation of the growing mandible with a disproportionate increase in anterior lower vertical face height. The dynamics of excessive clockwise growth can be reversed if the physical pressures placed on the craniofacial skeletal tissues are reversed. Such increases in anterior lower vertical face height are often associated with retrognathia (backward position of the mandible) and open bites. According to Nimela et al.,[25] children who had used a dummy had a greater risk of having recurrent attacks of otitis media than those who had not. Mouth breathing was significantly associated with otitis media, as was open bite, but other types of malocclusion, such as that caused by thumb sucking (Figure 4.7), were not. In conclusion, the switch from nasal to an oronasal breathing pattern induces functional adaptations that include an increase in total anterior height and vertical development of the lower anterior face resulting in a higher incidence of otitis media.[12,25,26]

There are many causes of a 'long face'. In our 'non-chewing' society (most food we eat is practically pre-chewed or pre-digested), the orofacial musculature is lacking in functional use. This condition further enhances the lack of full facial development because the necessary forces transmitted from the masticatory musculature to the facial skeleton are absent. Experimental

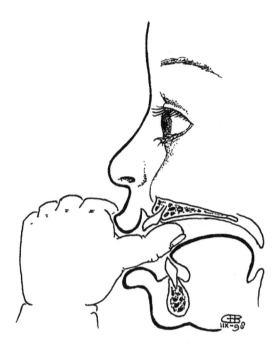

Figure 4.7 By thumb sucking the upper teeth are pushed forwards and the lower backwards, causing a malocclusion (open bite)

evidence suggests that altered muscular function can influence craniofacial morphology.

In summary, the reasons for the occurrence of disease early in life are likely to be a result of maturing anatomical, physiological, and immunological factors, some of which are identifiable (e.g. change in cranial configuration and vectors of the Eustachian tube, a development of protective antibodies to bacterial pathogens) but many of which are still to be defined.

Treatment of otitis media with effusion

Treatment with ventilation tubes has become the surgical intervention most practised for OME and, in fact, one of the most frequently performed operations upon chil-

dren in Europe and the USA (Figure 4.8). The traditional aims of treatment by ventilation tubes are to restore the hearing level, to modify the course of OME towards early resolution and to prevent long-term structural and functional sequelae of OME. Although tubes are very effective in improving hearing, there is no evidence as yet to support the attainment of the second aim and the extent to which the third aim can be achieved by surgical treatment is still unknown. Therefore, the current high rate of surgery for OME is questioned.

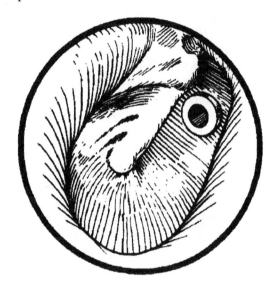

Figure 4.8 The ventilation tubes are inserted in an anterosuperior position in the tympanic membrane

These observations add to the evidence that OME experienced early in life is likely to affect a child's health later. Abnormalities of the tympanic membrane related to early OME were present in a large proportion of children and were most pronounced in children who had previously been treated with ventilation tubes. The degree of hearing loss associated with early OME was usually limited. In relation to auditory perception, language and educational skills at the age of 7.5–8 years, no substantial effect of early, persistent OME was found in this population. These results indicate that a conservative approach to surgical treatment of OME should be advocated. In general, a period of watchful waiting prior to surgical intervention is, therefore, recommended.

Between the ages of 3 and 7 years, ear disease was the most frequent complaint in our practice. Schilder[27] recently showed that placing ventilation tubes (over 50 000 each year) could indeed improve hearing capacity. However, no improvement was seen in the function of the middle ear and no long-term improvement was achieved, either structurally or functionally, in the consequences of OME.

Furthermore, analysis suggests that the correlation between middle ear infection and upper respiratory tract infection is much less than is often suggested in the literature.[28] Apparently there are other underlying factors influencing middle ear infections (the Eustachian tube function, the immunological status, allergy, environmental and social factors).[29] The conclusion is that chronic ear pain cannot be explained by the malfunction of the middle ear alone.

A different view on treatment of otitis media with effusion

A symptomatic middle ear effusion is relatively frequent in healthy children but usually resolves without medical or surgical intervention. Some physicians believe that antimicrobial therapy is used too frequently and should not be instituted for episodes of otitis media with minimal symptoms; that instead it should be reserved for severe cases, for otitis media associated with suppurative complications,

for effusions that become chronic, or for otitis media in certain high-risk children.

Considering the fact that paracentesis, tympanic tubes, tonsillectomy/adenoidectomy and antibiotics had no or moderate effect and passive movements of the craniofacial region did have effect, many children in our clinic have been treated by passive movements.

Does movement of the cranium exist?

Most parts of our skeleton allow movements between one piece and another: not just through our joints but also by mutual positional shifts of pieces of bones, which can move against each other. The cranium allows both kinds of movement: other than the temperomandibular joint there are many connections between bone structures, such as sutures and paradontia. The sutures act like joints that permit relative movement between bones and are therefore essential for movement of the cranium.

The sutures in the cranium have several more functions. They unite bones, absorb and transduce forces and play a role as growth sites in the growing cranium. All these functions together are important for movement of the cranium (see Chapters 1 and 2).

Few intrinsic genetic and local environmental factors occurring in the form of compressive and tensile forces control sutural growth.[30] There is a very close relationship between the mesenchyme from which the cranial dura is formed and that which is chondrified and ossified, or ossified directly, to form the cranium, and these layers are only clearly differentiated as the venous sinuses develop. The relationship between the developing cranium and the underlying dura mater continues during postnatal life while the bones of the calvaria are still growing.

It has been proposed that the control of suture morphogenesis was sited in the dura mater, and a variety of hypotheses have been generated to explain this process.[30]

The dura mater contains fibre tracts which extend from fixed positions in the cranial base to sites of dural reflection underlying each of the cranial sutures. The dural membrane is a tough, relatively inelastic sheath covering the central nervous system. The falx cerebri, falx cerebelli and the tentorium cerebelli are all formed by creases of the cranial dura. Distortion of the dural membranes may result from traumatic compression or plastic deformation of the osseous-articular cranium, and may seriously compromise venous drainage from the brain. The tensional forces so generated would dictate the position of the sutures and locally inhibit precocious ossification. The dura can also dictate the suture position in regeneration of the neonatal calvaria.[31,32]

The conclusion can be drawn that mutual movements between bony structures on each side of a suture depend on the mobility at the place of the suture itself and the growth of the sutures.

The presence of the fetal dura is not required for the initial suture morphogenesis, which appears to be controlled by mesenchymal cell proliferation and fibrous extracellular matrix synthesis induced by the overlapping of the advancing osteoinductive fronts of the calvarian bones.[33] Following overlap of the bone fronts, a signal is transferred to the underlying dura inducing changes in localized regions beneath the sutures. Once a suture has formed, it serves as a primary site for cranial bone growth but requires constant interaction with the dura to avoid ossiferous obliteration. For more information about this subject the reader is referred to Chapters 1 and 2.

A manual therapeutic approach in children with chronic ear disease

Assuming that motion of the cranium exists in children it is useful to establish its vulnerability. Some sutural structures are mathematically more vulnerable to traumatic compression. Interosseous compressive injury may reduce the natural plasticity of the bone. Such bony deformations are more likely to occur at junctions of centres of ossification. The occiput, which develops from five embryological parts, is especially vulnerable to this kind of injury.

There are a few joints in the cranium which are vulnerable to luxation; specifically, the pterygopalatine, petrojugular and temporomandibular joints. When the adaptive capacity of the system is exceeded by this loss of function, clinical expressions may take the form of cranial nerve malfunctions, postural/proprioceptive vestibular integrative malfunctions, cephalgia, orthodontal, periodontal and temporomandibular disease and a wide assortment of systemic illnesses. During prenatal life, birth and postnatal life there are many factors influencing the motion of the cranium.

Intrauterine forces can be aetiological in cranial dysfunction, but this information is hard to substantiate. It may be that the intrauterine position and diminished amniotic fluid are risk factors.

Moulding occurs during birth. This is a natural phenomenon rather than an injury. The cranial bones are able to override each other to reduce the diameter of the head. The frontal bones can slip under the parietal bones, which can slip under the occipital bone, so reducing the diameter of the head. Moulding is assessed by the degree of overlap at the sutures. If moulding is absent, the cranial bones are felt separately. With slight moulding, the bones just touch, then they override but can be reduced; finally they override so much that they cannot be reduced. Excessive moulding during labour indicates cephalopelvic disproportion and can result in intracranial damage. Intracranial haemorrhage is especially associated with difficult or fast labour and instrumental labour. Premature babies are especially vulnerable. Normally a degree of motility of intracranial contents is buffered by cerebrospinal fluid. Excessive moulding and sudden changes in pressure reduce this effect and are associated with trauma.[34]

During postnatal life, infections, using a dummy and thumb sucking are the main risk factors.

All the above-mentioned factors could result in a decrease of the motion of the cranium and an asymmetry of the growth of the cranium, resulting in bad draining and ventilatory function of the middle ear. The decreased function of the Eustachian tube, perhaps due to the asymmetry, is responsible for this. In evaluating and treating the neonatal cranium, it is important to remember that the occipitoatlantal joint is the only established cranial joint. The rest of the cranium is like a soft-shelled egg, containing the brain.[35]

Taking the view that motion of the cranium exists in children, the idea of treating children presenting with otitis media with effusion by means of passive movements of the cranium was formed. Passive movements restore and perhaps improve the natural position of the bones, resulting in a better draining and ventilation function of the middle ear. The outcome is an improved middle ear func-

tion, resulting in a recovery from otitis media with effusion. One suggestion would be to make the supplemental cranial examination of newborn babies a routine procedure.

The patient population

Over the past 10 years many children with a wide range of complaints have received treatment in our clinic. The number of children suffering from chronic ear pain was notable. Children ranging in age from 6 months to 10 years formed our study group. The largest part of this group consisted of children between 3 and 7 years of age (44 of the 60 children, Table 4.1).

Table 4.1 Division of children by sex and age

Age (years)	Females	Males	Total
1	4	1	5
2	3	2	5
3	3	4	7
4	8	5	13
5	5	5	10
6	3	5	8
7	2	4	6
8	4	0	4
9	0	0	0
10	2	0	2
Total	34	26	60

Most children suffering from ear disease are below 7 years of age (54/60). The eruption of permanent teeth, starting at the age of 6 years, could be an explanation. Eruption of teeth causes a better pneumatization of the mastoid air cells. The Eustachian tube function improves with advancing age, which is consistent with the decreasing incidence of otitis media from infancy to adolescence.[18]

In addition, the structure and function of the Eustachian tube and the child's immunity are usually more mature after they reach 6 years of age.

Outcome of investigation

The group of children with otitis media referred by general clinicians where standard treatments (tubes, paracentesis, tonsillectomy, adenoidectomy, and antibiotics) were not successful and where passive movement was effective is described in Table 4.2.

Table 4.2 Children with otitis media referred by general clinician where standard treatment was not successful and in whom passive movement was effective

Standard therapy (single or combination)	Total number of children	Good result passive movement	No result
No therapy	6	6	0
Tubes	13	10	3
Paracentesis	3	2	1
Antibiotics	3	2	1
Adenoidectomy/tonsillectomy	11	11	0
Tubes and adenoidectomy/tonsillectomy	12	9	3
Paracentesis and antibiotics	3	2	1
Paracentesis and adenoidectomy/tonsillectomy	3	2	1
Antibiotics and adenoidectomy/tonsillectomy	2	2	0
Tubes, paracentesis and antibiotics	1	1	0
Tubes, paracentesis and adenoidectomy/tonsillectomy	1	1	0
Paracentesis, antibiotics and adenoidectomy/tonsillectomy	1	1	0
Tubes, paracentesis and antibiotics and adenoidectomy/tonsillectomy	1	0	1
Total	60	49	11

Sixty children suffered from otitis media. The standard therapy for these children (antibiotics and/or paracentesis and/or tubes and/or adenoidectomy/tonsillectomy) was unsuccessful. Over the last 2 years 49 children with chronic ear pain have been treated successfully with manual therapy, 11 children showed no change.

The good results following treatment suggest that the ear pain cannot be explained by malfunction of the middle ear only, and the internal and external circulation and the motion of the cranium could be responsible for the pain.

It is suggested that passive movement of the cranium could restore the circulation and motion by which drainage of the middle ear is stimulated.

Relevant techniques used in children with chronic ear diseases

The Eustachian tube is situated between the ala major of the sphenoid and the pars petrosum of the temporal bone. It is supposed that a decrease in mobility of these bones could influence the ventilation function of the ear. According to the stress transducing forces (see Chapters 1 and 2), the temporal and occipital bones could influence the mastoid cells; the sphenoid and ethmoidal bones and the sphenoid and maxilla bones could influence the sinuses. It therefore seems very important to maintain the mobility of the cranium in the vulnerable first 6 years of its development. It is also suggested that the position and shape of the sulci and foramina formed by different cranial bones play an important role, allowing passage of the cranial nerve tissue and blood vessels (see Chapter 7). Before starting therapy it is useful to observe the cranium and look at symmetry or deformity, paying special attention to asymmetry, the orbital line, the level of ears related to the level of eyes, and the mastoids. Palpate the vault and position of the sutures, noting swelling and overlap and mobility. Test the condylar parts of the occiput and examine the occipitoatlantal mobility.

The techniques of passive motion testing

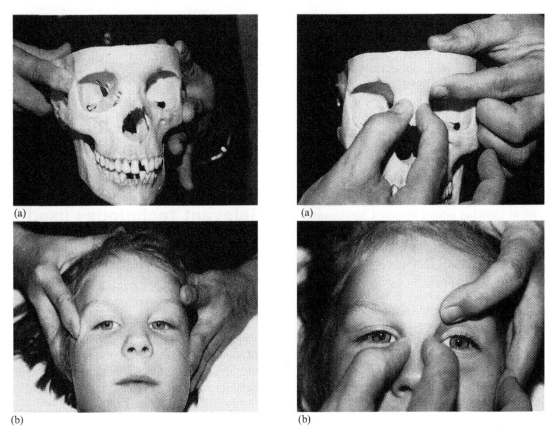

(a)

(b)

Figure 4.9 (**a**), (**b**) Transverse movement of the sphenoid

(a)

(b)

Figure 4.10 (**a**), (**b**) Nasal wiggle

are in our opinion also effective as therapeutic movements, with the application of
additional or sustained pressure. Place your
hands around the cranium as comfortably
as possible, be aware of where the sutures
are and keep the pressure minimal. Think
in grams rather than in kilos. There are
several different kinds of technique that can
have a positive influence on this patient
population. Some of these are described
below.

Transverse movement of the sphenoid

The patient lies with their head supported
on a firm pillow. The clinician sits behind

the head of the patient and puts the index
finger on the right sphenoid; the index
finger and the middle finger of the left hand
are above and beyond the left sphenoid on
the zygoma and the frontal bone. The right
hand pushes slightly to the left. The
sphenoid on the right side can be moved
in the same way. The right hand pushes the
right sphenoid to the left and the left
hand holds the left zygoma and parietal
bone or the left temporal bone and parietal
(Figure 4.9).

The effect is to move the sphenoid in a
horizontal plane (OME). All accessory
movements are possible. In our experience,
rotations around the transverse axis are
most useful.

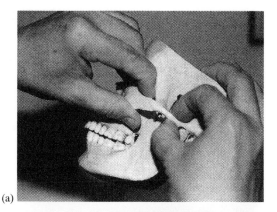

(a)

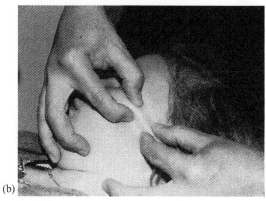

(b)

Figure 4.11 (a), (b) Movement of the zygoma-temporal region

Longitudinal movements of nasofrontal region (nasal wiggle)

The patient lies with their head supported on a firm pillow. The clinician stands at the side of the patient and uses the more cephalic hand to take a supraorbital contact with the soft tissue between the thumb and middle finger, then with the caudal hand pinches (the nasal bones) ever so lightly.

The technique is a longitudinal movement to caudal (distraction) of the nasofrontal region (Figure 4.10). It influences the frontal and maxillary sinuses and perhaps the sphenoid sinus (e.g. OME, sinusitis).

Transverse movement of zygoma-temporal and zygoma-maxilla regions

The patient lies with their head supported on a firm pillow. The clinician sits behind the head of the patient and places the first three fingers of each hand gently under the zygomatic arch close to the nose and with sufficient skin slack so as not to stretch the nose when the lift is applied.

- *Zygoma-temporal junction.* The clinician places the thumb and index finger of both hands on the bones near the joint line, and a gentle distraction between the two bones is made while the head is rotated to the opposite side (Figure 4.11).
- *Zygoma-maxilla junction.* The clinician places the thumb and index finger of one hand on the zygoma and the index finger of the other hand on the maxilla, and a gentle distraction will move the zygoma to lateral-cephalad and the maxilla to medial-caudal (Figure 4.12).

Technique: in time with the patient's breathing, the arches are gradually drawn up and backwards and then released again. This is repeated several times.

The effect is on the maxillary and frontal sinuses (e.g. OME, sinusitis).

Longitudinal movement of the petrous bone (mastoid lift)

The patient lies with their head supported on a firm pillow. The clinician sits behind the patient, the flexed finger of each hand is placed firmly under and around the mastoid process, and the arms are aligned with the long axis of the trunk (Figure 4.13).

Technique: the movement is in a cephalad

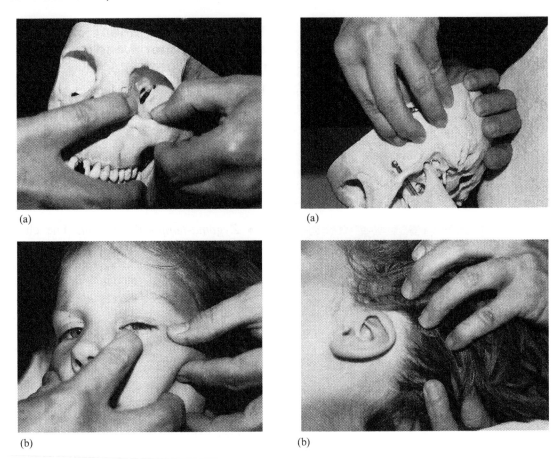

(a)

(b)

Figure 4.12 **(a)**, **(b)** Movement of the zygoma-maxilla region

(a)

(b)

Figure 4.13 **(a)**, **(b)** Longitudinal movement of the petrosal region

direction, parallel with the longitudinal axis, in time with breathing. The effect is obviously decompression, and traction on the petrosal region, which also influences the craniocervical region.

Rotation of forehead on hind-head

The patient lies with their head supported on a firm pillow. The clinician stands at the side and places a widespread cephalic hand under the posterior cranium with the fingers pointed caudally, and the other hand takes a supraorbital contact (Figure 4.14).

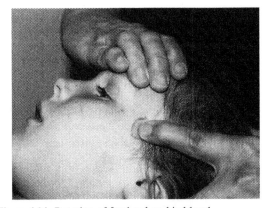

Figure 4.14 Rotation of forehead on hind-head

Technique: the hand under the cranium fixates, the one on the forehead rotates the

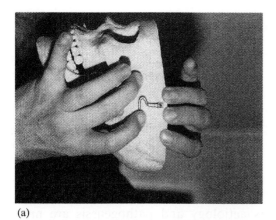

(a)

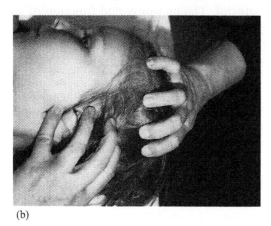

(b)

Figure 4.15 (a), (b) Distraction of parietal-temporal region

forehead in a clockwise and then a counter-clockwise direction. The effect is in general for headaches, OME and sinusitis.

Distractions of relevant sutures (suture gap)

Suture gap techniques can be applied to many of the sutures of the cranium.

These are in essence an attempt at 'gapping' distraction, a stretch across the suture line that moves all relevant sutures such as the zygoma/temporal; zygoma/maxilla; frontal/nasal; frontal/parietal; parietal/temporal (Figure 4.15). The patient lies on a firm pillow using either the pillow

or the clinician's abdomen as counter-pressure. The clinician sits or stands and places the middle fingers of each hand on either side of the suture, then with the skin slack over the suture presses in on the cranium to grip.

Technique: outward movement is made at right angles to the suture.

Opening the external auditory meatus

The patient is side lying with their head supported on a firm pillow and the clinician sits at the head of the table and uses the two middle fingers of each hand for contact. One pair contacts the easily palpated mastoid process and the other contacts a small raised area just in front of and cephalic to the external auditory meatus.

Technique: a rhythmic stretch of the area is performed between the contacts, gently at first and then progressing as follows:

* make the technique stronger
* have the patient swallow after a stretch
* have the patient swallow during a stretch
* do a Valsalva manoeuvre during a stretch.

Indication: for the relief of a sensation of 'blocked' ears of the nature that occurs after flying and experiencing a change in altitude pressure. Also on occasion it merits a trial where there has been a change in hearing following OME or other ear diseases.

Cranial examination and mobilization together with cranial soft tissue treatment such as skin stretch and deep frictions can be, in our opinion, a valid consideration in all headache and sinus conditions and possibly in moderate visual and auditory disturbances. It is however not familiar to many clinicians, who may be sceptical regarding its effectiveness (see also Chapters 1 and 2).

Discussion

Children with chronic ear diseases must be examined for abnormal craniofacial function by passive movements (see Chapter 10). Clinical reasoning helps to establish whether the dysfunction is relevant and will be a basis for further examination and treatment. There is still much research to be done in order to unravel the problems of the ear. The effect of the treatment itself provides additional confirmation. When we turn examination procedures into treatment techniques we must know that we influence many structures (joint, muscle, nerves).

Our feeling is that the link, especially in these children, between the cranial tissue and neurodynamics is of great clinical significance (see Chapter 7).

In our clinical opinion it is necessary that the cranium should be functioning as a mobile joint as rapidly as possible after birth. It is obvious why the cranial tissues are necessary prior to birth, but there is no reason why the cranium must become a solid encasement at any time. The same protective function would exist even with some mobility.

It is possible that further pathologies and symptoms are related to a dysfunction of the cranium. What is the cause of a craniosynostosis? Is it an infection, a dysfunction of the dura mater or is there a genetic factor? Is there a link with the KISS syndrome and those children with sleeping problems (see Chapter 3)?

Recognition of this clinical pattern could be a starting point for further examination and research, particularly in the newborn.

Conclusion

Otitis media with effusion (OME) is one of the most common diseases which affects young children. It is an inflammation of the middle ear in which a collection of liquid is present in the middle ear space. Improving the draining function of the middle ear is the key to health.

OME cannot be explained by poor function of the middle ear alone, because its aetiology and pathogenesis are multifactorial. The anatomy and function of the Eustachian tube and the mastoid air cells, the age of the child and the facial changes are key components.

- The Eustachian tube of the child is shorter than that of the adult and it lies at a lower angle to the horizontal plane. As a result, the function of the tube is less efficient in young children than in adults, and nasopharyngeal secretions may reflux more readily into the middle ear. The Eustachian tube function improves with advancing age.
- The mastoid cells are responsible for pneumatization of the middle ear. In the case of reduced middle ear pressure, when secretions can be aspirated in the middle ear, the mastoid air cells could act as a reservoir of gas. This would result in a higher pressure. Incomplete development of pneumatization has been associated with otitis media with effusion.
- The age of the child is one of the most important factors, since most studies of the epidemiology of otitis media with effusion show that the disease has a peak in infancy and declines rapidly after the age of about 6 years. In addition, the structure and function of the Eustachian tube and the child's

immunity are usually more mature after 6 years of age.

- After eruption of the teeth there is much more space within the maxillary sinuses and thus their ventilation function is improved. These cavities have particular influence on the increase of buffer capacity of our respiratory system and they also exert a mechanical effect on the growing facial part of the skeleton.

Treatment with ventilation tubes has become the surgical intervention most practised for OME. Although tubes are very effective in improving hearing, there is no evidence as yet to support their value in modifying the course of OME towards early resolution and in preventing long-term structural and functional sequelae of OME.

Assuming that motion of the cranium in children exists, the idea of treating children presenting with otitis media with effusion by means of passive movements of the cranium was formed. Manual therapy of the craniofacial region as a therapeutic approach in children with chronic ear pain can only be undertaken after studying the possibilities of movements of the cranium and trying to find the source of the symptoms.

Management by passive movements restores and perhaps improves the natural position of the bones, resulting in a better draining and ventilation function of the middle ear. The outcome is improved middle ear function, resulting in a recovery from otitis media with effusion.

In our practice 60 children suffered from otitis media; 49 of these children with chronic ear pain have been treated successfully with manual therapy, 11 children showed no change.

References

1 Berghaus, A., Rettinger, G. and Böhne, G. (1996). *Nasen–Ohren–Heilkunde*. Hippokrates Verlag, pp. 128–136.

2 Van der Bijl, G. (1986). *Het Individuele Functiemodel in de Manuele Therapie*. Tijdstroom.

3 Graves, G. O. and Edwards, L. F. (1944). The Eustachian tube: review of its descriptive, microscopic, topographic, and clinical anatomy. *Arch. Otolaryngol. Head Neck Surg.*, **39**, 359–397.

4 Proctor, B. (1967). Embryology and anatomy of the Eustachian tube. *Arch. Otolaryngol. Head Neck Surg.*, **86**, 503–526.

5 Sadé, J., Wolfson, S. and Sachs, Z. (1985). The human Eustachian tube in children. The isthmus. *Acta Otolaryngol.*, **99**, 305–309.

6 Swarts, J. D. and Rood, S. R. (1993). Preliminary analysis of the Eustachian tube. In: *Recent Advances in Otitis Media* (D. J. Lim, C. D. Bluestone *et al.*, eds), pp. 111–113. Decker Periodicals.

7 Sadler-Kimes, D., Siegel, M. and Todhunter, J. S. (1989). Age-related morphologic differences in the components of the Eustachian tube/middle ear system. *Otol. Rhinol. Laryngol.*, **98**, 854–858.

8 Ruah, C. B., Schachern, P. A. and Zelterman, D. (1991). Age-related morphologic changes in the human tympanic membrane: a light and electron microscopic study. *Arch. Otolaryngol. Head Neck Surg.*, **117**, 627–634.

9 Aoki, K., Esaki, S. and Honda, Y. (1990). Effect of middle ear infection on pneumatization and growth of the mastoid process. An experimental study in pigs. *Acta Otolaryngol. (Stockh.)*, **110**, 399–409.

10 Iwano, T., Kinoshita, T. and Hamada, E. (1993). Otitis media with effusion and Eustachian tube dysfunction in adults and children. *Acta Otolaryngol. (Suppl.) (Stockh.)*, **500**, 66–69.

11 Enlow, D. H. (1982). *Handbook of Facial Growth*, 2nd edn. WB Saunders Company.

12 Ayiomamitis, A and Parker, L. (1989). The differential diagnosis of nasal mucosal swelling and adenoidal hyperplasia using two- and three-parameter discriminant functions. *L. Arch-Otorhinolaryngol.*, **246**, 83–88.

13 Principato, J. J. (1991). Upper airway obstruction and craniofacial morphology. *Otolaryngol. Head Neck Surg.*, **104**, 881–890.

14 Bluestone, C. D. (1971). Eustachian tube obstruction in the infant with cleft palate. *Ann. Otol. Rhinol. Laryngol.*, **80**, 1–30.

15 Sakakihara, J., Honjo, L. and Fugita, A. (1993). Compliance of the patulous Eustachian tube. A. *Ann. Otol. Rhinol. Laryngol.*, **102**, 110–112.

16 Bluestone, C. D., Cantekin, E. L. and Beery, Q. (1975). Laryngoscopy Certain effects of adenoidectomy on Eustachian tube ventilatory function. *Ann. Otol. Rhinol. Laryngol.*, **85**, 113–127.

17 Paparella, M., Hiraida, F. and Juhn, S. (1970). Cellular events involved in middle ear fluid production. *Ann. Otol. Rhinol. Laryngol.*, **79**, 766–779.

18 Bylander, A., Tjernstrom, O. and Ivarsson, A. (1983). Pressure opening and closing functions of the Eustachian tube by inflation and deflation in children and adults with normal ears. *Acta Otolaryngol.*, **96**, 255–268.

19 Aoki, K., Esaki, S. and Morikawa, K. (1989). The size of the mastoid pneumatization and otitis media with effusion in children. *Nippon-Jibiinkoka-Gakkai-Kaiho.*, **92**, 893–898.

20 Kemaloglu, Y. K., Goksu, N. and Ozbilen, S. (1995). Otitis media with effusion and craniofacial analysis-II: 'mastoid–middle ear–Eustachian tube system' in children with secretory otitis media. *Int. J. Pediatr. Otorhinolaryngol.*, **32**, 69–76.

21 Fucsek, M. (1993). Attempt at prevention of chronic otitis media in childhood. *Orv-Hetil.*, **134**, 513–516.

22 Williams, P. L., Warwick, R., Dyson, M. and Bannister, L. H. (1995). *Gray's Anatomy*, 38th edn. Cranial characteristics at different ages, pp. 607–609. Churchill Livingstone.

23 Einstein, S. (1967). Minimal forces in tooth movement. *Am. J. Orthodont.*, **53**, 881–903.

24 Oudhof, H. R. J. (1986). Functional structure of the suture. *Nova Acta Leopoldina*, **262**, 459–464.

25 Nimela, M. and Uhari, M. (1994). Pacifiers and dental structure as risk factors for otitis media. *Int. J. Pediatr Otolaryngol.*, **29**, 121–127.

26 Tourne, L. P. (1990). The long face syndrome and impairment of the nasopharyngeal airway. *Angle Orthod.*, **60**, 167–176.

27 Schilder, A. G. M. (1993). *Long-term Effects of Otitis Media with Effusion in Children*. Cipdata Koninklijke Bibliotheek.

28 Hellsing, E. (1987). The relationship between craniofacial morphology, head posture and spinal curvature in 8, 11 and 15-year-old children. *Eur. J. Orthod.*, **9**, 254–264.

29 Bluestone, C. D. and Beery, Q. C. (1976). Concepts on the pathogenesis of middle ear effusions. *Ann. Otol. Rhinol. Laryngol.*, **85**, 182–186,.

30 Limborgh, J. (1970).The role of genetic and local environmental factors in the control of postnatal craniofacial morphogenesis. *Acta Morphol. Neerl. Scand.*, **10**, 37–47.

31 Wagemans, P. A. H. M. and Van de Velde, J. P. (1988). Sutures and forces. *Am. J. Orthod.*, **94**, 129–141.

32 Wagemans, P. A. H. M. (1986). The postnatal development of frontonasal suture. *J. Dent. Res.*, **65**, 558

33 Williams, P. L., Warwick, R., Dyson, M. and Bannister, L. H. (1989). *Gray's Anatomy*, pp. 257. Churchill Livingstone.

34 Collier, J. A. B., Longmore, J. M. and Hodgetts, T. J. (1998). *Oxford Handbook of Clinical Specialties*, 4th edn. Oxford University Press, pp. 86, 144.

35 Sutherland, W. G. (1948).Philosophy of osteopathy and its application by the cranial concept. Transcript of lecture by W. G. Sutherland. Second annual convention of the Osteopathic Cranial Association, July 18, Mass.

5

Cervicogenic headache: a clinician's perspective

P. Westerhuis

Introduction

Sternbach[1] states that every year in the USA, headache leads to more than 18 million visits to medical clinicians and 156 million days lost at work, costing an estimated $25 billion in lost productivity. Rasmussen *et al.*[2] state that approximately 16% of the population suffer from headaches. In the literature concerning headache, there is much debate over the importance of the cervical spine in its aetiology.[3,4,5] On the one hand there are authors like Nilsson,[6] who states: 'Cervicogenic headache appears to be a relatively common form of headache, similar to migraine in prevalence', and Sjaastad and Bovim,[7] who state that: 'in all probability several cervicogenic cases are at present being classified as cases of common migraine'. On the other hand there are authors like Edmeads,[8] who feels that: 'Cervicogenic headache requires much more substantial evidence before it can be accepted as a separate entity'.

The International Headache Society (IHS)[9] has produced criteria in order to classify the different types of headache (see Table 5.1).

At first glance it would seem that the cervical spine does not merit an important role as it is mentioned only in Section 11, while most studies of prevalence describe 80–90% of headache patients as suffering from migraine and/or tension-type headaches.[10,11]

Table 5.1 Classification and diagnostic criteria for headache disorders, cranial neuralgias and facial pain

1 Migraine
   1.1   Migraine without aura
   1.2   Migraine with aura etc.
2 Tension-type headache
   2.1   Episodic tension-type headache
   2.2   Chronic tension-type headache
   2.3   Headache of the tension-type not fulfilling above criteria
3 Cluster headache and chronic paroxysmal hemicrania
4 Miscellaneous headaches unassociated with structural lesion
5 Headache associated with head trauma
6 Headache associated with vascular disorder
7 Headache associated with non-vascular intracranial disorder
8 Headache associated with substances or their withdrawal
9 Headache associated with non-cephalic infection
10 Headache associated with metabolic disorder
11 Headache or facial pain associated with disorder of cranium, neck, eyes, ears, nose, sinuses, teeth, mouth or other facial or cranial structures
12 Cranial neuralgias, nerve trunk pain and deafferentation pain
13 Headache not classifiable

Adapted from: Headache Classification Committee of the International Headache Society[9]

Although these diagnostic criteria seem clear enough initially, the clinician will often have difficulty applying them in the clinical situation. Many studies describe three major problems with patient selection:

1 There is considerable overlap of symptoms between the different categories of headache. Sjaasstad and Bovim[7] for instance show that up to 50% of their patients with cervicogenic headache have associated symptoms such as nausea, vomiting and photophobia, while 27% describe a pulsating quality to their pain. These symptom descriptions are traditionally thought to represent a more vascular type of headache.

2 In the history the patient will often describe a change of the headache over the years. An initially predominant vascular type of headache may change into a more tension-type headache or vice versa.[12]

3 Many patients will not only complain of just one type of headache but on thorough questioning will be found to be suffering from different types of headache, which most importantly can be mutually enhancing.[12] Sanin *et al.*[13] classified 400 patients using the IHS criteria. The majority required more than two diagnoses, with some patients requiring up to four classifications (migraine headache, tension-type headache, drug-induced headache and chronic daily headache).

Cervicogenic headache criteria

The classification and diagnostic criteria which the International Headache Society have described are very strict.[9] The pain must be localized to the neck and occipital region, and may project into the forehead and orbital region. The pain has to be precipitated and/or aggravated by special neck movements and/or sustained positions. At least one of the three following factors has to be present. First, a limitation or restriction of passive movements; secondly, a change in neck muscle contour, texture, tone or response to active and passive stretching and contraction; and thirdly an abnormal tenderness of neck muscles. Also, radiological investigation must reveal at least one of the following three aspects: movement abnormalities in flexion/extension, an abnormal posture, and clear pathological findings like fractures etc.

Finally, the headache must disappear within 1 month of successful treatment or spontaneous remission of the underlying disorder.

To the clinician it will be apparent that, should a particular patient fulfil all the criteria, it is clear that the cervical spine is the cause for the headache. In clinical practice, however, only a minority will clearly fulfil all the criteria. There are many patients who are not as clear-cut, having concomitant other headache symptoms and/or only partly fulfilling all the above criteria. Vernon[14] investigated the cervical spine of patients who had been diagnosed as suffering from either migraine without aura or tension-type headache, and found that both groups demonstrated high rates of:

1 occipital and neck pain during headaches
2 tender points in the upper cervical region
3 greatly reduced or absent cervical curve
4 X-ray evidence of joint dysfunction in the upper and lower cervical spine.

Vernon[14] therefore states that: 'These findings support the premise that the neck plays an important role in the manifestation of adult benign recurring headaches.'

Finally, Watson and Trott[15] compared 30 asymptomatic controls with 30 headache sufferers with a history of at least 5 years duration. The headache group experienced at least one headache per month, but were not receiving treatment at the time of the study. Although the headache group was not specifically selected for cervical spine problems, the authors found that:

1 On investigation of passive accessory intervertebral movements (as described by Maitland[16]) of the upper three segments, all 30 patients had comparable joint signs (e.g. movement restrictions and production of local pain). Reproduction of symptoms was obtained in 12 cases, while the other 18 had only local joint signs in the form of movement restrictions and/or local pain.
2 Nineteen out of 30 patients described their pain as having a throbbing/pulsating quality.
3 Fifty per cent reported associated symptoms such as nausea, vomiting etc.
4 There was significant forward head posture.
5 There was decreased isometric strength and endurance of the upper cervical flexors.

As many of these patients would classically have been diagnosed as having migraine and/or tension-type headache, Watson and Trott state: 'The outcome of this study highlights the need to screen for cervical etiology in patients who are suspected of suffering from common migraine'.[15]

In conclusion it now becomes apparent that:

1 There seems to be reason to suspect that the criteria advocated in these schemes (including the IHS scheme) are inadequate when trying to distinguish between common migraine and cervicogenic headache.[7]
2 The cervical spine probably plays a more important role in the aetiology of headache than most prevalence studies will show. This can be either as the primary factor or as a secondary trigger factor.[7]
3 Furthermore, what is needed is a model which explains these overlaps, similarities etc. between the different types of headache and most importantly from which some guidelines can be drawn for the treatment and management of the headache patient.

Neuroanatomical basis for cervicogenic headache

Trigeminocervical nucleus

The neuroanatomical basis for cervicogenic headache may be found in the trigeminocervical nucleus.[17] Afferent fibres from the trigeminal nerve enter the pons and descend in the spinal tract to the level of C1 to C3. This pars caudalis of the trigeminal nerve and the dorsal horn of the upper three cervical nerves form a single functional nucleus (Figure 5.1).[18] This results in convergence of primary afferent fibres of cervical spinal nerves and the trigeminal nerve upon the same second order spinothalamic neuron (Figure 5.2).[18] This convergence of afferent fibres indicates that noxious upper cervical stimuli may cause referral of pain into the area normally

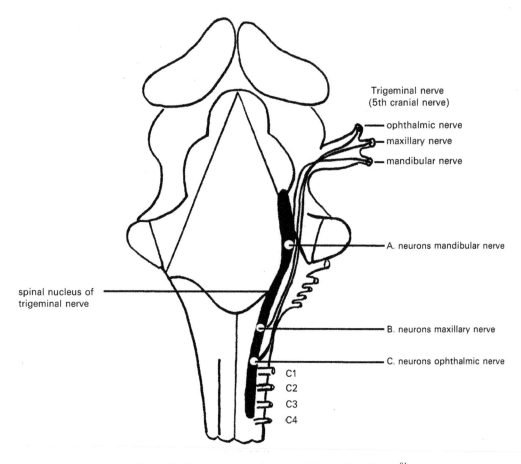

Figure 5.1 Trigeminocervical nucleus (adapted from Grieve[81])

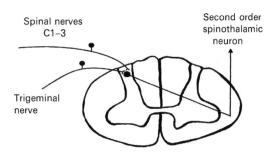

Figure 5.2 Convergence of primary afferent fibres of cervical spinal nerves and the trigeminal nerve upon the same second order spinothalamic neuron

innervated by the trigeminal nerve. Interestingly, it is primarily the ophthalmic division of the trigeminal nerve which

descends into the pars caudalis.[17] This branch innervates the area of the head where most cervicogenic headache patients complain of symptoms.

This suggests that all of the neuromusculoskeletal structures innervated by the upper three cervical nerves could cause headache.

1 Joints[19–24]

Dwyer *et al.*[20] and Dreyfuss *et al.*[21,23,24] have shown that injections of the atlanto-occipital, lateral atlantoaxial and C2–3 zygapophyseal joints are able to produce occipital headache.

Also Watson and Trott[15] were able to reproduce the patient's headache with passive accessory intervertebral movements (PAIVM) in 12 out of 30 subjects. Furthermore, the subjects with headache had significantly more joint signs in the upper cervical spine than the asymptomatic control group.

2 Nervous system

The nervous system consists of conductive tissue (neurons, etc.), vasculature (arteries and veins) and connective tissue (e.g. dura mater, epineurium, etc.).

The connective tissue has been shown to be innervated. Within the vertebral canal the dura mater is innervated by the sinuvertebral nerve.[25,26] The connective tissues of the peripheral nerves are innervated by the nervi nervorum and perivasale plexi.[27,28] This means that the nervous system itself can be a potential source of pain.[28]

Furthermore it has been shown that the nervous system undergoes considerable length changes during normal daily life activities. Louis,[29] for instance, has shown that the length of the vertebral canal (foramen magnum to the base of the sacrum) increases up to 6–9 cm when a subject moves from extension to flexion. Millesi[30] has shown that the median nerve has to adapt to up to 20% length changes during arm movements. In order to be able to adapt to these length changes, the nervous system has to be able to:

1 Slide within itself (e.g. dura mater versus arachnoidea; individual fascicles against each other[31])
2 Slide against the interfacing tissue. (e.g. dura mater against the vertebral bodies; median nerve against the biceps muscle with wrist extension[32])
3 Unfold and lengthen.[33,34]

However, should these dynamic capabilities of the nervous system be restricted, this may lead to the development of increased tension, pathological physiological responses (pain, paraesthesia etc.) and movement restrictions.[16,33,35–37]

Although nerve compression causing headache and neurological changes is relatively rare,[38] clinical observations indicate that the neurodynamics may be disturbed. This disturbance may be located inside the vertebral canal, leading to objective findings with straight leg raise and slump.[16,39]

Alternatively the greater occipital nerve may be involved.[40] Bovim et al.[41] and Gawel et al.[22,42] were able to relieve a selected group of cervicogenic headache sufferers of their pain by performing a greater occipital nerve block.

Vital et al.,[43] in describing the anatomy and dynamics of the greater occipital nerve, have shown that flexion of the upper cervical spine combined with contralateral rotation will lengthen the nerve. The clinician may differentiate symptoms by adding slump components.[16,35] For further description of the neurodynamic tests, see Chapter 7.

3 Muscle

Tension, tenderness and increased EMG-activity of the muscle are non-specific signs of many headache forms.[44] There is much debate about whether trigger points are a primary factor in the aetiology of headache, or merely secondary epiphenomena being maintained by other factors like joint dysfunction and secondary hyperalgesia.[45–47]

Recently the role of the upper cervical flexors has been the subject of research. Watson and Trott[15] have shown that patients with headache had significantly decreased isometric strength and endurance

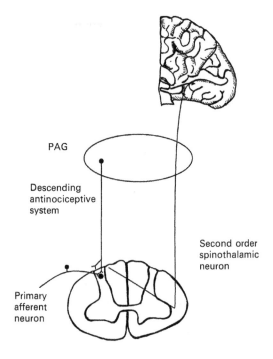

PAG

Descending
antinociceptive
system

Second order
spinothalamic
neuron

Primary
afferent
neuron

Figure 5.3 Descending neurons from brainstem nuclei have an inhibitory effect on both the first order sensory and the second order spinothalamic neurons. PAG; periaqueductal grey (adapted from Fields[49])

of the upper cervical flexors. Further research will have to show whether this is a primary or a secondary factor caused (for instance) by pain/disorder inhibition.[48]

Serotoninergic system

The transmission of incoming impulses in the dorsal horn may be modulated.[49] Descending neurons from brainstem nuclei have an inhibitory effect on both the first order sensory neuron and the second order spinothalamic neuron (Figure 5.3).[50] The main neurotransmitter released by this descending system is serotonin.[49,50]

In both migraine and tension-type headache, dysfunction in the serotoninergic system has been shown.[50] Hypofunctional serotonin activity leads to disinhibition, which will cause normal levels of afferent

stimuli to be elevated to suprathreshold levels and therefore be interpreted as pain. This disturbance of central pain-modulating systems could help to explain some of the inconsistent relationships between objective signs, structural changes and the occurrence of pain.

Sympathetic nervous system control centres like the hypothalamus and locus ceruleus are intimately related to and influence the serotoninergic system.[50] The clinical implication of this is that the clinician should include the sympathetic nervous system as a possible contributor to the problem, and not only restrict the assessment to the upper three cervical spinal nerves.

Trigeminovascular system

The mere peripheral nociceptive input of the afferent somatic fibres into the trigeminocervical nucleus cannot explain how, for instance, patients being classified as having migraine without aura, or patients complaining of an increase of their headache with weather changes, may benefit from treatment of the cervical spine.

Moskowitz[51] has shown that the trigeminal nerve also ipsilaterally innervates the most proximal segments of the anterior, middle and posterior cerebral arteries (especially the most proximal segments of the circle of Willis (Figure 5.4)). This is called the trigeminovascular system. This means that in the trigeminocervical nucleus there is convergence of input from somatic and vascular structures. As nociceptive input from one source may sensitize the wide-dynamic-range neurons in the dorsal horn to input from other sources, this could help to explain the throbbing quality of pain in cervicogenic headache patients and also how different types of headache can be mutually enhancing.

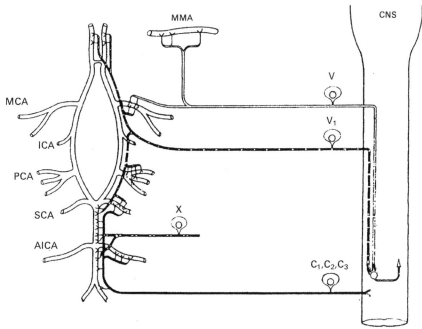

Figure 5.4 Innervation of the circle of Willis by the trigeminal nerve.

MCA	Middle Cerebral Artery	AICA	Anterior Inferior Cerebral Artery
ICA	Inferior Cerebral Artery	MMA	Middle Medullary Artery
PCA	Posterior Cerebral Artery	V	Trigeminal Nerve
SCA	Superior Cerebral Artery	V_1	Mandibular Branch

Neurogenic inflammation

In addition to transmitting nociceptive information from these vascular structures, Buzzi and Moskowitz[52,53] describe another role for the trigeminal nerve in the generation of headache. With activation there is orthodromic impulse traffic towards the trigeminocervical nucleus. There is however also antidromic impulse traffic, which leads to the release of vasoactive neurotransmitters (such as substance P) in the peripheral terminals. Released substance P leads to increased vascular permeability, vasodilation and sensitization of nociceptors (a process called neurogenic inflammation). Through this mechanism of neurogenic inflammation the trigeminal nerve may contribute to the afferent impulse traffic.[49]

The extent of neurogenic inflammation can be modulated by numerous factors (Table 5.2).[54]

Table 5.2 Modulation of blood vessel wall–sensory nerve interaction

1 *Biochemical*
  Hormones
  Mast cell constituents
  Alcohol and drugs
  Platelet contents
  Foods

2 *Mechanical*
  Stretch

3 *Ionic*
  Spreading depression

4 *Neural*
  Opiate-containing fibres
  Sympathetic
  Parasympathetic

Adapted from Moskowitz *et al.*[54]

Again there is an influence from the sympathetic nervous system, and it can now also be seen why certain patients seem to react to particular food products (e.g. cheeses with tyramine as a vasoactive

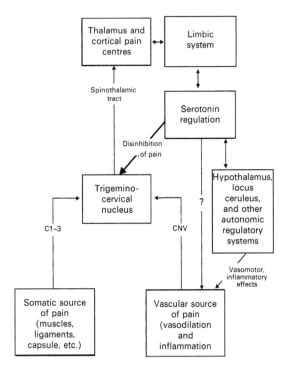

Figure 5.5 Scheme of benign recurring headache (adapted from Nelson[50])

substance). The clinical implication is that the clinician should screen for these contributing exogenous trigger factors as well.

Trigeminovascular transmission

Just as somatic input may be disinhibited, vascular input may be disinhibited.[50] The central modulation of trigeminovascular transmission has been shown to be influenced by for example periaqueductal grey modulation, special senses (light and sound), and altered physiological states like stress and sleep.[54] Authors like Diamond and Freitag[55] emphasize the importance for the patient to maintain regular sleep schedules and leisure management.

Continuum model

Olesen[56] has proposed a three-factor (vascular, supraspinal and myogenic) model for

chronic headache. Nelson[50] in modifying this model presents a continuum of benign recurring headache (Figure 5.5).

At the centre is the trigeminocervical nucleus, whose activity is dependent upon three main factors:

1 input from a somatic source (muscles, ligaments etc.)
2 input from a vascular source, which is probably responsible for the throbbing/pulsating quality of pain
3 whether or not the incoming input leads to pain, which is determined by the amount of inhibition by the serotoninergic system. (This is comparable to the pain mechanism which is dominantly related to the processing in the central nervous system as described by Gifford.[37])

The effect serotonin may have on the vascular source of pain is still debated,[49] being indicated by a question mark.

The autonomic system also plays an important role, first by regulating the serotoninergic system and secondly by influencing output by vasomotor activity and neurogenic inflammation (comparable to the pain mechanism which is related to output systems as described by Gifford;[37] see also Chapter 8).

Finally this model also helps to explain some of the affective changes so often encountered in headache patients. As serotonin has a strong effect upon the limbic system, disorders in the serotoninergic system will have mood-altering effects. (comparable to the pain mechanism which is related to the affective dimension as described by Gifford).[37] It is interesting that commonly used antidepressant medications in headache patients, such as amitriptyline and Prozac, are serotonin agonists.[49,57]

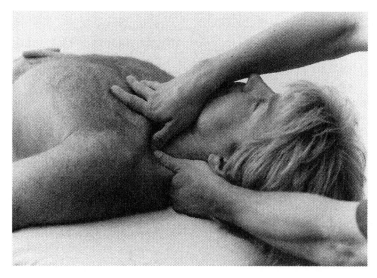

Figure 5.6 Mobilization of the first rib in a longitudinal caudal direction

Patients in whom the somatic component is dominant will fulfil all the necessary requirements for cervicogenic headache. Patients in whom the vascular component is dominant will be classified as having some form of migraine headache.

Most importantly, this model gives the clinician the rationale to search for contributing somatic trigger factors in patients exhibiting a mixed type of headache.

It also forces the therapist to leave pure mechanical thinking behind and to approach the headache patient with an overall management programme incorporating the following aspects:

- neuromusculoskeletal system-oriented treatment
- autonomic nervous system treatment
- lifestyle modifications
- detoxification
- patient information.

Overall management programme

Neuromusculoskeletal system

Boline *et al.*[57] reported on a randomized comparative trial of chiropractic manipulation versus amitriptyline in the treatment of tension-type headache. After 6 weeks and 12 treatments both groups had improved at similar rates. At the end of a further 4 weeks without treatment the manipulation group still had significantly less headache activity, while the amitriptyline group had returned to pre-treatment levels. It might be hypothesized that the amitriptyline therapy only treats symptomatically by compensating the serotonin deficits (it inhibits the uptake of serotonin in the synaptic cleft, thereby enhancing the antinociceptive effect of the serotonin). On the other hand, manipulation seems to treat the underlying disorder (causes of the symptoms), thereby having a more durable effect.

For further information see Vernon,[58] who reviews the literature on outcome studies of manipulation for tension-type and migraine headache. Beeton and Jull[59] and Schoensee *et al.*[60] present case histories of cervicogenic headache patients benefiting from treatment directed to neuromusculoskeletal tissues.

Autonomic nervous system

Treatment of the thoracic spine has been shown to be beneficial in patients suffering from symptoms like headache.[61] Harder[62] was able to ease symptoms in patients suffering from migraine by blocks of the superior cervical ganglion. Due to the close anatomical relationship of the cervical vertebrae and the first rib to the sympathetic chain, the rationale is provided for investigation of the effect of anteroposterior mobilizations of the cervical spine and mobilizations of the first rib (Figure 5.6).

Table 5.3 Treatment considerations of the mixed headache syndrome

Lifestyle modifications
1 *Dietary restrictions*
    Tyramine and other vasoactive amine-containing food
    e.g. Aged cheeses like Emmentaler, Cheddar
            Chicken liver
            Chocolate
            Citrus fruits
    Caffeine-containing products
    Alcoholic beverages (especially wine)
    Nitrites (e.g. colouring agents in processed meat)
    Monosodium glutamate (flavour enhancer in Chinese food)
    Aspartame ??
2 *Sleep habits*
    Adequate sleep
    Maintenance of scheduled sleeping and awakening times (compare longer sleeping in at weekends/holidays!)
3 *Stress management*
    Biofeedback
    Counselling (realistic goals)
    Relaxation and leisure management
4 *Detoxification* (withdrawal from)
    Analgesics with caffeine
    Narcotics
    Barbiturates
    Ergots

Adapted from Diamond and Freitag[55]

Overall management

As many patients complain of more than one kind of headache, and because these can be mutually enhancing, it becomes important to scan for other exogenous trigger factors. Diamond and Freitag[55] emphasize the importance of lifestyle modifications (Table 5.3).

Detoxification[55,63]

Edmeads[63] emphasizes that chronic daily analgesic abuse produces chronic daily headache (rebound headache); therefore it becomes important to monitor the amount of medication the patient uses, and it may be necessary to advise the patient to 'flush your pills to cure your ills'. This should only be done in liaison with the patient's physician if the medication is prescribed.

Patient information

Finally, but maybe most importantly, the clinician has the important task of educating and informing the patients. Bass *et al.*[10] investigated 272 patients presenting to family physicians with a new complaint of headache upon predictors of outcome after 1 year. Although there was some association between more severe pain, vomiting and poor outcome, 'the strongest predictor of resolution of headaches was the patient's statement, at the 6-week interview, that they had been able to discuss their headache and related problems with the doctor very fully'.

Contrary to most other neuromusculoskeletal problems, the aggravation of cervicogenic headache is not as clearly related to activities. This often leaves the patient with a feeling of insecurity, of not being in control over his or her own body. Furthermore, many headache patients are concerned over factors like having a brain tumour and/or being psychiatrically ill. This will lead to a destabilizing effect upon the limbic system and may therefore add to the serotoninergic dysfunction.[64]

Therefore it becomes essential for the clinician to try to relieve the anxiety feeling of the patient by:

1 thorough investigation in order to find the cause of the symptoms
2 explanation of the pain mechanism of the disorder with its contributing factors
3 trying to put the locus of control back with the patient by advising home exercises and dietary restrictions.

Clinical presentation of cervicogenic headache

Introduction

There are no laboratory tests which can positively assist diagnosis in the most common forms of benign recurring headache.[44] Plain X-rays are often inconclusive in differential diagnosis.[44] Therefore, diagnosis is primarily made on the clinical presentation of the symptoms, and is subsequently proven by finding comparable objective neuromusculoskeletal signs upon thorough physical examination.

The following cervicogenic headache profile is mainly based upon the work of the following authors: Edeling,[65] Fredriksen *et al.*,[66] Pfaffenrath *et al.*,[67] Sjaastad and Bovim,[7] Jull[44] and Watson.[68]

Localization and quality of symptoms

Although the pain may be located in any area of the head, the most common sites are the frontal, temporal, occipital and retro-orbital regions. The pain is often but not necessarily always accompanied by suboccipital and neck pain. As migraine patients may also complain of accompanying sub-occipital pain, Sjaastad[69] makes the important distinction that with cervicogenic headache the pain tends to start suboccipitally and subsequently spreads anteriorly, while with migraine patients the reverse tends to be the case. The pain may be unilateral and/or bilateral, but in contrast to migraine does not change sides.

The most commonly used descriptors of the symptoms are an ache or dull, boring pain. The patient may also complain of a tight band around the head or a pressing sensation. However, qualities like throbbing and pulsating may also be described.

Although the pain may reach severe levels of intensity, interfering with daily life activities in 20% of the cases,[44] it is seldom so excruciating that the only thing the patient can do is lie down.

Associated and neurological symptoms

All of the aforementioned authors describe cervicogenic headache patients complaining of associated symptoms like nausea, vomiting, dizziness, tinnitus, disturbance of vision and photo-/phonophobia etc. Most importantly, there was marked relief of these symptoms after successful treatment of the cervical spine.

As the pain in headache patients is usually a referred pain and not caused by compression of a nerve, neurological symptoms are seldom present.[17] Lance and Anthony[70] have described the so-called neck–tongue syndrome. This is a disorder where the patients complain of acute unilateral (sub) occipital pain in combination with a sensation of numbness in the homolateral half of the tongue. The symptoms are usually brought about by a sudden or uncontrolled movement (mainly rotation) of the head. Bogduk[71] hypothesizes that the symptoms are caused by excessive motion in the C1–2 joint leading to impingement and/or stretching of the C2 ventral ramus against the articular pillar of C2. The (sub) occipital pain is caused by fibres of C2 normally innervating the C1–2 joint, while the unilateral numbness is caused by compression of the proprioceptive afferents from the tongue which pass from the ansa hypoglossi into the C2 ventral ramus. Thorough assessment of the passive physiological intervertebral movements of the upper cervical spine[16] should reveal whether the problem is caused by a primary homolateral hypermobility/instability, or by a primary heterolateral hypomobility leading to secondary hypermobility on the symptomatic side.

Aggravating factors with a cervical component

The cervicogenic headache may be precipitated by neck movements. The patient may complain of headache with movements such as looking up (extension), reversing the car (rotation), shaving, etc. Most patients, however, will not have such a clear-cut presentation, and will describe sustained neck positions like working at a computer for a long time (forward head posture), waking up after having slept prone (rotation), riding a mountain bike (upper cervical extension) etc. In these instances it may not be as clear that the cervical spine is the culprit.

Further trigger factors

One of the implications of the continuum model is that other trigger factors may aggravate or even provoke a headache attack. The combination of a subclinical cervical joint dysfunction plus an exogenous trigger factor may be the cause of the headache.[55] It therefore becomes important to screen for other trigger factors. Trigger factors may be certain food products, a change in regular sleeping rhythm, stress, chronic daily use of analgesics, weather changes etc. (see Table 5.3).

The difficulty with food is first that no patient responds to all food products and secondly that the headache will often only start after a delay of up to 24 hours, and therefore the trigger factor is overlooked.

Easing factors

Cervicogenic headache patients will often have difficulty in describing factors which ease their symptoms. Relieving factors may be lying down, resting in a quiet (maybe even dark) room, trying to relax, massaging the temples/suboccipital area, stretching the suboccipital muscles etc. As these are the same factors many migraine patients will describe, this might be one of the reasons why a correct diagnosis is so often missed.

Special questions/general medical history

As headache could be the first symptom of more malignant disease, like tumours, it becomes imperative to screen for general medical conditions. Routine questions should incorporate general health, recent loss of weight, balance problems, other medication, blood pressure etc.

Although standard plain view radiographic examination is important to exclude more sinister pathology like fractures etc., it has been shown to be ineffective in the diagnosis of cervicogenic headache.[67,72] The reliability and clinical value of routine dynamic radiographic examination is still debated.[14,72,73]

History

It is often useful to ask the patient to keep a headache diary. This will give the clinician a temporal profile of the headache (which kind of headache, its intensity, how many hours/days it lasts and frequency). This diary will also enable a more realistic retrospective reassessment of a change in the condition. Furthermore, the diary helps to screen for the effect of possible exogenous trigger factors.

Most patients will present with a long history of headache, and it becomes important to ask for any recent change in their symptoms in order to assess the stability of the condition.

Only 50% of the cervicogenic headache patients are able directly to relate the onset of their problem to head or neck trauma,[44] and therefore accumulation of repetitive microtrauma (poor working postures) may play an important role.

Summary

Cervicogenic headache is a complex and often misdiagnosed syndrome.[7] It is usually caused by a combination of more than one type of pain mechanism (e.g. disturbance of input and processing, or disturbance of output and processing, etc.). Even in those patients where there is a dominance of neuromusculoskeletal problems one usually finds that there is not only one structure/ component involved but a combination (e.g. joint restrictions and disturbances of neurodynamics).[16]

As clinical diagnosis cannot be made based upon the subjective examination, thorough physical examination should aim to find abnormal physical signs in the neuromusculoskeletal system.[44]

Clinical management of the cervicogenic headache patient should incorporate all aspects of the different pain mechanisms involved and be aimed at all structures involved (see also Chapters 8 and 10).

References

1 Sternbach, R. A. (1986). Pain and 'hassles' in the United States: findings of the Nuprin report. *Pain*, **27**, 69–80.

2 Rasmussen, B. K., Jensen, R., Schroll, M. and Olesen, J. (1991). Epidemiology of headache in a general population – a prevalence study. *J. Clin. Epidemiol.*, **44**, 1147–1157.

3 Sjaastad, O. (1992). Cervicogenic headache: the controversial headache. *Clin. Neurol. Neurosurg.*, **94**, 147–149.

4 Pfaffenrath, V. and Kaube, H. (1990). Diagnostics of cervicogenic headache. *Funct. Neurol.*, **5**, 159–164.

5 Featherstone, H. J. (1985) Migraine and muscle contraction headaches: a continuum. *Headache*, **25**, 194–198.

6 Nilsson, N. (1995). The prevalence of cervicogenic headache in a random population sample of 20–59 year olds. *Spine*, **17**, 1884–1888.

7 Sjaastad, O. and Bovim, G. (1991) Cervicogenic headache: the differentiation from common migraine, an overview. *Funct. Neur.*, **6**, 93–100.

8 Edmeads, J. (1988) The cervical spine and headache. *Neurology*, **38**, 1874–1878.

9 Headache Classification Committee of the International Headache Society (1988). Classification and diagnostic criteria for headache disorders, cranial neuralgias and facial pain. *Cephalalgia*, **8** (suppl. 79), 1–96.

10 Bass, M. J., McWhinney, M. D., Dempsey, J. B. *et al.* (1986). Predictors of outcome in headache patients presenting to family physicians – a one year prospective study. *Headache*, **26**, 285–294.

11 Lance, J. W., Curran, D. A. and Anthony, M. (1965). Investigation into the mechanism and treatment of chronic headache. *Med. J. Aust.*, **2**, 909–914.

12 Marcus, D. A. (1992). Migraine and tension-type headaches: the questionable validity of current classification systems. *Clin. J. Pain*, **8**, 28–36.

13 Sanin, L. C., Mathew, N. T. and Bellmeyer, L. R. (1994). The International Headache Society headache classification as applied to a headache clinic population. *Cephalalgia*, **14**, 443–446.

14 Vernon, H., Steiman, I. and Hagino, C. (1992). Cervicogenic dysfunction in muscle contraction headache and migraine: a descriptive study. *J. Manipul. Physiol. Ther.*, **15**, 418–429.

15 Watson, D. H. and Trott, P. H. (1993). Cervical headache: an investigation of natural head posture and upper cervical flexor muscle performance. *Cephalalgia*, **13**, 272–84.

16 Maitland, G. D. (1986). *Vertebral Manipulation*, 5th edn. Butterworths.

17 Bogduk, N. (1994). Cervical causes of headache and dizziness. In: *Grieve's Modern Manual Therapy*, 2nd edn (J. D. Boyling and N. Palastanga, eds), pp. 317–331. Churchill Livingstone.

18 Grieve, G. P. (1988). *Common Vertebral Joint Problems*, 2nd edn. Churchill Livingstone.

19 Bogduk, N. and Marsland, A. (1988). The cervical zygapophysial joints as a source of neck pain. *Spine*, **13**, 610–617.

20 Dwyer, A., April, C. and Bogduk, N. (1990). Cervical zygapophyseal joint pain patterns I: a study in normal volunteers. *Spine*, **15**, 453–457.

21 Dreyfuss, P., Michaelsen, M. and Fletcher, D. (1994). Atlanto-occipital and lateral atlanto-axial joint pain patterns. *Spine*, **19**, 1125–1131.

22 Ehni, G. and Benner, B. (1984). Occipital neuralgia and the C1–2 arthrosis syndrome. *J. Neurosurg.*, **61**, 961–965.

23 Fukui, S., Ohseto, K., Shiotani, M. *et al.* (1996). Referred pain distribution of the cervical zygapophyseal joints and the dorsal rami. *Pain*, **68**, 79–83.

24 Star, M. J., Curd, J. G. and Thorne, R. P. (1992). Atlantoaxial lateral mass osteoarthritis. *Spine*, **17**, S71–76.

25 Bogduk, N. and Twomey, L. T. (1987). *Clinical Anatomy of the Lumbar Spine*. Churchill Livingstone.

26 Keller, J. T., Marfurt, C. F., Dimlich, R. W. and Tierney, B. E. (1989). Sympathetic innervation of the supratentorial dura mater of the rat. *J. Comp. Neurol.*, **290**, 310–321.

27 Hromada, J. (1963). On the nerve supply of the connective tissue of some peripheral nervous system components. *Acta Anat.*, **55**, 343–351.

28 Bove, G. M. and Light, A. R. (1997). The nervi nervorum. Missing link for neuropathic pain? *Pain Forum*, **3**, 181–190.

29 Louis, R. (1981). Vertebroradicular and vertebromedullar dynamics. *Anat. Clin.*, **3**, 1–11.

30 Millesi, H. (1986). The nerve gap: theory and clinical practice. *Hand Clin.*, **2**, 651–663.

31 Lundborg, G. (1988) *Nerve Injury and Repair*. Churchill Livingstone.

32 Mclellan, D. L. and Swash, M. (1976). Longitudinal sliding of the median nerve during movements of the upper limb. *J. Neurol. Neurosurg. Psychiatry*, **39**, 556–570.

33 Breig, A. (1978). *Adverse Mechanical Tension in the Central Nervous System*. Almqvist & Wiksell.

34 Doursounian, L., Alfonso, J. M., Iba-Zizen, M. T. *et al.* (1989). Dynamics of the junction between the medulla and the cervical spinal cord: an in vivo study in the sagittal plane by magnetic resonance imaging. *Surg. Radiol. Anat.*, **11**, 313–322.

35 Butler, D. S. (1991) *Mobilisation of the Nervous System*. Churchill Livingstone.

36 Shacklock, M. O., Butler, D. S. and Slater, H. (1994). The dynamic central nervous system: structure and clinical biomechanics. In: *Grieve's Modern Manual Therapy*, 2nd edn (J. D. Boyling and N. Palastanga, eds), pp. 21–38. Churchill Livingstone.

37 Gifford, L. S. (1998). *Whiplash: Science and Management. Fear-avoidance Beliefs and Behaviour. Topical Issues in Pain*. MOI Press.

38 Bogduk, N. (1980). The anatomy of occipital neuralgia. *Clin. Exper. Neurol.*, **17**, 167–184.

39 Hack, G. D., Koritzer, R. T., Robinson, W. L. *et al.* (1995). Anatomic relation between the rectus capitis posterior minor muscle and the dura mater. *Spine*, **20**, 2484–2486.

40 Bovim, G., Bonamico, L., Fredriksen, T. A. *et al.* (1991) Topographic variations in the peripheral course of the greater occipital nerve. *Spine*, **16**, 475–478.

41 Bovim, G., Berg, R. and Dale, L. G. (1992). Cervicogenic headache: anesthetic blockades of cervical nerves (C2–C5) and facet joints (C2/C3). *Pain*, **49**, 315–320.

42 Gawel, M. J. and Rothbart, P. J. (1992). Occipital nerve block in the management of headache and cervical pain. *Cephalalgia*, **12**, 9–13.

43 Vital, J. M., Grenier, F., Dautheribes, M. *et al.* (1989). An anatomic and dynamic study of the greater occipital nerve (n. of Arnold). *Surg. Radiol. Anat.*, **11**, 205–210.

44 Jull, G. A. (1994). Cervical headache: a review. In: *Grieve's Modern Manual Therapy*, 2nd edn (J. D. Boyling and N. Palastanga, eds), pp. 333–347. Churchill Livingstone.

45 Travell, K. G. and Simons, D. G. (1983). *Myofascial Pain and Dysfunction. The Trigger Point Manual*. Williams & Wilkins.

46 Langemark, M. and Olesen, J. (1987). Pericranial tenderness in tension headache. *Cephalalgia*, **7**, 249–255.

47 Quintner, J. L. and Cohen, M. L. (1994). Referred pain of peripheral nerve origin. An alternative to the 'myofascial pain' construct. *Clin. J. Pain*, **10**, 234–251.

48 Young, A., Stokes, M. and Iles, J. F. (1987). Effects of joint pathology on muscle. *Clin. Orthop. Rel. Res.*, **219**, 21–27.

49 Fields, H. L. (1990). *Pain Syndromes in Neurology*. Butterworths.

50 Nelson, C. F. (1994). The tension headache, migraine headache continuum: a hypothesis. *J. Manipul. Physiol. Ther.*, **17**, 156–167.

51 Moskowitz, M. A. (1990). Basic mechanisms in vascular headache. *Neurol. Clin.*, **8**, 801–815.

52 Buzzi, M. G. and Moskowitz, M. A. (1991). Evidence for 5-HT1B/1D receptors mediating the antimigraine effect of sumatriptan and dihydroergatamine. *Cephalalgia*, **11**, 165–168.

53 Buzzi, M. G. and Moskowitz, M. A. (1992). The trigeminovascular system and migraine. *Path. Biol.*, **40**, 313–317.

54 Moskowitz, M. A., Henrikson, B. M., Markowitz, S. and Saito, K. (1988). Intra- and extracraniovascular nociceptive mechanisms and the pathogenesis of head pain. In: *Basic Mechanisms of Headache* (J. Olesen and

L. Edvinsson, eds), pp. 429–437. Elsevier Science Publishers B.V.

55 Diamond, S. and Freitag, F. G. (1988). The mixed headache syndrome. *Clin. J. Pain*, **4**, 67–74.

56 Olesen, J. (1991). Clinical and pathophysiological observations in migraine and tension-type headache explained by integration of vascular, supraspinal and myofascial inputs. *Pain*, **46**, 125–132.

57 Boline, P. D., Kassak, K., Bronfort, G. *et al.* (1995). Spinal manipulation vs. amitriptyline for the treatment of chronic tension-type headaches: a randomized clinical trial. *J. Manipul. Physiol. Ther.*, **18**, 148–154.

58 Vernon, H. T. (1995). The effectiveness of chiropractic manipulation in the treatment of headache: an exploration in the literature. *J. Manipul. Physiol. Ther.*, **18,** 611–617.

59 Beeton, K. and Jull, G. (1994). Effectiveness of manipulative physiotherapy in the management of cervicogenic headache: a single case study. *Physiotherapy*, **80**, 417–423.

60 Schoensee, S. K., Jensen, G. J., Nicholson, G. *et al.* (1995). The effect of mobilization on cervical headaches. *JOSPT*, **21**, 184–196.

61 Oostendorp, R. A. B., Hagenaars, L. H. A., Meldrum, H. A. *et al.* (1986). De vertebrobasilaire insufficientie (deel IV). *Nederlands Tijdschrift voor Manuele Therapie*, **4**, 16–45.

62 Harder, H. J. (1981). Die Behandlung der Migraine Blanche und Opthalmique mit Blockaden des Gangion Cervicale Superius. *Reg. Anaesthesie*, **4**, 1–9.

63 Edmeads, J. (1990). Analgesic-induced headaches: an unrecognized epidemic. *Headache,* **30**, 614–615.

64 Sapolsky, R. M. (1994). *Why Zebras Don't get Ulcers. A Guide to Stress, Stress-related Diseases, and Coping.* WH Freeman and Company.

65 Edeling, J. (1988). *Manual Therapy for Chronic Headache.* Butterworths.

66 Fredriksen, T. A., Hovdal, H. and Sjaastad, O. (1987). 'Cervicogenic headache' clinical manifestations. *Cephalalgia*, **7**, 147–160.

67 Pfaffenrath, V., Dandekar, R. and Pollmann, W. (1987). Cervicogenic headache – the clinical picture, radiological findings and hypothesis on its pathophysiology. *Headache*, **27**, 495–499.

68 Watson, D. H. (1994). Cervical headache: an investigation of natural head posture and upper cervical flexor muscle performance. In: *Grieve's Modern Manual Therapy*, 2nd edn (J. D. Boyling and N. Palastanga, eds), pp. 349–359. Churchill Livingstone.

69 Sjaastad, O. and Fredriksen, A. (1989). The localization of the initial pain of attack. A comparison between classic migraine and cervicogenic headache. *Funct. Neurol.*, **4**, 73–78.

70 Lance, J. W. and Anthony, M. (1980). Neck–tongue syndrome on sudden turning of the head. *J. Neurol. Neurosurg. Psychiatry,* **43**, 97–101.

71 Bogduk, N. (1981). An anatomical basis for the neck–tongue syndrome. *J. Neurol. Neurosurg. Psychiatry*, **44**, 202–208.

72 Fredriksen, T. A., Fougner, R., Tangerud, A. and Sjaastad, O. (1989) Cervicogenic headache. Radiological investigations concerning head/neck. *Cephalalgia*, **9**, 139–146.

73 Pfaffenrath, V., Dandekar, R., Mayer, E. T. *et al.* (1988) Cervicogenic headache: results of computer-based measurements of cervical spine mobility in 15 patients. *Cephalalgia*, **8**, 45–48.

6

Cervicogenic headache: physical examination and management

P. Westerhuis and H. J. M. von Piekartz

Introduction

As there is considerable overlap in symptomatology between the different types of benign recurring headache,[1-4] the physical examination plays a crucial role in diagnosis. In order for a diagnosis of cervicogenic headache to be made, there have to be objective signs in the neuromusculoskeletal system of the upper cervical spine (see Chapter 5).[5,6] As the autonomic nervous system may also be involved, it is important to include the upper thoracic spine in the assessment.[7]

For possible involvement of the cranial tissue, the reader is referred to Chapters 2 to 7.

The aim of the physical examination is to support the hypothesis made in the subjective examination that the cervical spine is (one of) the cause(s) of the headache. During the physical examination, the clinician mainly assesses three factors, namely:

- behaviour of symptoms (local/referred pain, dizziness, tingling etc.)
- behaviour of resistance (stiffness, range of motion etc.)
- the occurrence of protective muscle spasm.

Abnormal behaviour of one of these factors is an objective physical sign.[8] The goal is to reproduce the abnormal symptoms of the patient, and/or produce physical signs in relevant joints which could be the cause of the symptoms (comparable signs).[8]

In planning the physical examination, the clinician must decide how much symptom provocation the condition allows and how vigorously the testing may be performed. Patient A complaining of severe headache provoked by minimal neck movements should be examined much more gently than patient B whose headache is only precipitated after having worked at the computer for more than 4 hours.

Neuromusculoskeletal system

All three components of the neuromusculoskeletal system must be assessed.

Articular dysfunction

Articular dysfunction is mainly evaluated by active movements, passive physiological intervertebral movements (PPIVMs) and passive accessory intervertebral movements (PAIVMs).

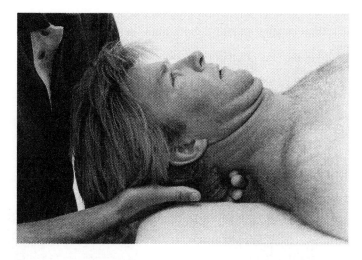

Figure 6.1 Upper cervical flexion (chin-tuck) without lifting the head off the occipital hand

For detailed descriptions of standard examination procedures the reader is referred to the work of Maitland,[8] Grieve[9] and Jull.[10]

Jull *et al.*[11] have shown that an experienced manipulative physiotherapist is able to detect whether or not a zygapophyseal joint is responsible for a patient's headache in a single-blind study. In a later study Jull *et al.*[12] went on to show that there was also excellent to complete agreement between six different examiners upon whether a subject had a painful joint dysfunction or not.

Patient example 1 (see p. 108) describes a headache patient with a predominant joint dysfunction.

Muscular dysfunction

Watson and Trott[13] have compared 30 cervicogenic headache sufferers with 30 asymptomatic subjects and found that the headache group had significant:

- forward head posture
- weakness of the deep cervical flexor muscles

- lack of endurance of the deep cervical flexor muscles.

It therefore becomes important to evaluate the function of these muscles. For a detailed description the reader is referred to the work of Watson,[14] Jull[5] and Sahrman.[15]

One simple test is described. The patient lies supine with the cervical spine in a neutral position. The clinician places one hand under the occiput and the other hand beneath the cervical spine. Subsequently the patient is asked to perform an upper cervical flexion movement ('chin-tuck') without lifting the head off the 'occiput hand' (Figure 6.1). On correct performance the clinician should feel a slight increase of pressure on the 'cervical hand' while the pressure on the 'occiput hand' should remain unchanged. Should, for instance, the patient substitute with an overactive sternocleidomastoid muscle, there will be a decrease of pressure on the 'occiput hand'. Endurance may be assessed by the amount of time before substitution or fatigue tremor occurs.

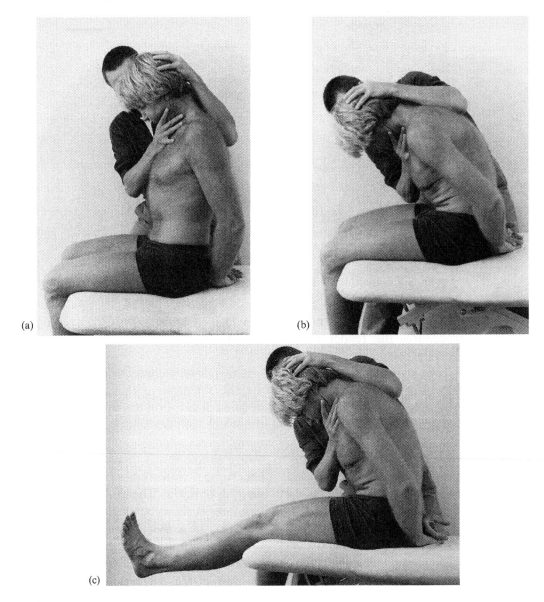

Figure 6.2 The slump test. **(a)** Upper cervical flexion in sitting; **(b)** flexion of the lumbar spine with a stabilized cervical spine; **(c)** extension of the left knee. The cervical and lumbar spine stay in flexion

Neurodynamics

The neurodynamics of both the neural tissue within the vertebral canal and the peripheral nerves (especially the greater occipital nerve) must be evaluated.

Neurodynamics within the canal may be assessed by variations of the slump test.[8,16]

If, for instance, on assessing the cervical flexion of patient A range is restricted by 50% and suboccipital pain is reproduced, this could be caused first by restricted mobility in the cervical joints, secondly by altered neurodynamics and/or thirdly by altered muscle length (Figure 6.2a). In order to increase the stress differentially

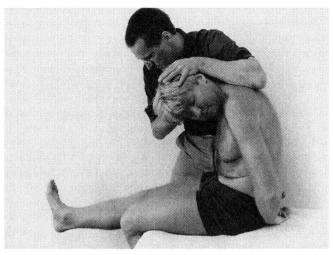

Figure 6.3 The slump test with emphasis on the right occipital nerve. The sequence of testing is upper cervical flexion, rotation to the left, side flexion to the left, mid to low cervical spine flexion, thoracic and lumbar flexion and knee extension

on the nervous system, the examiner holds the cervical spine absolutely stable while flexing the lumbar spine (Figure 6.2b). Extending the knee (Figure 6.2c) may increase the stress further. Should the symptoms increase, this indicates involvement of the nervous system.

In order to bias for the right greater occipital nerve, the sequence of testing is upper cervical flexion, rotation to the left, side flexion to the left, mid to low cervical spine flexion, thoracic and lumbar flexion and finally knee extension (Figure 6.3).

For further reading the reader is referred to the work of Maitland,[8] Elvey[17] and Butler.[18]

Principle of differentiation

Introduction

With most examination procedures, more than one structure is being stressed. In order to differentiate which of the structures is responsible for the symptoms, the clinician will change the stress on one structure only and evaluate the change in symptoms and or resistance (for example, compare 'slump' differentiation with restricted and painful cervical flexion).

The severity and/or irritability of the symptoms determines whether the differentiation procedure is performed in the painful position, or just before the onset of pain ('short of pain'). When cervical flexion produces only a slight pulling feeling in the neck, the slump differentiation may be performed while maintaining the cervical spine in the painful position. However, if the flexion movement reproduces a severe stabbing pain, the cervical spine is only flexed to a position short of the onset of pain, after which the slump procedure is added.

Assessment and 'clinical proof'

Another important principle of assessment is that one test in isolation is not enough on which to base a clinical diagnosis. It is only after several clues 'add up' that a final assessment can be made. If one test implicates a certain structure, the clinician should try to support this hypothesis by performing further tests which would also implicate this particular structure.[19,20] For example, if localized overpressure with the active spinal movements indicates that there is a dominant joint dysfunction in the upper cervical spine, this should be confirmed by the finding of comparable joint signs first by passive physiological intervertebral movements (PPIVMs) and secondly by passive accessory intervertebral movements (PAIVMs).

Final confirmation of the hypothesis is reached when retrospective reassessment shows that the condition has improved after treatment of the involved structure. For example, should the cervical flexion improve after careful straight leg raise mobilizations, this would further indicate the nervous system as being involved.

In the following pages, some selected examples of differentiation are described.

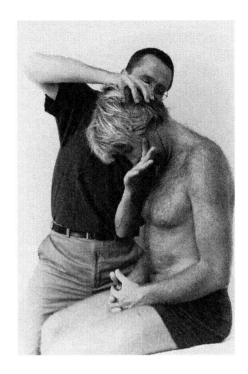

Figure 6.4 Overpressure of the upper cervical spine with the left hand on the maxillary bone to prevent stress on the TMJ

Pain on cervical flexion: temporomandibular joint versus upper cervical spine

In this example the patient complains of pain around the right mastoid process/temporomandibular joint (TMJ) area when performing a flexion movement.

The stress on the nervous system may be increased by slump manoeuvres. The stress on the upper cervical region may be increased by localized overpressure through the maxilla (Figure 6.4). Should there be any change in symptoms, this is followed up by PPIVMs and PAIVMs. It may also be useful to perform unilateral postero-anterior movements on C1/C2 in the position of flexion (Figure 6.5).

As cervical flexion normally leads to slight protrusion of the TMJ,[21,22] the movement is repeated after placing a 'spatula' between the teeth (Figure 6.6). The holding of the spatula decreases TMJ motion, while not changing the cervical spine. Any change of symptoms indicates TMJ involvement, which is further supported by performing, for example, postero-anterior mobilizations on the angle of the mandible in the position of cervical flexion.

In order to assess involvement of the cranial bony tissue, the flexion movement is repeated while performing a compression technique on the occipital bones (Figure 6.7).

Finally, should the differentiation clearly indicate the upper cervical spine to be the cause of the symptoms, only this structure is treated, after which a careful reassessment of the movement dysfunction should show some change.

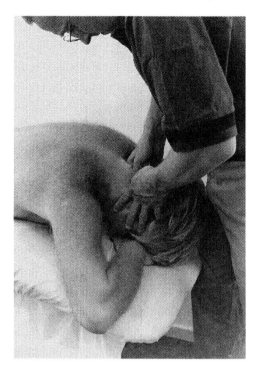

Figure 6.5 Unilateral postero-anterior movements on the right side of C1 and C2 in flexion of the head

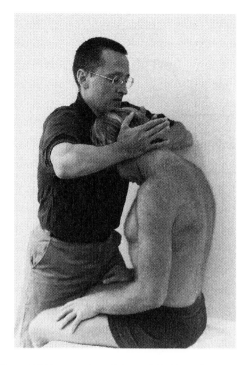

Figure 6.7 Compression of the occipital bone in upper cervical flexion. When the occipital bone manoeuvre changes the symptoms, a possible dysfunction of cranial tissue can be hypothesized

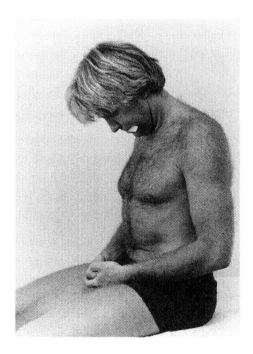

Figure 6.6 Head flexion without change of mandibular position by placing a 'spatula' between the teeth

Pain on cervical rotation: TMJ versus upper cervical spine

In this example the patient complains of pain around the right mastoid process/ TMJ area when performing a left rotation movement. The clinician can now try to differentiate whether the symptoms come from the rotation in the upper cervical spine or from the concomitant lateral gliding movement in the right TMJ. The differentiation consists basically of six tests. While the patient is in the painful position the mandible is fixed, after which the cervical rotation is increased (Figure 6.8a). Should the symptoms increase, this would lead to the hypothesis that the symptoms are being caused by the upper cervical spine. In the next test the same position is taken up, but now the cervical rotation only is decreased after which the

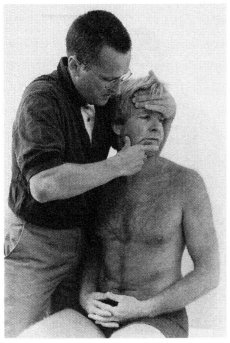

(a)

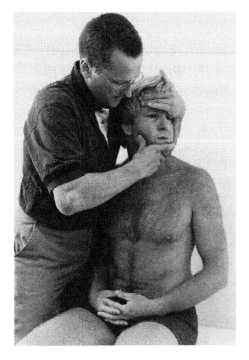

(b)

(c)

Figure 6.8 Differentiation on cervical rotation. **(a)** Mandible is fixed while cervical rotation is increased; **(b)** cervical spine is fixed and lateral deviation movement of the TMJ is increased/decreased; **(c)** isolated TMJ lateral deviation in neutral cervical spine position

symptoms should also decrease. In the third and fourth tests, the same position is taken up, but now the cervical spine is fixed and the lateral gliding movement of the TMJ is increased and decreased (Figure 6.8b).

Test five is isolated TMJ lateral gliding in the neutral cervical spine position (Figure 6.8c). Test six is isolated cervical spine rotation while maintaining the TMJ in the neutral position.

Further confirmation should come from other tests like repeating the movement with a spatula between the teeth, accessory movements on C1 in the rotated position, accessory movements on the mandible etc.

Differentiation of C1 versus TMJ versus cranium versus nervous tissue

In this last example the patient complains of a pulling, sometimes burning pain in the right suboccipital/mandibular angle region. The symptoms are provoked when talking on the telephone for long periods, especially when the phone is held between the left ear and shoulder. When the pain is severe, movements of both the head and the jaw aggravate it.

The patient is placed in left side lying with the upper cervical spine in slight side flexion to the left.

Occiput–C2

Initially the accessory movements of the upper cervical spine are performed. For instance if transverse movement to the right against the transverse process of C1 provokes symptoms, the clinician should vary the opening position of the mouth slightly. Any change in symptoms would indicate a contributory role of the TMJ to the problem.

Temporomandibular joint

Accessory movements, especially transverse to medial and in the postero-anterior direction are performed. When symptoms are provoked, the position of the upper cervical spine is slightly changed. Any change in symptoms would indicate a contributory role of the cervical spine to the problem.

Cranium bone tissue

Accessory movements, especially of the mastoid process (being a part of the temporal bone), and palpation of the styloid process are assessed. It is important to realize that pressure changes in this region also influence the foramina through which branches of cranial nerves exit the cranium (e.g. facial nerve canal in the temporal bone).[23] Therefore, when symptoms are provoked, the patient is placed in different cranial nerve positions (see Chapter 7).

Cranial nervous tissue

Apart from neurodynamic testing, further support for cranial nerve involvement comes from palpation of the individual branches. The clinician may, for instance, palpate the branches of the facial nerve and vagus nerve on the mastoid process (see Chapter 2).

Comparison of differentiation findings

In clinical practice, often more than one structure is involved. In these instances, the clinician will produce relevant physical signs in different structures.

The clinical decision about which structure to treat first in these cases is partly based upon comparison of the signs. For instance, in the last example of differentiation, if transverse movement of C1 is markedly restricted and reproduces the patient's symptoms, while transverse movement of the head of the mandible is only slightly restricted and produces only local pain, the initial treatment will be directed at the occiput–C1 joint.

Assessment and treatment/ management

Introduction

The following selected patient examples are described to outline the principles of physical examination and treatment. For

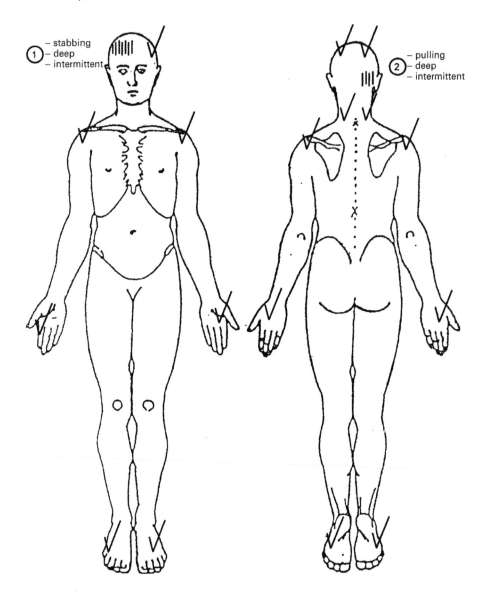

Figure 6.9 Body chart of a patient with unilateral headache

reasons of clarity, an abbreviated description of the main information is presented.

Patient 1

Subjective examination

Mr. X , aged 36 years, complains of right-sided frontal and temporal headache combined with 'pulling' in the right suboccipital area (Figure 6.9). The headache is brought on by sleeping prone (head rotated to the right) and riding a mountain bike for longer than 30 minutes. He furthermore feels that his right rotation is 'not as good as it used to be' when reversing the car. The symptoms slowly developed over the last year without any clear onset. In the last 3–4 weeks the symptoms have been present

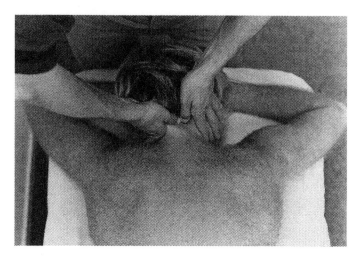

Figure 6.10 Differentiation between C1–C2 and C2–C3 and treatment techniques by unilateral postero-anterior movements in 30° head rotation

nearly every day. There are no contra-indications to manipulative treatment and medication gives only temporary relief.

Hypothesis

As the patient clearly relates the headache to cervical spine movements, and there is a concomitant feeling of suboccipital stiff-ness, this strongly implicates cervicogenic headache. If this hypothesis is correct then there should be clear signs on neuromuscu-loskeletal examination.

Physical examination

There is 30° of movement restriction of cervical extension. With localized over-pressure of the upper cervical region there is reproduction of the suboccipital pain (see Figure 6.9). Furthermore, rotation to the right and side flexion to the left are restricted. At the C1–C2 region rotation is coupled with contralateral side flexion, whereas in the C2–C7 region it is coupled with ipsilateral side flexion.[24] Therefore, an

initial hypothesis is formed that there is C1–C2 involvement. This is supported by the 20° of movement restriction found on the occiput–C2 rotation test. Here the clinician fixates the spinous process of C2 and assesses the amount of head rotation the patient has. Further confirmation should come from the passive accessory intervertebral movements (PAIVMs). Right-sided unilateral postero-anterior mobilizations on C2 are painfully re-stricted. As C1–2 or C2–3 may cause this, the patient is asked to rotate his head 30° to the right (Figure 6.10). In this manoeuvre the postero-anterior stress on C1–2 is increased and as his symptoms also in-crease, this implicates a C1–2 joint involve-ment.

There is no neural and/or muscular involvement.

Treatment

As this is mainly a stiffness–dominant joint problem, the initial treatment consists of mobilization of the C1–2 joint with

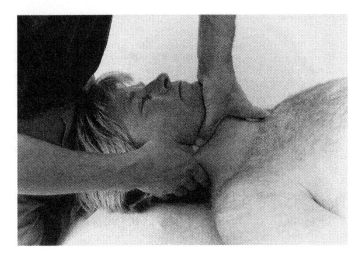

Figure 6.11 Unilateral antero-posterior mobilization on the right side of C2

PAIVMs and rotation to the right (see Figure 6.10). In the later stages, side flexion mobilization to the left of the upper cervical spine is added (heterolateral coupling of side flexion and rotation).

Furthermore, ergonomic advice concerning the position of the cervical spine on the mountain bike is given.

Patient 2

Subjective examination

A male patient aged 42 complains of right-sided occipital pain spreading to the top of the head. The pain can be both stabbing and pulling. There are no associated symptoms. He has difficulty defining aggravating activities, but there is a slight tendency for increased symptoms with flexed positions, such as reading for more than 30 minutes. The symptoms have developed over the last 2 years with a gradual increase of intensity. He does not recall any major trauma.

Physical examination

With the active movements there is restriction of cervical flexion producing subocci-pital 'pulling'. Rotation to the right is full, while to the left there is 15° of movement restriction. As isolated active movements do not reproduce the patients' symptoms it is decided to combine upper cervical flexion with rotation to the left, which reproduces the occipital pain. Neurodynamic testing biasing towards the greater occipital nerve (GON) reproduces the pain in the top of the skull. Further indication for GON involvement is found when palpation of the nerve on the base of the head (approximately 3 cm lateral from the midline) reproduces a stabbing sensation.[25] Further examination of cranial tissue is inconclusive (see Chapter 7).

Although unilateral postero-anterior accessory movements on C2 are slightly painful, there is no movement restriction. It is therefore decided to evaluate the antero-posterior accessory movement of C2, which also reproduces the occipital symptoms.

Treatment

This patient shows both neural and joint signs. The GON mainly consists of fibres from the C2 spinal nerve. Bogduk[26] has

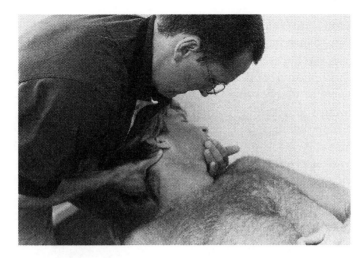

Figure 6.12 Cervical rotation mobilization in slight flexion position of the head

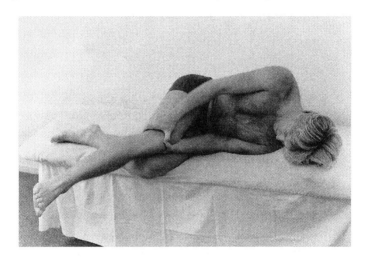

Figure 6.13 Automobilizing in side lying of the right SLR in slump position

shown the close anatomical relationship between the C2 dorsal ganglion and the C1–2 joint. This could mean that the pathoneurodynamics are secondary, caused by a primary joint dysfunction. The initial treatment therefore consists of anteroposterior mobilizations of C2 (Figure 6.11). In the later stages upper cervical rotation in flexion position is added (Figure 6.12). After three treatments there are no remaining joint signs, although the greater occipital nerve slump test is still able to reproduce some of the patients' symptoms. It is therefore decided to add mobilization of the nervous system by performing SLR movements in a slumped position. This movement is also integrated into a home exercise (Figure 6.13).

Patient 3

Subjective examination

A 37-year-old female keyboard operator complains of a right-sided pulsating pain in the temporal region and bilateral retro-orbital pressure in combination with a 'burning feeling' in the eyes. Associated symptoms are photophobia and nausea. There is no suboccipital or neck pain, but on closer questioning she describes a tight feeling in the interscapular region. There is an absence of aura.

The symptoms are not related to movements of the cervical spine and are mainly aggravated by stress, weather changes and long bouts of sitting at the computer.

Over the last 3 months, due to an increase in workload, the symptoms have slowly increased to chronic daily headache, forcing her to take medication at least 5 days per week. Although MRI of the skull is normal, she is also worried about having a brain tumour.

Hypothesis

This patient clearly does not fulfil the criteria the International Headache Society has defined for cervicogenic headache. It will probably not be possible to find clear joint signs in the upper cervical region. There is, however, some indication of sympathetic involvement with this patient. Furthermore, there seems to be a pain management deficit.

Physical examination

On inspection a flat thoracic spine (especially T2–8) with a slightly accentuated dowager's hump is seen. The skin between the scapulae is 'pulled in' and its mobility is markedly restricted. The active movements of the cervical spine are normal, and even inclusion of tests for the upper cervical spine, such as upper cervical quadrant,[8] provokes only some local discomfort. Therefore, it is decided to evaluate the thoracic spine. Extension is normal but

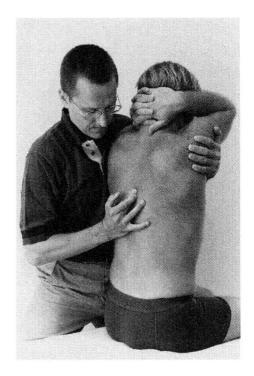

Figure 6.14 Passive physiological movement of the thoracic region

flexion and both right and left rotations are markedly restricted, reproducing strong interscapular pulling.

The same pulling is reproduced with slump and can be influenced by knee extension or upper cervical flexion.

Passive physiological intervertebral movements of the mid-thoracic region (Figure 6.14) show segmental restriction of flexion. Accessory movements of the vertebral joints are relatively normal, but there are marked movement restrictions of the costovertebral and costotransverse joints.

Treatment

The first session primarily consists of explaining to the patient that although it is not possible to reproduce her symptoms, there are enough 'comparable' joint signs in

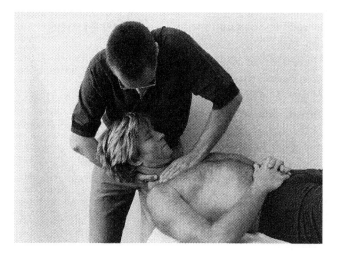

Figure 6.15 Anterior-posterior mobilization of the upper thoracic spine through the sternum

the thoracic spine to justify treatment. Furthermore, the patient is asked to keep a headache diary. In the second treatment she volunteers that the symptoms on their own are unchanged, but that she feels a little 'less threatened' by them. As thoracic flexion is the most restricted movement, initial treatment mainly consists of increasing flexion by means of anteroposterior mobilization through the sternum (Figure 6.15). Thoracic soft tissue mobilization is added to influence sympathetic outflow.[27,28] The costovertebral and costotransverse joints are mobilized by means of 'screw' mobilization with the hands placed laterally on the ribs (Figure 6.16).

Home exercises consist of thoracic flexion automobilization in sitting and slump in side-lying.

After eight treatments over 6 weeks the chronic daily headache has disappeared, and the patient is reassured that she does not have a brain tumour. She only complains of an occasional temporal pulsating pain, which has decreased in intensity by 50%. On comparing the occurrence of this headache with the intake of food products

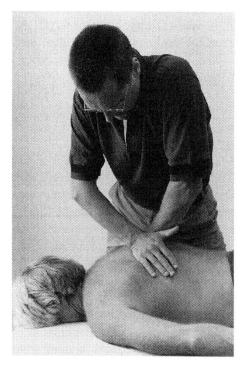

Figure 6.16 Mobilization of the costovertebral and costotransverse joints by the 'screw'

(headache diary) it is found that there seems to be a correlation with the consumption of chocolate.[29] Treatment is paused for 4 weeks, during which the patient is not allowed to consume any chocolate products. After 10 days the patient telephones because she is suffering from a very severe headache, which she has not experienced before. The hypothesis is that this a 'withdrawal' headache. She is therefore asked to take medication and to report back should the symptoms not subside within 4 hours. After another 5 weeks she reports again to describe reduction of symptoms to a level of 5%. There has not been another 'withdrawal' attack.

Conclusion

This example nicely emphasizes the need for an overall management programme consisting of patient education (explanation, headache diary, home exercises etc.), a neuromusculoskeletal system approach (in this case mainly sympathetic nervous system) and dietary restrictions.

Conclusion

Physical examination (especially of the upper cervical spine) is the mainstay in the diagnosis of cervicogenic headache.[5,30] The finding of relevant/comparable physical signs in the neuromusculoskeletal system is the foundation upon which rationale for treatment/management is based.

Retrospective reassessment showing relief of symptoms after successful treatment of the physical signs is the final clinical proof for neuromusculoskeletal system involvement in the headache syndrome.[19]

However, successful treatment cannot be based upon a monostructural approach, but should include overall management strategies[29,31,32] (see also Chapters 8 and 11).

References

1 Featherstone, H. J. (1985). Migraine and muscle contraction headaches: a continuum. *Headache*, **25**, 194–198.

2 Marcus, D. A. (1992). Migraine and tension-type headaches: the questionable validity of current classification systems. *Clin. J. Pain*, **8**, 28–36.

3 Sanin, L. C., Mathew, N. T. and Bellmeyer, L. R. (1994). The International Headache Society headache classification as applied to a headache clinic population. *Cephalalgia*, **14**, 443–446.

4 Sjaastad, O., Fredriksen, T. A. and Stolt-Nielsen, A. (1986). Cervicogenic headache, C2 rhizopathy, and occipital neuralgia: a connection? *Cephalalgia*, **6**, 189–195.

5 Jull, G. A. (1994). Cervical headache: a review. In: *Grieves Modern Manual Therapy*, 2nd edn (J. D. Boyling and N. Palastanga, eds), pp. 333–347. Churchill Livingstone.

6 Lord, S. M., Barnsley, L., Wallis, B. J. and Bogduk, N. (1994). Third occipital nerve headache: a prevalence study. *J. Neurol. Neurosurg. Psychiatry*, **57**, 1187–1190.

7 Jänig, W. and Stanton-Hicks, M. (1996). *Reflex Sympathetic Dystrophy: a Reappraisal*. IASP Press.

8 Maitland, G. D. (1986). *Vertebral Manipulation*, 5th edn. Butterworths.

9 Grieve, G. P. (1988). *Common Vertebral Joint Problems*, 2nd edn. Churchill Livingstone.

10 Jull, G. A. (1994). Examination of the articular system. In: *Grieves Modern Manual Therapy*, 2nd edn (J. D. Boyling and N. Palastanga, eds), pp. 511–528. Churchill Livingstone.

11 Jull, G. A., Bogduk, N. and Marsland, A. (1988). The accuracy of manual diagnosis for cervical zygapophyseal joint pain syndromes. *Med. J. Aust.*, **148**, 233–236.

12 Jull, G., Zito, G., Trott, P. *et al.* (1997). Inter-examiner reliability to detect painful upper cervical joint dysfunction. *Aust. Physiother.*, **43**, 125–129.

13 Watson, D. H. and Trott, P. H. (1993). Cervical headache: an investigation of natural head posture and upper cervical flexor muscle performance. *Cephalalgia*, **13**, 272–84.

14 Watson, D. H. (1994). Cervical headache: an investigation of natural head posture and upper cervical flexor muscle performance. In: *Grieves Modern Manual Therapy*, 2nd edn (J. D. Boyling and N. Palastanga, eds), pp. 349–359. Churchill Livingstone.

15 Sahrman, S. A. (1988). Postural applications in the child and adult. Neurodevelopmental aspects. In: *TMJ Disorders. Management of the Craniomandibular Complex* (S. L. Kraus, ed.), pp. 295–309. Churchill Livingstone.

16 Maitland, G. D. (1979). Negative disc exploration: positive canal signs. *Aust. J. Physiother.*, **25**, 129–134.

17 Elvey, R. L. (1994). The investigation of arm pain: signs of adverse responses to the physical examination of the brachial plexus and related neural tissues. In: *Grieves*

Modern Manual Therapy, 2nd edn (J. D. Boyling and N. Palastanga, eds), pp. 577–586. Churchill Livingstone.

18 Butler, D. S. (1991). *Mobilisation of the Nervous System.* Churchill Livingstone.

19 Jones, M. A. (1994). Clinical reasoning process in manipulative therapy. In: *Grieves Modern Manual Therapy*, 2nd edn (J. D. Boyling and N. Palastanga, eds), pp. 471–490. Churchill Livingstone.

20 Schon, D. A. (1983). *The Reflective Clinician.* Basic Books.

21 Kraus, S. L. (1995). *Temporomandibular Disorders*, 2nd edn. Churchill Livingstone.

22 Rocabado, M. (1988). Biomechanical relationship of the cranial, cervical and hyoid regions. *Physical Therapy*, **1**, 62.

23 Lang, J. (1996). *Skull Base and Related Structures. Atlas of Clinical Anatomy.* Schattauer.

24 White, A. A. and Panjabi, M. M. (1978). *Clinical Biomechanics of the Spine.* J. B. Lippincott.

25 Vital, J. M., Grenier, F., Dautheribes, M. *et al.* (1989). An anatomic and dynamic study of the greater occipital nerve (n. of Arnold). *Surg. Radiol. Anat.*, **11**, 205–210.

26 Bogduk, N. (1981). An anatomical basis for the neck–tongue syndrome. *J. Neurol. Neurosurg. Psychiatry*, **44**, 202–208.

27 Oostendorp, R. A. B., Hagenaars, L. H. A., Meldrum, H. A. *et al.* (1986). De vertebrobasilaire insufficientie (deel IV). *Nederlands Tijdschrift voor Manuele Therapie*, **4**, 16–45.

28 Sato, A. and Swenson, R. S. (1984). Sympathetic nervous system response to mechanical stress of the spinal column in rats. *J. Manipul. Physiol. Ther.*, **7**, 141–147.

29 Diamond, S. and Freitag, F. G. (1988). The mixed headache syndrome. *Clin. J. Pain*, **4**, 67–74.

30 Treleaven, J., Jull, G. and Atkinson, L. (1994). Cervical musculoskeletal dysfunction in post-concussional headache. *Cephalalgia*, **14**, 273–279.

31 Beeton, K. and Jull, G. (1994). Effectiveness of manipulative physiotherapy in the management of cervicogenic headache: a single case study. *Physiotherapy*, **80**, 417–423.

32 Schoensee, S. K., Jensen, G. J., Nicholson, G. *et al.* (1995). The effect of mobilization on cervical headaches. *JOSPT*, **21**, 184–196.

7

Neurodynamics of cranial nervous tissue (cranioneurodynamics)

H. J. M. von Piekartz

Introduction

Shacklock[1] encouraged the use of the term 'neurodynamics' when he discussed the mechanics and physiology of the nervous system and their relationship to each other. Nervous tissue is required to undergo complicated movements of elongation, sliding and compression (Figure 7.1). These loading phenomena, which occur during normal daily movements, involve physiological effects such as changes in blood circulation and axonal transport in both autonomic and somatic systems.[1-3] Changes in neural mechanics and physiology may lead to abnormal neurodynamics or neural pathodynamics. These changes are strongly related to the environment directly surrounding the nervous tissue, which is referred to as the mechanical interface or neural container. Every part of the body has its typical neurodynamics and neural containers, including the craniofacial region. The facial canal of the temporal bone is a good example of a neural container – in this instance of the facial nerve – which contacts the canal for about 2.5 cm.[2] How might the facial nerve influence head–neck and mandibular move-

ments? The testing of neurodynamics is not only a useful tool for examining the health of the nervous tissue and its containers, but also provides information about pain mechanisms in order to classify pain.[3,4] Nowadays, neurodynamic testing has to be seen within a larger framework and gives the clinician clues for further refined management, which is discussed in Chapter 8. Hopefully this chapter will convey the message that cranioneurodynamics, that is the neurodynamics of the head, neck and face region, is no different to the neurodynamics of the rest of the body. The only difference is the region. Both behave in similar ways and have an influence on each other (Figure 7.2).

The lack of research in this area and the absence of good standardization in the literature coupled with personal observation led to my interest in this subject. For a better understanding of what is meant by cranioneurodynamic testing, I refer the reader to the section describing craniodynamic tests later in this chapter (p. 131).

Up-to-date, relevant biomedical knowledge is included to ensure an understanding of the neurodynamics of the head, neck and facial region. The main emphasis is on

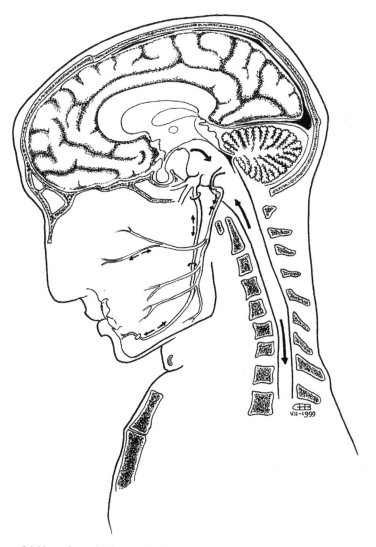

Figure 7.1 Neurodynamic changes during sliding, elongation, compression, convergence and divergence of craniocervical and craniofacial nervous tissue on altered head movements in this figure of the spinal cord and branches of the mandibular nerve

mechanics in order to facilitate a clear understanding of the neurodynamic testing of cranial nerves.

Physiological features of cranial nerve tissue during movement

Normal nerves exhibit properties which allow stretching, elongation, compression, adaptation and a continuance of normal physiology.[5,6]

Abnormal mechanical events lead to the development of pathophysiological responses, such as a change of blood supply related to inflammation, healing and repair or minor pain states.[6,7] Most pathophysiological features of peripheral nerves seem to be the same for cranial nervous tissue, although the literature is less specific in this area. Some general features are discussed here.

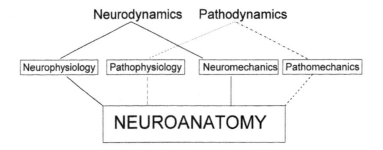

Figure 7.2 Cranioneurodynamics is a part of neurodynamics of the whole body and can be divided into the neurophysiological and neuromechanical components. Pathological changes are expressed in pathophysiological and pathomechanical qualities (pathodynamics). The mechanical part can be clinically tested by (cranio) neurodynamics, which also give an impression about altered physiology of the nervous system and clues regarding the pain scale of the patient. (Adapted from Shacklock, 1995[1])

Blood supply

Uninterrupted blood supply to cranial nervous tissue is important for the metabolic demands of the nerve trunks and axons and especially for providing power for axonal transport and impulse generation.[2,3,6,7] The intracranial part of the nervous system has an especially high vascular permeability, which supports the physiological enhancement of cranial blood vessels.[8,9] Lack of blood supply can cause neurophysiological and mechanical changes of the cranial nerves which can lead to vascular headache.[10] Cerebral blood vessels, especially the venous sinuses, may play a part in vasodilatation and inflammation of the cerebral arteries and nerves. This is due to the release of substance P and the calcitonin gene-related peptide (CGRP) and is not, as formerly thought, attributable to problems in the dura.[11,12] Physiological processes result from sustained stress and compression of the venous sinuses, which in turn impact on the brain, dura connective tissue and skull.[13] It is possible to hypothesize that the physiological impact on the venous sinuses may be the cause of such a high incidence of vascular headache post-head injury.[14]

'After' effect of vascular decompression

Varying results of neurosurgical decompression and excision of tumours are reported. For example, such procedures can give total symptom reduction,[15–17] or slow recovery over a long period.[18,19]

Where there is total symptom reduction, physiological effects such as disturbances in bidirectional axonplasmic flow and antidromic impulses often linger or remain and have repercussions for the nervous tissue itself as well as for the target tissue it supplies. Therefore this will slow down the healing process.[19] Another pattern to emerge is that of the postoperative symptoms which are due to ectopic neural discharges. Schlessel[20] reported that 63.7% of patients who underwent surgery to the cerebellopontine angle by a suboccipital approach complained of local discomfort and headache postoperatively (Figure 7.3). Local nerve blocks, acupuncture, and cervical manipulations were ineffective. Sections of specimens show the adherence of several tissues such as the nuchal musculature to the dura, which can be a relevant source of these postoperative symptoms.

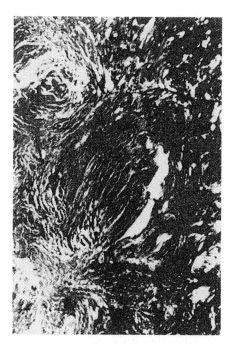

Figure 7.3 Scarring of the dura in the suboccipital region after surgery to the cerebellopontine angle by a suboccipital approach (from Schlessel *et al.* 1992[20] with kind permission of Lippincott-Raven)

Cranial neurogenic inflammation and blood circulation

Neurogenic inflammation is followed by plasma leakage. This stimulates the trigeminal ganglion by a complicated physiological process to release neuropeptides like substance P and CGRP from perivascular unmyelinated C-fibres. This influences the neurophysiology of the cranial blood vessels, and is proposed as a pathogenic mechanism for migraine, cluster and cervical headache and pathodynamic changes of cranial nerve tissue.[10,21,22] Serotonin as a neurotransmitter in the body can inhibit the peptide release and block the neurogenic inflammation.[23] For more detailed information related to this clinical pattern, see Chapter 5.

Neurodynamics of cranial nerve tissue designed for movement

Looking at the functional anatomical features of cranial nervous tissue it is clear that movements of elongation, sliding, and compression in a relatively small space are a normal adaptation to altered head neck or body movements.[24,25] Zones and structures which most probably play an important role in the process of adaptation to (ab)normal movements are discussed here.

Design of intracranial neurons

Neural tissue from the cortex to the brainstem has a different design to cranial nerves. It is a well-organized complex of neurons, which runs to the brainstem (Figure 7.4). Neural tissue distal to the brainstem (tissue which organizes into cranial nerves) changes and has the same quality and design features as peripheral nerves, which arise from the spinal cord.[26,27,28] This includes the lower motor neuron (LMN) for the motor pathway and the primary and secondary neurons for the secondary pathways. The cell bodies are located outside the central nervous system in sensory ganglia which have the same features as dorsal root ganglia and the grey matter of the brainstem.[26,27,29] The sensory ganglia of cranial nerves are highly active when pain is related to vascular changes such as migraine and cluster headaches.[30] General cranial nervous tissue moves and slides much as other nervous tissue,[26] but it is not certain if it has the same mechano- and chemosensitivity as the dorsal root ganglion.[31]

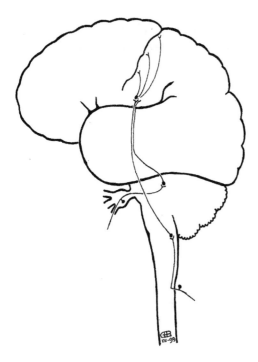

Figure 7.4 The design of the sensory pathways, which are composed of three major neurons. The primary neuron is located outside the central nervous system in sensory ganglia. The secondary neurons are in the dorsal grey matter of the brainstem and project on the thalamus where the tertiary neurons are housed. Their axons project to the sensory cortex

Connective tissue design (internal dural layer, falx cerebellum, cerebri and cranial nerve connections)

Cranial nerves and other neural tissues in the cranium are surrounded by connective tissue with visco-elastic properties, similar to ligament and tendon.[5,32,33] This tissue commonly has a protective role. Cranial nerve roots are often seen as vulnerable zones and have a higher density of connective tissue. For example:

- the external layer of the dura and part of the internal layer such as the falx cerebri and falx cerebelli

- the oculomotor (III), trigeminal (V), facial (VII), vestiblocochlear (VIII), hypoglossal (XII), vagus (X) and glossopharyngeal (IX) nerves, which have close connection with the internal layer of the dura, falx cerebri and falx cerebellum.[26,27]

Clinical findings and literature suggest the mechanical continuous design of the cranial nervous tissue. For example, hydrocephalus caused by impingement of the corpus callosum shows that cranial nervous tissue such as the dura of cranial nerves adapts to compression and stretch throughout the skull.[34,35] Also, during head movement, sliding, elongation and compression changes occur in the falx cerebri and dura, cranial nerves and tentorium. Connective tissue has been shown to limit extreme movement and compression of the brain.[36] Changes in cranial connective tissue have often been noted in conjunction with diseases that target multiple structures. For example, diabetic neuropathy, which changes the physiology of different cranial nerves, can provoke severe facial pain, numbness and dysfunction such as (minor) facial pareses and dysphagia.[37]

Tumours around the brainstem and transitional areas of the skull such as the foramina are often structurally involved with cranial connective tissue, causing changes in anatomical positions and pathological loading on neural structures.[38–40]

- Some cranial nerves (CN) have the same intracranial topography and are richly connected by connective tissue in different zones, which are continuous and share the same dural sleeves. This design has the advantage that many different structures (including

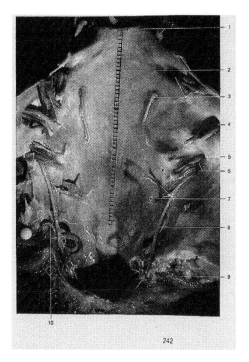

Figure 7.5 Dural openings at the clivus together with the anatomical connections of several cranial nerves. (From Lang 1995[27] by kind permission of Schattauer)

1. Dorsum sellae and IIIrd cranial nerve
2. Millimeter pater and IVth cranial nerve
3. Openings of VIth and Vth cranial nerves
4. Internal acoustic meatus
5. Opening of IXth cranial nerve.
6. Openings of Xth and XIth cranial nerves
7. Opening of XIIth cranial nerve
8. Spinal part of XIth cranial nerve
9. Vertebral artery, atlantal part
10. Meningeal branch from intracisternal segment of PICA (variation)

cranial nerves) can be housed in a relatively small space like the cranium (Figures 7.5 and 7.6).[24,41]

On the other hand, when mechanical forces and neural container changes occur, such as aneurysms, vascular anomalies, and tumours, physiological changes such as neural ischaemia also occur. This results in multiple clinical patterns. In general, neck and cranial bone movements are techniques by which one can change cranial neurodynamics. Because of the short dis-

tance from the brainstem to vulnerable zones like the cavernous sinus (see critical cranial zones, below), connections with the dura mater and the exit foramina of the cranium, it may be difficult to specify which part of the intracranial nervous tissue is related to the patient's problem, when relevant dysfunctions are found.

Brainstem topography

For explanation of the cranial neurodynamic tests it is useful to know that the cranial nerves come from the dorsal or lateral side of the brainstem and lie dorsal to the flexion/extension axis of the head (Figure 7.7).[24,41,42] Head movements such as flexion, extension and lateral flexion can probably change elongation, compression, and sliding of nervous tissue in the head and also in the rest of the body.[24] For more information see Movement of cranial nervous tissue (p. 129).

Critical intracranial zones

Nerve entry zones (NEZ)

Most cranial nerves arise from the dorsolateral part of the brainstem (nerve entry zones) (Figure 7.8). In this region they are mostly very close to each other (for example the facial and vestibulocochlear and the glossopharyngeal, vagus and accessory nerves).[26,43] Most cranial nerve entry zones are surrounded with connective tissue and arteries. Vascular anomalies such as vascular 'loops' can cause vascular compression followed by cranial nerve neuralgia[44–47] and paralysis.[48] Neurosurgeons have noted that different head positions such as flexion and side flexion change the localization and the compression of these loops. This can make neurosurgery less difficult because movement

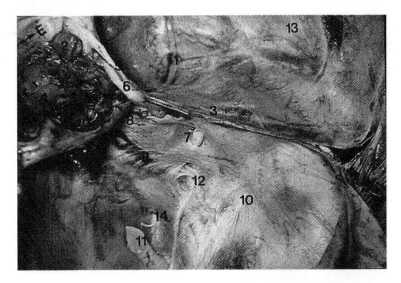

Figure 7.6 Superior surface of right temporal bone in a skull with dura attached. Note the rich connections of the cranial nerves (see numbers 6, 7 and 12 with the dura)

1. Middle meningeal artery
2. Internal carotid artery
3. Superior petrosal sinus
4. Pituitary fossa
5. Petroclinoid ligament
6. Oculomotor (III) cranial nerve
7. Internal auditory meatus with VII and VIII cranial nerves
8. Petrous bone apex
9. Inferior petrosal sinus
10. Superior bulb of the internal jugular vein
11. Vertebral artery
12. Cranial nerves IX, X, XI
13. Middle cranial fossa
14. Hypoglossal nerve (XII)

allows a better position of the nerve tissue which is to be operated upon.[49] The anatomical features described above have consequences for neurodynamics. Head movements such as flexion and also side bending load the nerve entry zones more on one side, and during this manoeuvre the neurodynamics of most cranial nerves are influenced.[24]

Cerebellopontine angle (CPA)

The cerebellopontine angle is a cerebrospinal fluid-filled space bounded by the pons, cerebellum, and the petrous and temporal bones. The CPA contains arteries, veins and cranial nerves such as the trigeminal (V), facial (VII), vestibulocochlear (VII) (VIII), glossopharyngeal (IX) and vagus (X) nerves (Figure 7.9).[27,42,50] Pathophysiological changes and symptoms mostly

occur due to an abnormal neural container, such as when aneurysms or vascular compression on the cranial nerves are present.[50–56] Also, minor arterial compression or distortion of, for example, the trigeminal nerve in the CPA results in demyelination and stimulates abnormal impulse generating sites (AIGS) which may contribute to minor cranial nervous tissue neuralgia.[53–59]

The vascular system of the CPA is extensive and has many loops and anastomoses.[60,61] For example, the anterior inferior cerebellar arteries (AICA) loop around the facial and acoustic nerve branches; the posterior-inferior cerebellar artery (PICA) loops around the medulla oblongata and has anastomoses with the cerebellum; and the superior petrosal veins occupying the superior part of the CPA

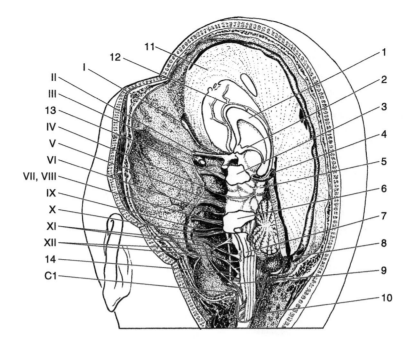

Figure 7.7 Most cranial nerves come from the dorsal or lateral side of the brainstem. The brainstem itself lies dorsal to the flexion, extension axis of the head (adapted from E. Pernkopf [1963] *Atlas of Topographical and Applied Human Anatomy*. Saunders)

1. Callous corpus
2. Fornix
3. Cerebral pedunculus
4. Greater cerebral vein
5. Quadrigeminal layer
6. Cerebellar pedunculus
7. Cuneate tubercle
8. Confluenting sinuses
9. Enticulate ligament
10. Dura mater
11. Cerebral falx
12. Anterior cerebral artery
13. Internal carotid artery
14. Vertebral artery

loop around the trigeminal nerve. These are important for the blood supply of the nerves.[62,63] The design of these arterial blood vessels often leads to minor or major compression of nervous tissue, and can lead to neurogenic inflammation, pain and dysfunction, for example, glossopharyngeal neuralgia, hemifacial spasm, tic douloureux, tinnitus, vertigo, trigeminal neuralgia and cluster headache.[49,51,64,65]

Microsurgical vascular decompression techniques by thermorhizotomy, stretching, and positioning of the arterial loops shows good results and less recurrence of the symptoms, especially those coming from the trigeminal, facial and hypoglossal nerves.[49,50,53,54,56,66,67] Upper cervical flexion and contralateral flexion also change the compression or decompression of the arterial loops on the cranial nerves in the cerebellopontine angle. Neurosurgeons often use this position during surgical intervention (Figure 7.10).[68,69]

As a clinician one can use this knowledge during examination, neurodynamic testing and treatment to influence the cerebellopontine angle region.

Examples of pathology around the cerebellopontine angle and their clinical relevance

The CPA is a critical neural container for

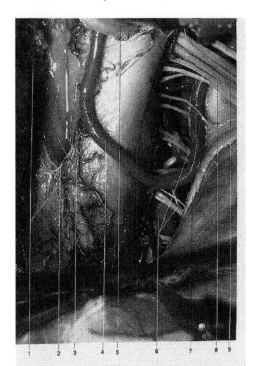

Figure 7.8 Nerve entry zones (NEZ) in the dorsolateral region of the brainstem. Note how the posterior inferior cerebellar artery (5) loops and can be a predisposition for compression of the NEZ of the hypoglossal (6), accessory (8) and vagus nerves (9)

1. Choroid plexus of fourth ventricle and left tuberculum gracile
2. Area postrema and obex
3. Triangles of the vagal and hypoglossal nerves
4. Posterior inferior cerebellar artery and dorsal medullary branch
5. Cerebellar tonsil, shifted upward, and caudal cerebellar peduncle
6. Root bundle of XIIth cranial nerve and vertebral artery
7. Spinal root of XIth cranial nerve
8. Cranial roots of XIth cranial nerve
9. Tenth cranial nerve
(From Lang[27] by kind permission of Schattauer)

several cranial nerves as described earlier, because there is less space for the many different structures which have to adapt on movement, elongation and compression of this region. It is particularly critical when there are real structural (pathological) changes. Some examples described in the literature are lipomas, cysts, meningiomas and neuromas. Lipomas and cysts are uncommon occurrences at the cerebello-pontine angle around the cranial nerves, and surgery often has a good prognosis.[70–73] Meningiomas of the CPA are the second most frequent type of tumour in this region and constitute more than one-third to one-half of all meningiomas of the posterior cranial fossa.[74] In a fundamental clinical study by Matthies,[73] the cranial nerves V (19%), VII (11%) and VIII (67%) and the caudal nerves (6%) have features which can lead to pathophysiological changes. An example is a neuroma, which develops over years and where the signs and symptoms are slowly progressive.[66–77] For example, a glossopharyngeal neuroma often presents as a long history of headache (years), vomiting, progressive hearing loss, tinnitus, and dizziness.[15,28]. One must be aware of the slowly progressive increase of a complex of symptoms. A wise course of action is to refer the patient for further differential diagnosis. Recent advances in computerized tomography and MRI scans have yielded better anatomical details such as the temporal and cerebellopontine angle, which have contributed enormously to better diagnosis.[67,78–82]

Of course, not all abnormalities are necessarily the cause of the symptoms the patient is suffering! There must be a strong correlation with the patient's clinical presentation. Surgery in most cases of lipomas, cysts and tumours has a good prognosis.[83–89] Postoperative pain after surgery is acknowledged to occur, especially after the suboccipital approach to the cerebello-pontine angle, but is rarely taken seriously. Schlessel[20] and Resnick[90] reported that 63.7% of patients complained of 'cervical discomfort' and 'headache' after CPA surgery (using the suboccipital approach). Also Sekiya[91] reported neck pain and headache in patients, caused by extreme movements and/or avulsions of the nerves

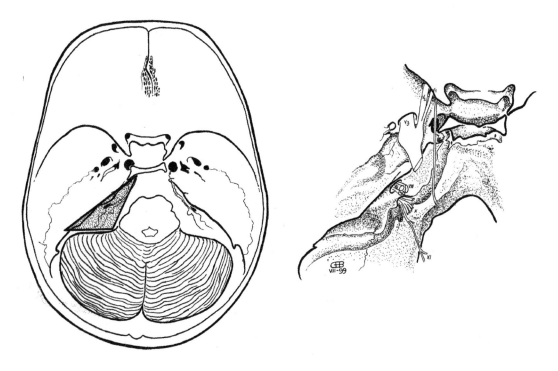

Figure 7.9 A major grouping of cranial nerves is found in the cerebellopontine angle (CPA), a shallow triangle lying dorsal to the flexion/extension axis of the head, between the cerebellum, the lateral pons and the inner third of the petrous ridge. The right part of the figure shows the foramina and their cranial nerves in the CPA

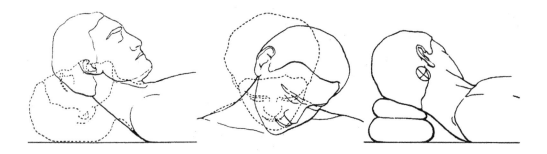

Figure 7.10 Manoeuvres used to position patients for the approach to the trigeminal nerve for microvascular decompression (from Barba and Alksne[69] with kind permission of the *Journal of Neurosurgery*, Virginia)

at the cerebellopontine angle. Schlessel[92] suggests that the adherance of nuchal soft tissue to the underlying dura following suboccipital surgery could also contribute to the postoperative pain.

Perhaps gentle movement of the neural tissue of the cranium and neck could be a method of preventing or relieving the patient of symptoms after a major craniotomy. Minor pathophysiological and dynamic changes in the CPA, such as minor neurogenic inflammation, arterial loops and fibrosis, have not been mentioned and are not discussed in the literature. A real possibility is that these minor changes can lead to undiagnosed cranio-cervical and facial dysfunction and pain. Neurodynamic examination and treatment of cranial nervous tissue maybe employed by the clinician. For more detailed information on this exciting area, the reader is referred to the description of cranioneurodynamic tests (p. 131).

Cavernous sinus

The cavernous sinus lies on the same side as the body of the sphenoid bone and extends from the superior orbital fissure to the apex of the petrous temporal bone. The internal carotid artery, the oculomotor nerve, trochlear nerve and ophthalmic and maxillary divisions of the trigeminal nerve, which is surrounded by dural connective tissue, also run through it (Figure 7.11).[28,41] Four venous spaces have been identified in the cavernous sinus (CS). These spaces are formed by the contents of the CS.[93–95] Aneurysms, meningiomas, neuromas and fistulas may occupy these spaces and thereby alter neurodynamic properties.[95–109] These authors reported signs and symptoms such as oculomotor and trochlear nerve palsies, ocular congestion, ptosis, nausea, diplopia, ataxic gait, tinnitus, dysphagia, chronic otitis media, and trigeminal neuralgia.

Microsurgery for occulomotor dysfunction,[110] for example occlusion of the cavernous carotid artery,[111–113] trigeminal neuromas,[105,114,115] and optic nerve dysfunction,[116] in the region of the cavernous sinus has had good results, but still has a predisposition to damage the dura.[117] Maxillofacial trauma, even minor head trauma, as a result of direct or indirect forces can lead to fistulae in the region of the cavernous sinus and provoke symptoms such as those described above.[118–122] From anatomical studies it is well known that the CS has many sympathetic fibres, which are grouped in a plexiform configuration surrounding the internal carotid artery, together with neural and venous tissue,[123] the ophthalmic and the maxillary branches of the trigeminal, the superior cervical and sphenopalatine ganglia and many veins.[28] Moskowitz reported that small pathophysiological changes of all these structures could lead to the most severe and debilitating form of vascular headache called 'cluster headache'.[124] Ruskell[125] found in his detailed anatomical studies of the cavernous sinus plexus in monkeys that the CS plexus provides a concentration of different cranial nervous tissue with autonomic fibres. These studies were modified by Moskowitz, who found that afferent fibres originate from the ophthalmic trigeminal divisions and supply the vessels of the circle of Willis, explaining these direct relationships.[124] Further neuroanatomy of this region is complex but may provide an answer to some of the unusual symptoms of which patients complain. The following neuroanatomical examples may explain certain symptom presentations:

- The maxillary branches receive branches from the orbitociliary nerve. The orbitociliary nerve is connected with other ganglia, for example, the ciliary and sphenopalatine ganglia, which have a dominant parasympathetic function.
- Sympathetic fibres supplying the cervical plexus project via the superior cervical ganglion to the internal carotid nerve, which follows the course from proximal to distal of the cavernous carotid artery which supplies the eye and the circle of Willis.[28,126–128]
- The sphenopalatine parasympathetic contributions reach the cervical plexus

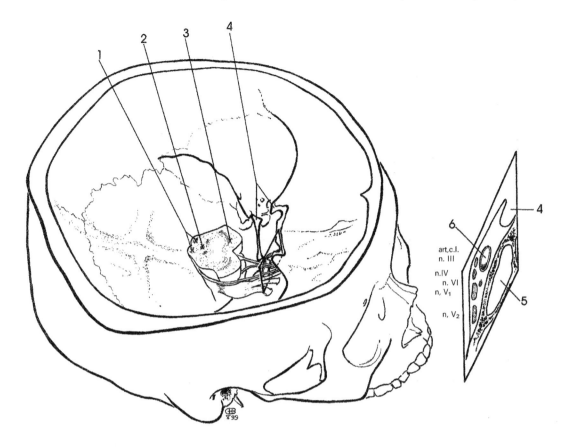

Figure 7.11 The localization of the cavernous sinus and the cranial nerves (III, IV, VI, V1 and V2) which run through it.

1. Quadrigeminal corpuscles
2. Cerebral aquaduct
3. Cerebral peduncle

4. Turk saddle
5. Sphenoid sinus
6. Internal carotid artery

via the rami orbitalis and also project onto the circle of Willis (Figure 7.12).[124,125,127]

From these three examples it is probably reasonable to hypothesize that pathophysiological changes in one nerve structure lead to changes in other structures, which can be expressed in different symptom presentations. Clinically one will suspect different underlying causes in different regions. For example, changes of the neural container around the cavernous sinus, such as carotid narrowing or occlusion of the veins, activate the trigeminovascular system resulting in neurogenic inflammation which probably starts in the dura mater.[11,124,126] The inflammation can obliterate the venous outflow from the cavernous sinus on one side and injure the right sympathetic fibres which run through the eyelid, skin of the forehead, and the intracranial internal carotid artery and its branches. These pathophysiological events probably create an imbalance between sympathetic and parasympathetic activity,[29,123,129–131] and are expressed in symptoms such as severe unilateral orbital, supraorbital and/or tem-

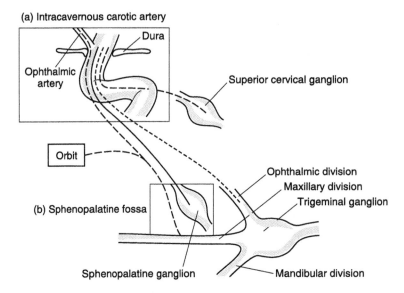

Figure 7.12 A single focus within the complicated anatomy of the superior aspect of the cavernous sinus plexus could explain: the parasympathetic symptoms of lacrimation, rhinorrhoea and nasal congestion; Horner's syndrome, facial and forehead sweating (via activation of sympathetics in the superior cervical ganglion); and the peri- and retro-orbital pain (from Moskowitz[124] with kind permission of *Headache*)

poral pain. These symptoms are often associated with the following signs: conjunctival infection, lacrimation, nasal congestion, rhinorrhoea, forehead and facial sweating, miosis, ptosis and eyelid oedema.[126,128,132] Therapeutic interventions such as anti-inflammatory medication reduce the neurogenic inflammation and oedema. Iced water also relieves the pain, and this is probably related to cooling of afferent fibres within the cavernous sinus by venous blood. Drainage from the periorbital plexus[124] and afferent stimulation within the area to which the pain is referred may be relevant for management.[126,130,132–134]

Neurodynamic treatment approaches where drainage of the cavernous sinus is evident might include gentle cranial movement of the sphenoid, temporal and petrosal bones, avoiding excessive load on nervous tissue, which is discussed in Chapter 2. Cranial neurodynamic treat-

ment might also help to recover normal physical health of the tissue, which allows the cranial nervous system to stretch and to glide in tunnels during movement for optimal electrochemical function.[135] Cluster headache can be a challenge to 'hands on' treatment. Other vascular headaches where the cavernous sinus and other more complex pain-sensitive structures of the upper cervical nerves, posterior fossa, trigeminal system and the autonomic system are involved can also be challenging for the clinician.[131,136,137]

The foramina of the skull, transitional areas for cranial nervous tissue

Most of the cranial nerves (with the exception of the olfactory and optic nerves) run, with connective tissue of the internal and external layers of the dura, through the

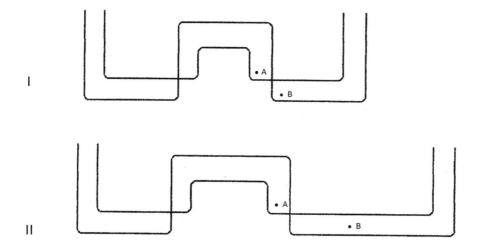

Figure 7.13 A schematic diagram depicting the cranial base growth (adapted from Enlow, 1986).
I. The process of normal growth in the cranial base. An average adaptation of the blood vessels and cranial nerves and cranial nerves from A to B.
II. The process of asymmetrical cranial base growth. The cranial base develops. Abnormal growth processes, asymmetrically different cranioneurodynamics can take place, which can be a predisposition finding during (minor) neuropathies and abnormal cranioneurodynamic testing

foramina of the skull. Growth of different individual skull areas stops at a variable period after birth.[27,138,139] The skull floor has many foramina and a high growth rate in different regions during the first 10 years of life.[139] For example, the posterior cranial fossa has the highest growth rate in the first 5 years and the middle cranial fossa in the first 8 years, respectively 97.5% and 98% of the adult value.[27,140] The planum sphenoidale can still grow 27% after the first 9 years. The skull normally functions as a container for emerging neural tissue. Hence when there is abnormal (asymmetrical) skull growth, as seen in the case of KISS children (kinematic imbalance suboccipital strain,[141] TMJ anomalies,[125] craniosynostosis and facial paralysis[141]), the skull is predisposed to an abnormal load, pressure and sliding which in turn can result in physical dysfunction and neuropathies (Figure 7.13).

Movement of cranial nervous tissue

Head and neck movements

It is possible to look at the effects of movement and sustained position on the neuraxis. The term neuraxis was first introduced by Bowsher[143] and is used instead of the 'central nervous system' so as to emphasize the nervous system from a biomechanical perspective.[2] The neuraxis consists of all the nervous tissue and connective tissue housed in the bony structure of the vertebral canal and cranium. The enormous variations in thickness and interconnections of connective tissue sheaths around the brain structures, cranial nerves and skull betray the extensive dynamic potential of this part of the neuraxis. Hopefully this portrays a picture of the nervous system as one organ, which spreads out like a cobweb in the body so

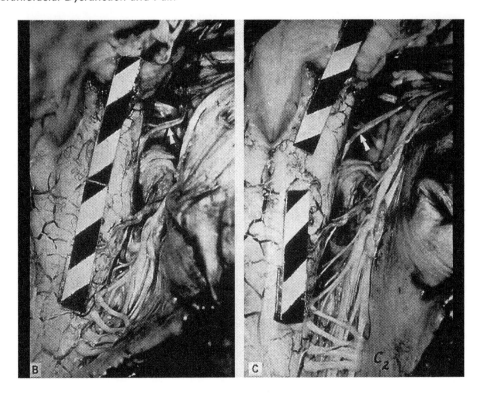

Figure 7.14 Effect of flexion and extension of intracranial tissue and the cervical spine in the region of the pons and brainstem. After removal of cranial and cervical tissue in the right suboccipital region, neurodynamic changes can be noted from full neck extension (L) to full neck flexion (R).
Left: the markers have been inserted so that their ends are in contact pons, brainstem, cranial nerves and cervical nerve roots are shortened and slackened. Right: the ends of the markers have moved apart pons, brainstem, cranial nerves and cranial roots adapt to the movement by elongation and stretching to their maximum physiological extent

that symptoms can be referred anywhere. During clinical observation I found that immobility of the neural tissue in the suboccipital region can be related to distal symptoms. From the literature it is known that cranioneurodynamics (such as upper cervical flexion and side flexion) influence the neurodynamics of the upper limbs,[134] and that subjects who are symptom free demonstrate the following during neck/head flexion:

- An increased tension in the tissues of the brainstem, cord, cranial nerves, and internal and external layers of the dura[144,145]

- Adaptation of the brainstem and fourth ventricle. Both become smaller and 1.5 cm longer in their maximal range of shortening and elongation (Figure 7.14)[146]

- Movement and loading of cranial nerves such as the trigeminal, hypoglossal, facial and the accessory nerve by at least 5–7 mm.[24]

In his book *Adverse Mechanical Tension in the Central Nervous System*, Breig[24] urged that neck/head flexion must be considered as an integral part of any general examination or rehabilitation routine, often shedding new light on clinical action. Recent clinical data support this.[142]

Lateral flexion of the head, for example:

- changes the neurodynamics of nerve tissue in the masticatory system, especially the auriculotemporal nerve.[147] These changes are also emphasized by mandible movements, which are mostly decreased.[29]
- moves the hypoglossal nerve in the suprahyoid region and the facial nerve in the region of the mastoid. Again these changes (in my experience) decrease the opening and/or lateral glide (away) of the mandible.[148]
- during mandibular movements, especially from maximum closing to maximum opening, causes the lingual nerve in the adult mandible to adapt in its nerve bed by an average of 0.8 cm.[148]

Cranial pathology and neurodynamics

Clinical patterns in patients with dysfunctions such as dural adhesions or entrapment of cranial nerves often have the same pathodynamics as clearly diagnosed pathology in the craniocervical and craniofacial region.[20,24] The following features are some examples of pathology, which give an idea that when one examines or treats a patient with cranioneurodynamics, one must be sure that serious pathology is excluded.

- Children with neuroblastoma of the cranial neuraxis have difficulty extending and flexing the neck.[149]
- Patients with foramen magnum and high cervical cord lesions can have bizarre neurological signs and symp-

toms, such as bilateral leg numbness, and spasm, during upper cervical head extension.[150]

- A posterolateral neurosurgical approach in an extended position for dural lesions provides less risk of cerebrospinal fluid leakage and is more likely to relax the cranial blood vessels and nerves.[151]
- The general test for acute meningitis is flexion of the head or the neck, whereby range of motion and the reaction of the patient is assessed.[152]

Description of some cranioneurodynamic tests

Introduction

This section gives an overview of the physical examination by neurodynamics of two cranial nerves, the mandibular branch of the trigeminal nerve and the facial nerve, which are often involved in craniocervical and craniofacial dysfunction and pain.[10] The tests and some clinical comments on the mandibular and facial nerves are discussed to give the principles of testing cranial tissue. The tests are in most cases a basis for treatment and for further management.[5,25,68] Treatment and ongoing management are not described in this chapter, and the reader is referred to previous literature.

A brief overview of anatomy is given, followed by a description of the test and some clinical comments. The examiner is referred to as 'clinician' or 'she', and the subject as patient or 'he'. The starting position during the tests is with the clinician positioned on the right side of the plinth, and the right cranial nerves are tested.

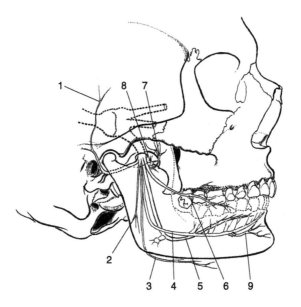

Figure 7.15 The mandibular nerve and its branches

1. Auriculotemporalis n.
2. Massetericus n.
3. Mylohyoideus n.
4. Alveolaris inferior n.
5. Lingualis n.
6. Buccalis n.
7. Temporali profundi n.
8. Ganglion oticum n.
9. Mentalis n.

The neurodynamic test of the mandibular nerve (V3)

Relevant neuroanatomy

The mandibular nerve (V3) travels laterally from the trigeminal ganglion through the foramen ovale, which is a hole roughly 1 cm in diameter and 2–3 mm in length located in the greater wing of the sphenoid bone (Figure 7.15). Because of the variation in the way the many different branches spread out as it exits different neurodynamic loading is possible. The branches are:

- buccal nerve: not to be confused with the nerve to buccinator, a motor branch of the seventh cranial nerve, the buccal nerve runs a deep course through the cheek to the masseter and pierces the lateral pterygoid muscle to join the main trunk of the mandibular nerve

- lingual nerve: this nerve runs from the trigeminal ganglion downwards between the mandible and the medial pterygoid muscle. This branch curves here to join the main trunk of the mandibular nerve at some depth in the lateral pterygoid muscle

- auriculotemporal nerve: a branch of the mental nerve, which runs below the head of the mandible to the ventral part of the acoustic meatus

- mental nerve: the mental nerve enters the mandibular foramen into the mandibular canal, which has a length of about 4–6 cm. Within the canal some branches run to the lower teeth. The end of the nerve passes through the mental foramen.

Mandibular division (V3)

Site of test	Positions of hands	Type of movement	Figure
Cervical spine	Both hands laterally cup the occiput	Upper flexion, side flexion away	7.17a
Mandible - lingual, mental nerves	Right index and middle finger grasp around mandible	Depression and lateral glide away	7.17b
- buccal, auriculo-temporal nerves	Right thumb and index finger on the mandibular condyl	Transverse movement medially of the mandibular head	7.17c
Cranium - sphenoid	Right thumb and index finger on the wings of sphenoid bone	Accessory movements of sphenoid	

Figure 7.16 Overview of neurodynamic testing of the mandibular nerve (V3)

Neurodynamic test

Upper cervical flexion and contralateral side flexion of the cervical spine is the first manoeuvre for changing neurodynamics around the brainstem. Depression (about 1 cm) and contralateral deviation of the mandible is needed for the lingual and mental nerves. For the buccal and auriculotemporal branches, passive transverse movement of the mandible medially or laterally is added (Figure 7.16). In particular, movements of the sphenoid can influence the foramen ovale where the mandible runs through.

Starting position

The patient lies supine and is comfortable and relaxed with his head over the end of the plinth and his hands on his abdomen. The clinician grasps around the occiput with both hands. Both thumbs are on the mandibular angles and she rests the patient's head against her abdomen without compression. The patient must relax the mandible. She asks the patient to bring the tip of his tongue against the palate with the mouth slightly open, and to follow this by relaxing the tongue back again in the floor of the mouth. The mandible will then stay in this position (a mouth opening of about 1.5 cm measured from the upper to the lower incisors).

Method

For the upper cervical spine the clinician flexes the head on the patient's neck (Figure 7.17a). This is upper cervical flexion through an imaginary transverse axis which runs through the first and second vertebrae. The second movement is side flexion away from the upper cervical spine (head on neck movement), where the imaginary sagittal

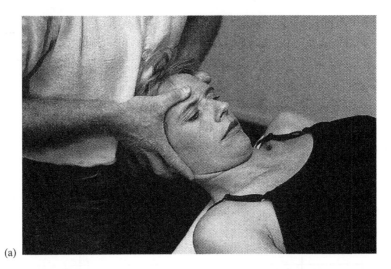

(a)

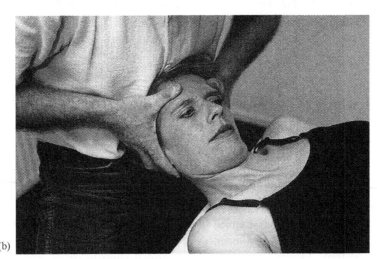

(b)

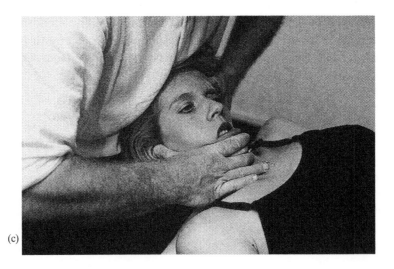

(c)

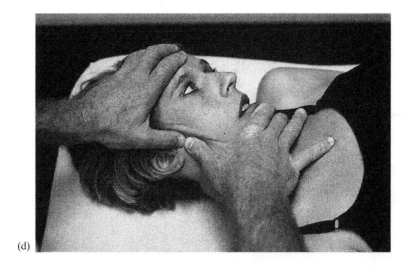

(d)

Figure 7.17(a) Upper cervical flexion; (b) side flexion away of the upper cervical spine; (c) lateral glide away of the mandible; (d) transverse movement medially of the head of the mandible

axis also runs between the first and second vertebrae (Figure 7.17b). She guides both movements with her hands followed by a small trunk movement in the direction to be examined. Both movements are performed to the maximal permitted resistance and/or pain, because of the optimal load on the intracranial tissue, which is necessary for testing of the extracranial branches of the mandible nerve. In this position, the lateropulsion or lateral glide away (here to the left) has to be executed. With her left hand she holds the patient's head in this combined upper flexion position. Her right hand moves slowly to the right side of the mandible and the right index finger is positioned on the superior part of the mandible with the metacarpal joint lying under the right corner of the mouth. The right middle finger contacts the mandible inferiorly so that the right side of the mandible is resting between these two fingers. Before the manoeuvre, she checks if the mouth of the patient is still relaxed and the tongue is still on the floor of the mouth. If not, she asks the patient to relax

the mandible by taking the tip of the tongue back against the palate again, followed by relaxing the tongue in the floor of the mouth. After checking this she can perform the lateral excursion to the left. Be aware that lateral glide is not a linear movement but a curve-like movement.

A small body movement without increasing pressure in the right hand (Figure 7.17c) causes lateral glide of the mandible. The clinician registers any qualities such as resistance, endfeel, noises, range and symptom reproduction for further interpretation.

An alternative way of influencing the neurodynamics is to move the head of the mandible – for example, a transverse movement medially (Figure 7.17d) or accessory movements of the sphenoid bone such as transverse glide and rotation around a sagittal axis.

Comment

Mandibular nerve neuropathy

The rich variation of sensory branches in

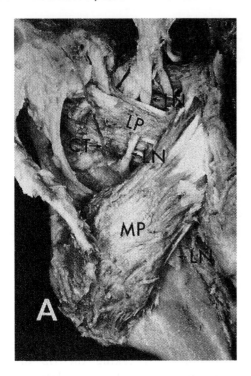

Figure 7.18 Medial view of lingual nerve entrapment by lateral pterygoid muscle in lingual nerve. LP: lateral pterygoid muscle; MP: medial pterygoid muscle; A: angle of mandible (with permission of Isberg, A.M., Isacsson, G., Williams, W.N. and Loughner, B.A. (1987). Lingual numbness and speech articulation deviation associated with temporomandibular joint disk displacement. *Oral Surg. Oral Med. Oral Pathol.*, **64**, 12, Figures 1 and 2)

the craniofacial region and motor innervation of the masticatory muscles suggest that loading changes in the trigeminal nerve can influence neuropathies. This includes orofacial pain, TMJ dysfunction, tinnitus, vertigo, eye and ear aches, atypical facial pain and other neuropathies such as trigeminal neuralgia or tic douloureux.[10,153] Some examples where dynamic changes in the nerve might change symptoms from a minor trigeminal neuropathy include the following:

- The widespread projection of primary afferents of the first neuron in the trigeminal brainstem complex.[154,155] Directed loading of the nerve branches can create neurophysiological and neurobiological changes in the caudal nucleus of the trigeminal brainstem complex and the possibility of convergence with other neurons, for example from the cervical spine.[10,156]

- Ectopic discharges, which occur at the sites of nerve injury, were shown to increase mechanosensitivity and chemosensitivity of the nerve as observed by Devor.[157] Rappaport and Devor[158] saw that demyelination of the trigeminal ganglion is the first sign of damage to the rest of the trigeminal nerve. This reminds us that we must be alert to the nature of the morphological changes that are presenting. Pathophysiological processes such as the setting up of a circuit between excitatory and inhibitory synapses that continues indefinitely, or so-called autorhythmic firing, starts in the trigeminal ganglion and sets off the whole activity, especially in the mandibular division.[159] Pain or other symptoms may affect all three divisions of the trigeminal nerve. White and Sweet,[160] in their study, looked at 8124 patients with craniofacial pain and found that 32% of symptoms were related to the trigeminal nerve and that the mandibular branch was dominant and 17% had mixed disturbances with the other trigeminal branches. Zakrzewska and Nally[161] found, in patients with facial pain who had undergone cryotherapy of the peripheral nerve branches, that most pain was reduced by cryotherapy of the mandibular nerve branches and that 38% was mixed with the other trigeminal branches.

- The difference between the functional

Facial Nerve (VII)

Site of test	Positions of hands	Type of movement	Figure
Cervical spine	Both hands grasp the occiput	Upper flexion side flexion away, rotation towards the examined side	7.20a 7.20b
TMJ	Right index finger and middle finger contact mandible	Depression lateral pulsion away (Buccal branch)	7.20c
Cranium • temporal bone	Right thumb index, middle and little finger contact temporal bone	Temporal bone movements (mech., int.)	7.20b
• petrosal bone	Right thumb and index finger	Petrosal movements	
• hyoid	Right thumb and index finger	Hyoid movement (cervical branch)	7.20d

Figure 7.19. Overview of neurodynamic tests of the facial nerve (VII)

anatomy and dynamics of the mandibular nerve branches might alone provide a clue to symptoms that present in this area. The auriculotemporal, inferior alveolar and lingual nerves have three main differences to the other nerve division. First, all three have longer extracranial branches than the other cranial nerves.[26,162] Secondly, they have a wide variety of extracranial tunnels, anastomoses and fixation points, more so than in other divisions, and thus they must adapt to the resulting dynamic interface.[43,163–165] Spasm in the medial pterygoid and/or lateral pterygoid muscles from craniomandibular dysfunction is an example of where the lingual nerve has an influence on neuropathy (Figure 7.18).[163] Another is the case of mandibular growth spurts in youth, where the inferior alveolar nerve and the lingual nerve must adapt vertically and horizontally, respectively.[166] The intraosseous anterior loop of the inferior alveolar nerve is another often forgotten branch where functional neuroanatomy and dynamics might be implicated. It extends beyond the mental foramen, and anatomical and radiological studies show that variations in this branch are relatively common, with the average length being 6.95 mm and consistent findings of a 2 mm loop.[167] The third and final factor which might realistically provide some insights into mandibular nerve neuropathies is the enormous range of movement of the TMJ (50–60 mm maximum opening), to which the mandibular nerve has to adapt.[168,169]

The neurodynamic test for the facial nerve (VII)

Relevant neuroanatomy

Cranial nerve VII emerges from the brainstem dorsolateral to the pons and has four components which run laterally and enter

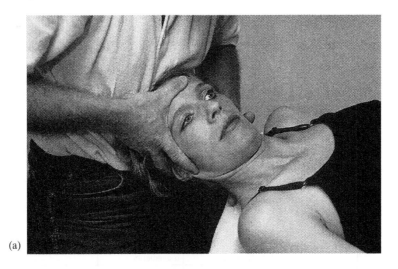

(a)

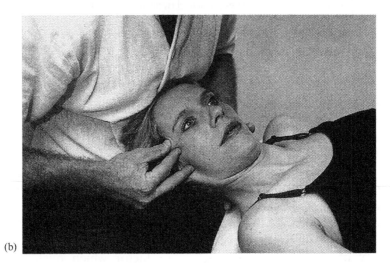

(b)

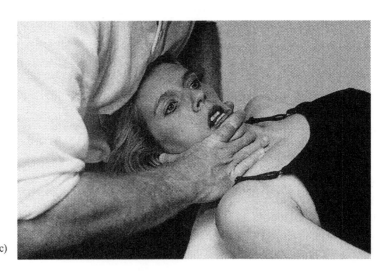

(c)

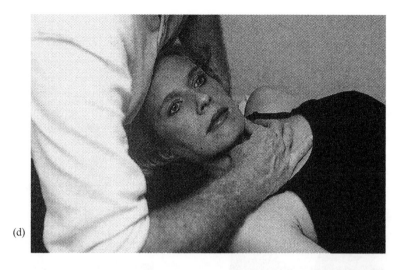

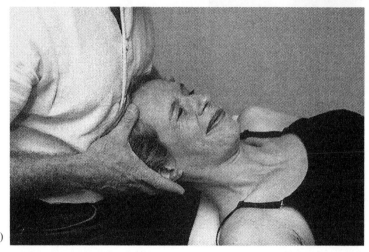

Figure 7.20 The neurodynamic test for the facial nerve (nl): (**a**) Upper cervical flexion, side flexion away and rotation of the head to the same side; (**b**) movement of the temporal bone in flexion and side flexion away of the cervical spine; (**c**) lateral deviation of the mandible to load the buccal branch; (**d**) movement of the hyoid bone to have more influence on the suprahyoid branches; (**e**) facial expression on the examined side

the internal auditory meatus of the temporal bone together with the vestibulocochlear nerve (VII). This meatus leads to the facial canal of the temporal bone, which runs laterally for about 2 cm, then turns 90°, runs posteriorly/inferiorly for 5 cm and terminates at the stylomastoid foramen, which is located behind the base of the styloid process. A further six branches are formed, which run in the facial muscle and are relatively superficial. The six branches are named for the regions where they run. The nerves are the temporal nerve, the zygomatic nerve, the buccal nerve, the mandibular nerve, the cervical nerve and the posterior auricular nerve.

Neurodynamic test

The cervical spine is positioned in upper cervical flexion and lateral flexion away

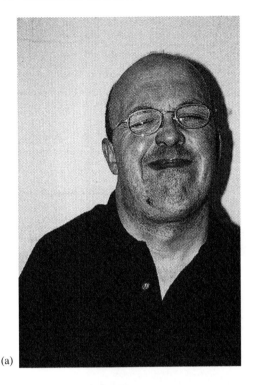

(a)

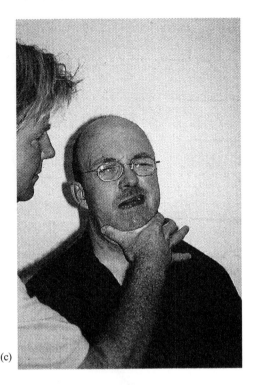

(c)

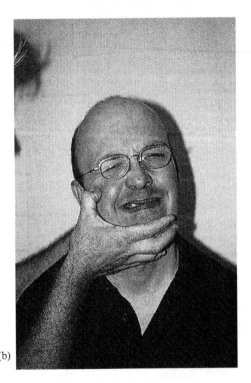

(b)

Figure 7.21 (a) Facial muscle contraction is easier in a relaxed neurodynamic position of the facial nerve; (b) palpation of the buccal branch facilitates the facial muscles; (c) in neurodynamic position of the facial nerve the facial muscle contraction is more difficult than in an 'unload' position

from the examined side and in ipsilateral rotation to get more load on the branches, which are directly extracranial and run parallel with the sternocleidomastoid. Temporal bone movements are possible to influence the intra-auditory meatus and facial canal. Petrosal bone movement produces changes in the stylomastoid foramen region. One possibility is to move the mandible into depression and deviation to the left (for the mandibular buccal branch), and to move the left facial muscles, which produces loading of the examined side. Contraction of the right facial muscles can produce compressive loading of the side being examined. When the cervical branch of the facial nerve is examined, a longitudinal caudad movement of the hyoid can be useful (Figure 7.19).

Starting position

The patient lies comfortably in a relaxed position. The clinician sits or stands at the top of the plinth facing the patient's head. Both the clinician's hands are cupped around the lateral side of the head, avoiding extreme compression on the cranium. An alternative position is to place the left hand on the occipital region and the right hand on the frontal bone when the nasal or orbital regions are to be examined or treated.

Method

The clinician moves her body as little as possible with both forearms on the table for the upper cervical flexion, side flexion away and rotation of the head to the same side (Figure 7.20). Movement of the temporal or petrosal bone can be added by moving the right hand to the lateral side of the head and making contact with, for example, the temporal bone (Figure 7.20b). For mandibular movement, the clinician's right hand grasps around the lateral side of the mandibular angle, her right index finger lies on the superior part and the middle finger contacts the inferior part of the chin. In this position she can perform a slight depression and lateral deviation of the mandible to the left to emphasize the mandibular buccal branch (Figure 7.20c). When hyoid movement is needed, the right index finger and thumb grasp around the hyoid and perform the longitudinal movement (Figure 7.20d). Active facial expression by the patient can be initiated in any position to change the neurodynamics (Figure 7.20e).

Are neurodynamics of the facial nerve useful in rehabilitation?

Testing in functional positions such as sitting and standing is more comparable, especially for patients with neurological facial paresis. An example is given in Figure 7.21 of a patient with congenital hemiparesis and facial paresis. The patient has an upper motor neuron lesion (UMNL). Lower motor neuron lesion (LMNL) components may also play a role in his facial motor dysfunction with regard to articulation and eating. In an unloaded position of the facial nerve (upper cervical extension, lateral flexion towards and rotation away from the examined side), facial muscle contraction can be improved and the dysfunction therefore decreased (Figure 7.21a). Palpation of the branch of the facial nerve stimulates the activity even more (Figure 7.21b). More loading (cervical flexion, side bending away and rotation towards the examined side) gives the same patient less expression (Figure 7.21c). This neurodynamic principle is in my opinion very useful for mobilization and for integration into neurological exercise therapy. Cranial nerves are richly innervated by their own nerves called nervi nervorum and by the autonomic nervous system, which regulates the vascularization of these nerves.[170] Changes of the neural container because of spasm of the facial muscles due to chronic pain[18] and neurological diseases (facial pareses) can change the physiological mechanisms of the nerve (pathodynamics) and can be a source of symp-toms.[6] Alleviating pain and normalizing muscle tone of the muscles of facial expression using neurodynamic movements can in my opinion be a reason why the symptoms of patients with orofacial pain and facial pareses can change. The application of the neurodynamic concept in the craniofacial region is still at an early stage. Good description and standardization of testing of cranial nervous tissue is needed and can be a challenge for further research in this area.

Summary and conclusion

- Cranial nervous tissue is designed for movement. There are different intracranial vulnerable zones such as nerve entry zones, the cerebellopontine angle (CPA), the cavernous sinus and the skull foramina. The cranial nervous tissue together with the intracranial connective tissue as a continuum is strongly linked to vital organs (e.g. cerebrum, cerebellum) and pain-sensitive structures (e.g. cranial nerves and dura mater), and injury or pathology can make the nervous tissue mechanosensitive.
- During clinical observation, atypical dysfunctions and pain patterns in the craniocervical and craniofacial regions, with or without a clear diagnosis, can be recognized and perhaps linked with abnormal cranioneurodynamics.
- Biomedical and clinical knowledge of this relatively new and exciting area is needed. This is particularly so for those clinicians who want to understand and manage patients with long-term, sometimes undiagnosed, dysfunction and pain in the head and neck region.
- Clinical reasoning is a useful approach, which opens doors to the recognition of new clinical patterns and makes the clinician creative in developing new tests and treatment techniques.

- Good standardization and further research such as reliability studies and clinical randomized trials are probably the next steps which will help the patient and the clinician to further unravel craniocervical and craniofacial dysfunction and pain.

References

1 Shacklock, M. (1995). Neurodynamics. *Physiotherapy*, **81**, 9–16.
2 Counter, R. T. (1989). *A Colour Atlas of Temporal Bone. Surgical Anatomy.* Wolfe Medical Publications Ltd.
3 Lundborg, G. (1988). Intraneural microcirculation. *Orthop. Clin. North Am.*, **19**, 1–12.
4 Wall, P. D. and Melzack, R. (1994). *Textbook of Pain.* Churchill Livingstone.
5 Kwan, M. K., Wall, E. J., Massie, J. and Garfin, S. R. (1992). Strain and stress and stretch of peripheral nerve. Rabbit experiments in vitro and in vivo. *Acta Orthop. Scand.*, **63**, 267–272.
6 Gifford, L. (1998). *Topical Issues in Pain. Whiplash Science and Management. Fear-avoidance Beliefs and Behaviour.* NOI Press.
7 Lundborg, G., Dahlin, L. B., Danielsen, N. and Nachemson, A. K. (1986). Tissue specificity in nerve regeneration. *Scand. J. Plast. Reconstr. Surg.*, **20**, 279–283.
8 Walksman, B. H. (1961). Experimental study of diphtheric plyneuritis in the rabbit and guinea pig. III The blood–nerve barrier in the rabbit. *J. Neuropath. Exper. Neurol.*, **21**, 35–77.
9 Nakao, Y., Sakihama, N., Matshumoto, K. *et al.* (1994). Vascular permeability to sodium fluorescein in the rabbit cranial nerve root; possible correlation with normal cranial nerve enhancement on gadolinium-enhanced magnetic resonance imaging. *Eur. Arch. Otorhinolaryngol.*, **251**, 457–460.
10 Okeson, J. P. (1994). *Bell's Orofacial Pains.* Quintessence Publishing Co. Inc.
11 Markowitz, S., Saito, K. and Moskowitz, M. A. (1987). Neurogenically mediated leakage of plasma protein occurs from blood vessels in dura mater but not brain. *J. Neurosci.*, **59**, 648–666.
12 Geppetti, P., Del Bianco, E., Santicioli, P. *et al.* (1990). Release of sensory neuropeptides from dural venous sinuses of guinea pig. *Brain Res.*, **510**, 58–62.
13 McCullock, J., Uddman, R., Kingman, T. A. and Edvinsson, L. (1986). Calcitonin gene-related peptide: functional role in cerebrovascular regulation. *Proc. Natl. Acad. Sci. USA*, **83**, 5731–5735.
14 Penfield, W. and McNaughton, F. (1992). Dural

headache and innervation of the dura mater. *Arch. Neurol. Psychiatry*, **44**, 43–75.

15 Sindou, M. and Mertens, P. (1993). Microsurgical vascular decompression (MVD) in trigeminal and glosso-vago-pharyngeal neuralgies. A twenty-year experience. *Acta Neurochir. Suppl. (Wien)*, **58**, 168–170.

16 Jannetta, P. J. (1981). Hemifacial spasm. In: *The Cranial Nerves: Anatomy, Pathology, Pathophysiology, Diagnosis, Treatment* (M. Samii and P. J. Jannetta, eds), pp. 486–493. Springer-Verlag.

17 Adams, C. B. T. (1989). Microvascular compression: an alternative view and hypothesis. *J. Neurosurg.*, **70**, 7–12.

18 Baldwin, N. G., Sahni, K. S., Jensen, M. E. *et al.* (1991). Association of vascular compression in trigeminal neuralgia versus other 'facial pain syndromes' by magnetic resonance imaging. *Surg. Neurol.*, **36**, 447–452.

19 Colletti, V., Fiorino, F. G., Policante, Z. and Bruni, L. (1996). New perspectives in intraoperative facial nerve monitoring with antidromic potentials. *Am. J. Otol.*, **17**, 755–762.

20 Schlessel, D. A., Nedzelski, J. M., Rowed, D. and Feghali, J. G. (1992). Pain after surgery for acoustic neuroma. *Otolaryngol. Head Neck Surg.*, **107**, 424–429.

21 Buzzi, M. G., Moskowitz, M. A., Peroutka, S. J. and Byun, B. (1991). Further characterization of the putative 5-HT receptor which mediates blockade of neurogenic plasma extravasation in rat dura mater. *Br. J. Pharmacol.*, **103**, 1421–1428.

22 Moskowitz, M. A. (1992). Cluster headache: evidence for a pathophysiologic focus in the superior pericarotid cavernous sinus plexus. *Headache*, **28**, 584–586.

23 Feniuk, W., Humphrey, P. P. and Perren, M. J. (1991). Rationale for the use of 5-HT 1-like agonists in the treatment of migraine. *J. Neurol.*, **238**, 57–61.

24 Breig, A. (1978). *Adverse Mechanical Tension in the Central Nervous System*. Almqvist & Wiksell.

25 Butler, D. S. (1991). *Mobilisation of the Nervous System*. Churchill Livingstone.

26 Wilson-Pauwels, L., Akesson, E. and Stewart, P. (1988). *Cranial Nerves, Anatomy and Clinical Comments*. BC Decker Inc.

27 Lang, J. (1995). *Skull Base and Related Structures. Atlas of Clinical Anatomy*. Schattauer.

28 Patten, J. (1995). *Neurological Differential Diagnosis*. Springer.

29 Jones, M. A. (1994). Clinical reasoning in manual therapy. *Phys. Ther.*, 72, 875–884.

30 Hardebo, J. E. (1991). On pain mechanisms in cluster headache. *Headache*, **31**, 91–106.

31 Dubner, R. (1991). Neuronal plasticity and pain following peripheral tissue inflammation or nerve injury. In: *Proceedings of the VIth World Congress on Pain* (M. R. Bond, J. E. Charlton and C. J. Woolf, eds), pp. 264–276. Elsevier.

32 Sunderland, S. and Bradley, K. (1961). Stress–strain phenomena in human peripheral nerve trunks. *Brain*, **84**, 102–119.

33 Bora, F. W., Richardson, S. and Black, J. (1980). The biomechanical responses to tension in a peripheral nerve. *J. Hand Surg.*, **5**, 21–25.

34 Jinkins, J. R. (1991). Clinical manifestations of hydrocephalus caused by impingement of the corpus callosum on the falx: an MR study in 40 patients. *Am. J. Neuroradiol.*, **12**, 331–340.

35 Xiong, L., Rauch, R. A., Hagino, N. and Jinkins, J. R. (1993). An animal model of corpus callosum impingement as seen in patients with normal pressure hydrocephalus. *Invest. Radiol.*, **28**, 46–50.

36 Ruan, J. S., Kahalil, T. and King, A. L. (1991). Human head dynamic response to side impact by finite element modeling. *J. Biomech. Eng.*, **113**, 276–283.

37 Hagen, N. A., Stevens, J. C. and Michet, C. J. Jr (1990). Trigeminal sensory neuropathy associated with connective tissue diseases. *Neurology*, **40**, 891–896.

38 Kaga, A., Isono, M., Mori, T. *et al.* (1991). Cavernous angioma of falx cerebri; case report. *No Shinkei Geka*, **19**, 1079–1083.

39 Iwamoto, Y., Mizukawa, N., Sekimoto, T. and Nakahara, Y. (1993). A case of cervical vagus neurinoma with hypoglossal palsy. *No To Shinkei*, **45**, 567–570.

40 Patel, S. J., Sekhar, L. N., Cass, S. P. and Hirsch, B. E. (1994). Combined approaches for resectionof extensive glomus jugulare tumors. A review of 12 cases. *J. Neurosurg.*, **80**, 1026–1038.

41 Williams, P. L., Warwick, R., Dyson, M. and Bannister, L. H. (1989). *Gray's Anatomy*, 37th edn. Churchill Livingstone.

42 de Slegte, R. G. M., Valk, J., Lohman, A. H. M. and Zonneveld, F. W. (1986). *Cisternographic Anatomy of the Posterior Cranial Fossa*. Van Gorcum.

43 Leblanc, A. (1965). *The Cranial Nerves*. Springer.

44 Aksik, I. (1993). Microneural decompression operations in the treatment of some forms of cranial rhizopathy. *Acta Neurochir. (Wien)*, **125**, 64–74.

45 Greene, K. A., Karahalios, D. G. and Spetzler, R. F. (1995). Glossopharyngeal neuralgia associated with vascular compression and choroid plexus papilloma. *Br. J. Neurosurg.*, **9**, 809–814.

46 Pamir, M. N., Zirh, T. A., Ozer, A. F. *et al.* (1995). Microvascular decompression in the surgical management of trigeminal neuralgia. *Neurosurg. Rev.*, **18**, 163–167.

47 Miller, N. R. (1996). The ocular motor nerves. *Curr. Opin. Neurol.*, **9**, 21–25.

48 Lunardi, P., Mastronardi, L., Farah, J. O. *et al.* (1996). Spinal accessory nerve palsy due to neurovascular compression. Report of a case diagnosed by magnetic resonance imaging and magnetic resonance angiography. *Neurosurg. Rev.*, **19**, 175–178.

49 Jannetta, P. J. (1982). Treatment of trigeminal neuralgia by micro-operative decompression. In: *Neurological Surgery* (J. R. Youmans, ed), pp. 3589–3603. W B Saunders.

50 Smirniotopoulos, J. G., Yue, N. C. and Rushing, E. J. (1993). Cerebellopontine angle masses: radiologic–pathologic correlation. *Radiography*, **13**, 1131–1147.

51 Rowed, D. W. (1990). Chronic cluster headache managed by nervus intermedius section. *Headache*, **30**, 401–406.

52 Sindou, M., Amrani, F. and Mertens, P. (1990). Microsurgical vascular decompression in trigeminal neuralgia. Comparison of 2 technical modalities and physiopathologic deductions. A study of 120 cases. *Neurochir.*, **36**, 16–26a.

53 Møller, A. R. (1991a). The cranial nerve vascular compression syndrome: I. A review of treatment. *Acta Neurochir. (Wien)*, **113**, 18–23. Møller, A. R. (1991b). The cranial nerve vascular compression syndrome: II. A review of pathophysiology. *Acta Neurochir. (Wien)*, **113**, 24–30.

54 Stenglein, C. and Cidlinsky, K. (1992). Neurovascular makes contact with the inner ear canal and cerebello-pontine angle. An ethodologic comparison between CT with pneumocisternomeatography and MR angiography. *HNO*, **40**, 381–385.

55 Matthies, C., Carvalho, G., Tatagiba, M. *et al.* (1996). Meningiomas of the cerebellopontine angle. *Acta Neurochir. Suppl.*, **65**, 86–91.

56 Tancioni, F., Gaetani, P., Villani, L. *et al.* (1995). Neurinoma of the trigeminal root and atypical trigeminal neuralgia: case report and review of the literature. *Surg. Neurol.*, **44**, 36–42.

57 Dubner, R. and Basbaum, A. I. (1994). Spinal dorsal horn plasticity following tissue or nerve injury. In: *Textbook of Pain* (P. D. Wall and R. Melzack, eds), pp. 225–241. Churchill Livingstone.

58 Jannetta, P. J. and Rand, R. W. (1967). Arterial compression of the trigeminal nerve at the pons in patients with trigeminal neuralgia. *J. Neurosurg.*, **26**, 159–162.

59 King, W. A., Black, K. L., Martin, N. A. *et al.* (1993). The petrosal approach with hearing preservation. *J. Neurosurg.*, **79**, 508–514.

60 Braun, J. P., Tournadec, A. and Adynowski, J. (1984). A comparative anatomical CT study of the vascular and nervous structures of the cerebello-pontine angle. *Neurorad.*, **26**, 3–7.

61 Shore, R. M., Rao, B. K. and Berg, O. B. (1988). Massive jugular and dural sinus reflux associated with cerebral death. *Pediatr. Radiol.*, **18**, 164–166.

62 Daniels, D. I., Schenck, J. F., Foster, T. *et al.* (1985). Magnetic resonance imaging of the jugular foramen. *AJNR*, **6**, 699–703.

63 Brain, S. D., Cambridge, H., Hughes, S. R. and Wilsoncroft, P. (1992). Evidence that calcitonin gene-related peptide contributes to inflammation in the skin and joint. *Ann. N. Y. Acad. Sci.*, **30**, 412–419.

64 Petty, P. (1977). Vascular compression of lower cranial nerves. *Aust. N. Z. J. Surg.*, **46**, 314–320.

65 Morales, F., Mostacero, E., Marta, J. and Sanchez, S. (1994). Vascular malformation of the cerebellopontine angle associated with 'SUNCT' syndrome. *Cephalalgia*, **14**, 301–302.

66 Pitty, L. F. and Tator, C. H. (1992). Hypoglossal–facial nerve anastomosis for facial nerve palsy following surgery for cerebellopontine angle tumors. *J. Neurosurg.*, **77**, 724–731.

67 Schwarze, H. P., Hirsch, B. E. and Johnson, P. C. (1995). Oculostapedial synkinesis. *Otolaryngol. Head Neck Surg.*, **113**, 802–806.

68 Maitland, G. D. (1986). *Vertebral Manipulation*, 5th edn. Butterworths.

69 Barba, D. and Alksne, J. F. (1984). Success of microvascular decompression with and without prior surgical therapy for trigeminal neuralgia. *J. Neurosurg.*, **60**, 104–107.

70 Nakase, H., Ohnishi, H., Touho, H. and Karasawa, J. (1994). Large ependymal cyst of the cerebello-pontine angle in a child. *Brain Dev.*, **16**, 260–263.

71 Kato, T., Sawamura, Y. and Abe, H. (1995). Trigeminal neuralgia caused by a cerebello-pontine angle lipoma: case report. *Surg. Neurol.*, **44**, 33–35.

72 Hotta, J., Kubokura, T., Ozawa, H. *et al.* (1996). Cerebellopontine angle epithelial cyst presenting as hemifacial spasm. *No To Shinkei*, **48**, 281–285.

73 Matthies, C., Carvalho, G., Tatagiba, M. *et al.* (1996). Meningiomas of the cerebello-pontine angle. *Acta Neurochir. Suppl. (Wein)*, **65**, 86–91.

74 Mohsenipour, I., Deusch, E., Ortler, M. and Pallua, A. (1993). Meningiomas of the cerebello-pontine angle. *Neurochir. (Stuttg.)*, **36**, 90–92.

75 Kojima, Y., Tanaka, N. and Kuwana, N. (1990). Massive hemorrhage in acoustic neurinoma after minor head trauma – case report. *Neurol. Med. Chir. (Tokyo)*, **30**, 972–976.

76 Quester, R., Menzel, J. and Thumfart, W. (1993). Radical removal of a large glossopharyngeal neurinoma with preservation of cranial nerve functions. *Ear Nose Throat J.*, **72**, 600–611.

77 Mason, R. B., Cook, L. E. and Hargraves, R. W. (1996). Delayed diagnosis of large cerebellopontine angle tumors, despite hearing conservation training. *Mil. Med.*, **161**, 108–112.

78 Bellet, P. S., Benton, C. Jr, Matt, B. H. and Myer, C. M. III (1992). The evaluation of ear canal, middle ear, temporal bone, and cerebellopontine angle masses in infants, children, and adolescents. *Adv. Pediatr.*, **39**, 167–205.

79 Mark, A. S. and Fitzgerald, D. (1994). MRI of the inner ear. *Baillieres Clin. Neurol.*, **3**, 515–535.

80 Rhee, B. A., Kim, T. S., Kim, G. K. and Leem, W. L. (1995). Hemifacial spasm caused by contralateral cerebellopontine angle meningioma: case report. *Neurosurg.*, **36**, 393–395.

81 Casselman, J. W. (1996). Temporal bone imaging. *Neuroimaging Clin. North Am.*, **6**, 265–289.

82 Lavezzi, P., Bondioni, M. P., Chiesa, A. and Ettore, G. C. (1996). The anatomy of the temporal region viewed by magnetic resonance. *Radiol. Med. (Torino)*, **91**, 33–38.

83 Wigand, M. E., Aurbach, G., Haid, C. T. *et al.* (1991). Topographical anatomy of the internal auditory canal. Implications for functional surgery in the cerebellopontine angle. *Acta Otolaryngol. (Stockh.)*, **111**, 269–272.

84 Cohen, M. M. and Kreiborg, S. (1993). Cranial base and face in mandibular dysostosis. *Am. J. Med. Genet.*, **47**, 753–760.

85 Prasad, S., Kamerer, D. B., Hirsche, B. E. and Sekhar, L. N. (1993). Preservation of vestibular nerves in surgery of the cerebellopontine angle: effect on hearing and balance function. *Am. J. Otolaryngol.*, **14**, 15–20.

86 Andrews, D. W., Silverman, C. L., Glass, J. *et al.* (1995). Preservation of cranial nerve function after treatment of acoustic neurinomas with fractionated stereotactic radiotherapy. Preliminary observations in 26 patients. *Stereotact. Funct. Neurosurg.*, **64**, 165–182.

87 Patil, A. A. and Chand, A. (1995). Modifications of transnasal and transoral stereotactic procedures – technical notes. *Acta Neurochir. (Wien).*, **134**, 46–50.

88 Grey, P. L., Baguley, D. M., Moffat, D. A. *et al.* (1996). Audiovestibular results after surgery for cerebellopontine angle meningiomas. *Am. J. Otol.*, **17**, 634–638.

89 Yamakami, I., Yamaura, A., Ono, J. and Nakamura, T. (1996). Anatomical aspects of posterior fossa affecting lateral suboccipital approach: evaluation by bone-window CT. *No Shinkei Geka*, **24**, 157–163.

90 Resnick, D. K., Jannetta, P. J., Lunsford, L. D. and Bissonette, D. J. (1996). Microvascular decompression for trigeminal neuralgia in patients with multiple sclerosis. *Surg. Neurol.*, **46**, 358–362.

91 Sekiya, T., Iwabuchi, T. and Okabe, S. (1990). Occurence of vestibular and facial nerve injury following cerebellopontine angle operations. *Acta. Neurochir. (Wien)*, **102**, 108–113.

92 Schlessel, D. A., Rowed, D. W., Nedzelski, J. M. and Feghali, J. G. (1993). Postoperative pain following excision of acoustic neuroma by the suboccipital approach: observations on possible cause and potential amelioration. *Am. J. Otol.*, **14**, 491–494.

93 Hoang, T. D. (1987). Cavernous branches of the internal carotid artery: anatomy and nomenclature. *Neurosurg.*, **20**, 205–210.

94 Fox, J. L. (1988). Microsurgical treatment of ventral (paraclinoid) internal carotid artery aneuryms. *Neurosurg.*, **22**, 32–39.

95 Sadasivan, B., Ma, S. H., Dujovny, M. *et al.* (1991). The anterior cavernous sinus space. *Acta Neurochir. (Wien)*, **108**, 154–158.

96 Sekhar, L. N., Lanzino, G., Sen, C. N. and Pomonis, S. (1992). Reconstruction of the third through sixth cranial nerves during cavernous sinus surgery. *J. Neurosurg.*, **76**, 935–943.

97 Brazis, P. W. (1991). Localization of lesions of the oculomotor nerve: recent concepts. *Mayo Clin. Proc.*, **66**, 1029–1035.

98 Civantos, F., Ferguson, L. R., Hemmati, M. and Gruber, B. (1993). Temporal meningiomas presenting as chronic otis media. *Am. J. Otol.*, **14**, 403–406.

99 Bellet, P. S., Benton, C. Jr, Matt, B. H. and Myer, C. M. III (1992). The evaluation of ear canal, middle ear, temporal bone, and cerebellopontine angle masses in infants, children, and adolescents. *Adv. Pediatr.*, **39**, 167–205.

100 Majoie, C. B., Verbeeten, B. Jr, Dol, J. A. and Peeters, F. L. (1995). Trigeminal neuropathy: evaluation with MR imaging. *Radiograph.*, **15**, 795–811.

101 Brazis, P. W. (1993). Palsies of the trochlear nerve: diagnosis and localization – recent concepts. *Mayo Clin. Proc.*, **68**, 501–509.

102 De Jong, T. and Matricali, B. (1990). Asymptomatic occlusion of the internal carotid artery at the skull base. *Neurosurg.*, **34**, 21–27.

103 Yamada, M., Miyasaka, Y., Kitahara, Y. *et al.* (1994). Dural arteriovenous malformation involving the inferior petrosal sinus – case report. *Neurol. Med. Chir. (Tokyo)*, **34**, 300–303.

104 Ganesan, V. Lin, J. P., Chong, W. K. *et al.* (1996). Painful and painless ophthalmoplegia with cavernous sinus pseudotumour. *Arch. Dis. Child.*, **75**, 239–241.

105 Yamasaki, T., Nagao, S. and Kagawa, T. (1996). Therapeutic effectiveness of combined microsurgery and radiosurgery in a patient with a huge trigeminal neurinoma. *No To Shinkei*, **48**, 845–850.

106 Selky, A. K. and Purvin, V. A. (1994). Isolated trochlear nerve palsy secondary to dural carotid–cavernous sinus fistula. *J. Neuro-ophthalmol.*, **14**, 52–54.

107 Cerillo, A., Bianco, M., Narciso, N. *et al.* (1995). Trigeminal cystic neurinoma inthe cavernous sinus. Case report. *J. Neurosurg. Sci.*, **39**, 165–170.

108 Larson, J. J., van Loveren, H. R., Balko, M. G. and Tew, J. M. Jr (1995). Evidence of meningioma infiltration into cranial nerves: clinical implications for cavernous sinus meningiomas. *J. Neurosurg.*, **83**, 596–599.

109 Pérez Sempere, A., Martinex Menéndez, B., Cabeza Alvarez, C. and Calandre Hoenigsfeld, F. (1991). Isolated oculomotor nerve palsy due to cavernous sinus fistula. *Eur. Neurol.*, **31**, 186–187.

110 Nutik, S. L. (1988). Removal of the anterior clinoid process for exposure of the proximal intracranial carotid artery. *J. Neurosurg.*, **69**, 529–534.

111 Perneczky, A., Knosp, E., Vorkapic, P. and Czech, T. (1985). Direct surgical approach to infraclinoidal aneurysms. *Acta Neurochir. (Wien)*, **76**, 36–44.

112 Sekhar, L. N., Sen, C. N. and Jho, H. D. (1990). Saphenous vein graft bypass of the cavernous internal carotid artery. *J. Neurosurg.*, **72**, 35–41.

113 Linskey, M. E., Lunsford, L. D., Flickinger, J. C. *et al.* (1992). Stereotactic radiosurgery for acoustic tumors. *Neurosurg. Clin. North Am.*, **3**, 191–205.

114 Regis, J., Manera, L., Dufour, H. *et al.* (1995). Effect of the gamma knife on trigeminal neuralgia. *Stereotact.*

Funct. Neurosurg., **64**, 182–192.

115 Kato, T., Sawamura, Y. and Abe, H. (1995). Trigeminal neuralgia caused by a cerebellopontine angle lipoma: case report. *Surg. Neurol.*, **44**, 33–35.

116 Aurbach, G., Ullrich, D. and Mihm, B. (1991). Surgical anatomy of the optic nerve and the internal carotid artery in the laeral wall of the sphenoid sinus. An anatomic study of the cranial base. *HNO*, **39**, 467–475.

117 Schick, B., Weber, R., Mosler, P. *et al.* (1996). Duraplasty in the area of the sphenoid sinusi. *Laryngorhinootol.*, **75**, 275–279.

118 Chang, C. J., Chen, Y. R., Noordhoff, M. S. *et al.* (1990). Facial bone fracture associated with carotid–cavernous sinus fistula. *J. Trauma*, **30**, 1335–1339.

119 Keiser, G. J., Zeidman, A. and Gold, B. D. (1991). Carotid cavernous fistula after minimal facial trauma. Report of a case. *Oral Surg. Oral Med. Pathol.*, **71**, 549–551.

120 Kunz, U., Mauer, U., Waldbaur, H. and Oldenkott, P. (1993). Early and late complications of craniocerebral trauma. Chronic subdural hematoma/hygroma, carotid–cavernous sinus fistul, abscess formation, meningitis and hydrocephalus. *Unfallchirurg.*, **96**, 595–603.

121 Roland, J. T. Jr, Hammerschlag, P. E., Lewis, W. S. *et al.* (1994). Management of traumatic facial nerve paralysis with carotid artery cavernous sinus fistula. *Eur. Arch. Otorhinolaryngol.*, **251**, 57–60.

122 Kuno, R. and Robertson, W. D. (1995). Cavernous sinus air following orbital trauma. *Am. J. Roetgenol.*, **164**, 980.

123 van Overbeeke, J. J., Dujovny, M. and Troost, D. (1995). Anatomy of the sympathetic pathways in the cavernous sinus. *Neurol. Res.*, **17**, 2–8.

124 Moskowitz, M. A. (1988). Cluster headache: evidence for a pathophysiologic focus in the superior pericarotid cavernous sinus plexus. *Headache*, **28**, 584–586.

125 Ruskell, G. L. and Simons, T. (1987). Trigeminal nerve pathways to the cerebral arteries in monkeys. *J. Anat.*, **155**, 23–37.

126 Mayberg, M. R., Zervas, N. T. and Moskowitz, M. A. (1988). Trigeminal projections to supratentorial pial and dural blood vessels in cats demonstrated by horseradish peroxidase histochemistry. *J. Comp. Neurol.*, **223**, 46–56.

127 Arnold, F. (1851). *Handbuch der Anatomie der Menschen*. Freiburg in Breisgau.

128 Lyon, D. B., Lemke, B. N., Wallow, I. H. and Dortzbach, R. K. (1992). Sympathetic nerve anatomy in the cavernous sinus and retrobulbar orbit of the cynomolgus monkey. *Ophthal. Plast. Reconstr. Surg.*, **8**, 1–12.

129 Hardebo, J. E., Arbab, M., Suzuki, N. and Svengaard, N. A. (1991). Pathways of parasympathetic and sensory cerebrovascular nerves in monkeys. *Stroke*, **22**, 331–342.

130 Hardebo, J. E. (1994). How cluster headache is explained as an intracavernous inflammatory process lesioning sympathetic fibers. *Headache*, **34**, 125–131.

131 Hannerz, J., Hellström, G., Klum, T. and Wahlgren, N. G. (1990). Cluster headache and 'dynamite headache': blood flow velocities in the middle cerebral artery. *Cephalagia*, **10**, 31–38.

132 Davis, K. D. and Dostrowsky, J. O. (1988). Responses of feline trigeminal spinal tract nucleus neurons to stimulation of the middle meningeal artery and sagittal sinus. *J. Neurophysiol.*, **59**, 648–666.

133 Solomon, S. (1986). Cluster headache and the nervus intermedius. *Headache*, **26**, 3–8.

134 Hardebo, J. E. and Elner, A. (1987). Nerves and vessels in the pterygopalatine fossa and symptoms of cluster headache. *Headache*, **27**, 528–532.

135 Butler, D. S. (1997). The dynamic nervous system. Analysis and treatment of pathodynamics in neural tissues. In: *Proceedings IFOMT Manual Therapy Congress, Lillehammer Norway*, pp. 66–67.

136 Sjaadstad, O. and Bovim, G. (1991). Cervicogenic headache. The differentiation from common migraine. An overview. *Funct. Neurol.*, **6**, 93–100.

137 Sanin, L. C., Mathew, N. T. and Ali, S. (1993). Extratrigeminal cluster headache. *Headache*, **33**, 369–371.

138 Profitt, W. R. (1993). Concepts of growth and development. In: *Contemporary Orthodontics* (W. R. Profitt and H. W. Fields, eds), pp. 18–55. Mosby Year Book.

139 Harzer, W. (1982). Biologische Grundlagen der Schädelentwicklung. In: *Lehrbuch der Kieferorthopädie* (W. Harzer, ed), pp. 7–34. Carl Hanser Verlag.

140 Gefferth, K. (1976). The growing skull. Part I. Neurocranium, statistical considerations. *Acta Paediatr. Acad. Sci. Hung.*, **17**, 43–50.

141 Biedermann, H. and Koch, L. (1996). Zur Differentialdiagnose des KISS-Syndroms. *Manuel. Med.*, **34**, 73–81.

142 Davies, P. M. (1994). *Starting Again. Early Rehabilitation after Traumatic Brain Injury or Other Severe Brain Lesion*. Springer-Verlag.

143 Bowsher, D. (1988). *Introduction to the Anatomy and Physiology of the Nervous System*. Blackwell.

144 Brieg, A., Turnbull, I. and Hassler, O. (1966). Effects of mechanical stresses on the spinal cord in cervical spondylosis: a study on fresh cadaver material. *J. Neurosurg.*, **25**, 45–56.

145 Doursounian, L., Alfonso, J. M., Iba-Zizen, M. T. *et al.* (1989). Dynamics of the junction between the medulla and the cervical spinal cord: an in vivo study in the sagittal plane by magnetic resonance imaging. *Surg. Radiol. Anat.*, **11**, 313–322.

146 Breig, A. (1960). *Biomechanics of the Central Nervous System*. Almqvist and Wiksell.

147 Costen, J. B. (1934). Syndrome of ear and sinus symptoms dependent upon disturbed functions of the temporomandibular joint. *Ann. Otol. Rhinol. Laryngol.*, **43**, 112–118.

148 Slegter, R. G. M., Arzouman, M. J. *et al.* (1993). Observation of the anterior loop of the inferior

alveolar carnal. *Int. J. Oral Maxillofac. Implants*, **8**, 295–300.

149 Kellie, S. J., Hayes, F. A., Bowman, L. *et al.* (1991). Primary extracranial neuroblastoma with central nervous system metastases: characterization by clinicopathologic findings and neuroimaging. *Cancer*, **68**, 1999–2006.

150 Abbott, K. H. (1950). Foramen magnum and high cervical cord lesions simulating degenerative disease of the nervous system. *Ohio State Med. J.*, **46**, 645–650.

151 Crockard, H. A. and Sen, C. N. (1991). The transoral approach for the management of intradural lesions at the craniovertebral junction: review of 7 cases. *Neurosurgery*, **28**, 88–98.

152 Spillane, J. (1995). *Birkerstaff's Neurological Examination in Clinical Practice*. Blackwell Science.

153 Zakrzewska, J. M. (1995). *Trigeminal Neuralgia, Major Problems in Neurology*. WB Saunders Company.

154 Sessle, B. J. (1993). Neural mechanisms implicated in the pathogenesis of trigeminal neuralgia and other neuropathic pain stated. *Am. Pain Soc. J.*, **2**, 17–20.

155 Fields, H. L. (1990). *Pain Syndromes in Neurology*. Butterworth.

156 Hu, J. W. and Sessle, B. J. (1981). Functional properties of neurons in cat trigeminal subnuclear caudales (medially dorsal horn) I: response to oral facial noxious and non noxious stimuli and projection to tralatum and subnucleus oralis. *J. Neurophys.*, **45**, 173–192.

157 Devor, M., Goorin-Lipperman, R. and Angelides, K. (1993). Na$^+$ channel immunolocalization in peripheral mammalion axons and changes following nerve injury and neuroma formation. *J. Neurosci.*, **13**, 1976–1992.

158 Rappaport, Z. H. and Devor, M. (1994). Trigeminal neuralgia: the role of self sustaining discharge in the trigeminal ganglion. *Pain*, **56**, 127–138.

159 Connor, J. A. (1985). Neural pacemakers and rhythmicity. *Ann. Rev. Physiol.*, **47**, 17–28.

160 White and Sweet, W. H. (1969). Pain and the neurosurgeon. In: *A 40-year Experience* (C. Thomas, ed), pp. 123–256. Springfield.

161 Zakrzewska, J. M. and Nally, F. F. (1988). The role of cryotherapy (cryoanalgesia) in the management of paraxysmal trigeminal neuralgia: a six year experience. *Br. J. Oral. Maxillofac. Surg.*, **26**, 18–25.

162 Soeira, G. (1994). Microsurgical anatomy of the trigeminal nerve. *Neurosurg. Res.*, **16**, 210–227.

163 Isberg, A. M., Isacsson, G., Williams, W. N. and Loughner, B. A. (1987). Lingual numbness and speech articulation deviation associated with temporomandibular joint disk displacement. *Oral Surg. Oral Med. Oral Pathol.*, **64**, 9–14.

164 Shinichi, A., Tetsuya, I., Yoshinobu, I. and Chikara, S. (1997). An anatomical study of a muscle bundle separated from the medial pterygoid muscle. *J. Craniomand. Prac.*, **15**, 341–344.

165 Loughner, B. A., Larkin, L. H. and Mahan, P. E. (1990). Nerve entrapment in the lateral pterygoid muscle. *Oral Surg. Oral Med. Oral Pathol.*, **69**, 299–306.

166 Enlow, R. H. (1982). *The Human Face*, 2nd edn, pp. 116–130. WB Saunders Company.

167 Misoh, C. E. and Crawford, E. A. (1990). Predictable mandibular nerve location. A clinical zone of safety. *Today*, **9**, 32–35.

168 Palla, S. (1998). *Myoarthropathien des Kausystems und Orofaziale Schmerzen*. Fotoplast AG.

169 Kraus, S. L. (1994). Cervical spine influences on the management of TMD. In: *Temporomandibular Disorders* (S. L. Kraus, ed), pp. 325–413. Churchill Livingstone.

170 Hromada, J. (1963). On the nerve supply of the connective tissue of some peripheral nervous system components. *Acta Anatom.*, **55**, 343–351.

8

Experience of pain and the craniofacial region

D. S. Butler

Introduction

Pain has become a popular and almost trendy subject. Since the head and face are very common sites of pain, these areas have been extensively studied. There are journals and societies devoted to head and facial pain, however, readers should also be aware there are many journals and societies devoted to the pain phenomenon in general, not caring so much where it is, but how it emerges and its effect on the body as a whole.

Gate control theory[1] is widely recognized as the beginning of a pain revolution which continues to gather momentum as witnessed by the journals, conferences and the growth of the International Association for the Study of Pain (IASP) and other pain special interest groups. Gate control challenges the still widely held view that pain is an electrically dominant process which begins peripherally from an injuring stimulus and then travels to the brain. A more modern biologically evidence-based view is that pain is an electrochemical event which can be altered at many levels of the nervous system including pathways which descend from the brain.

Thirty-five years have passed since the gate control work was published. Despite the years, though, there is little evidence to show that patients are benefiting, particularly those with spinal and head pain. The scientific revolution has been slow to herald a much needed clinical revolution. For example, approximately one person in every ten in western society suffers a persistently painful problem,[2] one in seven according to Magni.[3] Pain clearly deserves better analysis. This should not only involve a closer look at the tissues which appear to house pain, but also at the phenomenon of pain itself.

What is pain?

Pain in the foot is not much different to pain in the head. Geographical differences and tissue components apart, the pathobiological processes are very similar. Perhaps it is a worthwhile thing for readers to take time to attempt a personal definition of this thing called pain. It will have a slightly different meaning to each person. I suggest that clinicians seek a broad answer and read widely in pathophysiological areas[4,5] and also in sociocultural areas.[6,7]

The IASP definition has survived some

years of argument. This association defines pain as, '*an unpleasant sensory and emotional experience associated with actual or potential tissue damage or described in terms of such damage*'.[8] Experience is a key word here. It takes away the instant link between pain and injuring peripheral stimuli that most clinicians make or seek. Potential tissue damage means that a threat or fear can also be considered a painful event. Some of the biochemical changes which occur from potential tissue damage also occur after injury.

If the pain experience was all related to input, it would be easy to understand and should be easy to manage by altering or stopping the input. This would make pain a passive process, a registering of impulse trains in the central nervous system following alterations of input. However, it is more accurate to consider it as something a person creates or processes actively and highly reliant on endogenous processes.[9] Pain in the head frequently lacks a traumatic peripheral initiating stimulus. Precipitating factors are more likely, for example, stress, posture and intake of various foods,[10] although sometimes precipitating factors cannot be identified. This suggests that there may be existing 'headache pathways' already established in the CNS which, depending on circumstances, are activated by the various precipitating factors. It is as though the head pain is there already, only subclinically. This does not deny, however, the potential for a close correlation between injury and pain which exists, for example, in dental pain, the most common facial pain.

Classifications of pain in the face and head

All clinicians and researchers use clinical categorizations, sometimes unknowingly. It is natural to attempt to make some sense out of the chaotic blend of injury and society. There have been attempts to classify head and facial pain. In 1988 a detailed classification was published by the International Headache Society (IHS).[11] This classification, based on pain patterns and available tests, includes 13 categories and many subcategories providing a worthwhile attempt to group the most common presenting complaints to doctors' offices. There is much 'blurring' of categories. The IASP has also proposed slightly different classifications,[8] although focusing more on chronic pain. There is much literature related to the classifications for head and facial pain.[10,12–15] (See also Chapter 5.)

This chapter is also about categorization. I wish to introduce and discuss the concept of mechanisms or processes of pain, that is, to look at the 'big picture' of pain in order to dissect it in pathobiological terms. Essentially the pathobiological processes driving the pain experience can be predominantly input-based, more CNS processing-related, or a result of activity in CNS output systems such as the motor or the autonomic systems.[16–18] The proposal here is to try to reason which pathobiological mechanisms are dominant in a particular patient's presentation. This call to consider pain mechanisms is not new.[19–21] Examples of input-based mechanisms include nociceptive pain from target tissues of nerve, for example muscle, ligament, bone, tendon and fascia, and peripheral neurogenic pain, for example from trigeminal or occipital nerve injury. Central mechanisms emerge from maladaptive processing in the central nervous system and the output systems include the autonomic, motor, immune and endocrine systems along with various coping behaviours.

An absolutely vital part of this is that all

pain states, including acute pain, will involve various combinations of these mechanisms. In some, one particular mechanism may stand out. For example, in acute pain from a neck strain or acute toothache an input mechanism will probably predominate, whereas in a long-standing facial pain state when damaged tissues have had an adequate time to heal, the biological processes behind the pain state may be more central in origin.

activity and conscious processing of the pain experience. Clinicians should consider what therapies are available for all dimensions of the pain experience.

In my view, clinicians can make reasoned attempts to diagnose pain in terms of these pathobiological categories. Though not pathognomic, these will be dynamic clinical diagnoses which may allow better and more biologically appropriate therapies than those which are currently delivered.

Multiple mechanisms lead to multiple dimensions of pain

Pain arises from combinations of the mechanisms discussed above. To the patient it is just pain, hopefully to the clinician the contributing mechanisms can be reasoned. The pain will be expressed in three interacting dimensions – sensory–discriminative, cognitive–evaluative and motivational–affective.[22,23] This categorization is useful to assist clinicians and patients to grasp the entire pain experience. The sensory dimension is the intensity, location, quality and behaviour of pain. The cognitive dimension relates to thoughts about the problem and will be influenced by previous experiences and knowledge. Finally, affective is the negative emotional response that motivates or governs responses to the pain (e.g. fear, anxiety or anger).[24] All dimensions are essential parts of all pain experiences, not just responses to injury, and all dimensions interact to produce altered behaviour. For example, negative thoughts about the pain state may arouse negative emotions, which may then arouse the autonomic and neuroendocrine response systems, potentially impacting again on the sensory system. Simultaneously, altered levels of activity occur under the influence of subconscious reflex

The moving, recurring nature of head and face pain demands that classification should be a dynamic process

Perhaps pains in the head are normal – in one large study fewer than 10% of a non-clinical population denied ever having a headache.[25] The fury and intensity of some headaches is undoubted, although the intensity does not seem to match up to whether the headache is benign or malignant. Most are benign. Fewer than 10% of the population with a pain in the head seek medical attention, presumably a far greater number must prefer self-treatment or no treatment. A small number go on to neurologists and although headache accounts for 25% of visits to neurologists,[26,27] less than 1% of those who visit them have intracranial pathology.[28]

The rare serious pathologies apart, most head pain is common, recurrent, and self-limiting. It may not be so much the head pain which is the problem, but the fact that it keeps returning. There are two issues here. Biopsychosocial triggers for recurrence are as worthy of study, as is the search for the actual pathoanatomy. Secondly, recurrence means that the pathobiological processes involved in the pain state may change over time. Symptoms which initially have been associated with a traumatic event to tissues, but which reappear over time, should raise the suspicion that different mechanisms may be involved. Over time, the pain mechanisms may become dominated by maladaptive plastic changes in the CNS. This is discussed further below. Recurrence will also relate to the development of negative emotions such as anger and frustration. There may be spillover into work and family. It would be a tragedy for the clinician just to focus on the head pain aspects, without taking pain in its larger dimension as discussed above. In addition, head and facial pain is often associated with other symptoms such as vertigo, visual alterations and nausea. These symptoms may be of greater concern to the patient than the actual headache.

All pain is in the head

The title is not meant in the derogatory sense which unfortunately is so often applied to patients whose injuries do not heal in the expected time frame of current medical models. It is meant more in the sense of a biological appreciation that all pain is ultimately in the brain.[29] A painful experience does not only involve the firing of high threshold A-beta or C fibres. All a general anaesthetic does is take away an awareness of pain, these high threshold fibres will still fire. Pain is dependent on the excitatory and inhibitory currents in operation in higher level neurons at the time of stimulation. Patients with severe head and neck trauma will often say there was no pain at the time of injury. This points to powerful control systems in the central nervous system. Any pain classification must therefore include brain-related mechanisms.

The concept of primary and secondary sensitivity – the start of pain diagnosis

If the cervical spine or the temporomandibular joint (TMJ) are injured or if the sinuses or a tooth are inflamed, then the tenderness which nearly always arises is referred to as primary hyperalgesia. It means tissue-based sensitivity to input. It is very common. However, tenderness (or hypoaesthesia) often spreads after local injury and sometimes persists or increases over time, when tissue healing has apparently taken place. This is referred to as secondary hyperalgesia. This may be due in part to a local seeping of pain-producing chemicals through tissues, but there is now strong evidence that the spread of tenderness and sensitivity is much more related to changes in spinal and supraspinal circuitry.[30–33] Take the example of a patient who has a persistent headache. Sometimes light touch, even of the hair, evokes or increases pain. Here, an input which enters the CNS via A-beta fibres is now painful. Somehow the CNS must have acquired novel abilities to upregulate the input.

Although secondary hyperalgesia has not entered the pain lexicon,[8] many clinicians and researchers discuss it.[31,34–38] Secondary hyperalgesia is often discussed in the research community under the broad label of central sensitization. The challenge of secondary hyperalgesia is that the tissues at the site of input are normal or only slightly damaged or unhealthy. This is likely to elicit many false positives with physical examination of musculoskeletal and neural tissues.[34] It is not an easy thing for patients and clinicians alike to accept that the tender tissues touched may not be the actual source of the problem. Nor is it easy to accept that a relentless diagnostic and therapeutic search for a solely tissue source

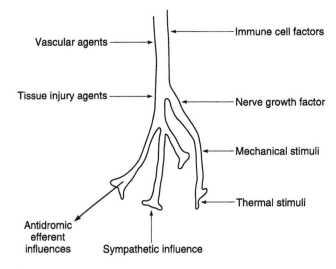

Figure 8.1 Stimuli for nociceptive pain (adapted from Dickensen, A. H. (1996). Pharmacology of Pain Transmission and Control. In: *Pain – An Updated Review* (J. N. Campbell, ed) IASP Press

of pain may make a problem worse by enhancing concepts of tissue damage and thus encouraging disability.

Further pain diagnosis – the mechanisms of pain

As discussed, the proposal is that the pathobiological basis of the pain experience can be categorized into input, processing or output dominant mechanisms. Clinically, two input dominant pain mechanisms – nociceptive and peripheral neurogenic pain – can often be recognized.

Nociceptive pain – pain originating from target tissues

The head contains a wide variety of specialized sensory structures, thus presenting a great potential for a variety of face and head pain.[39] When nerve endings in these structures are stimulated by mechanical and physiological processes, A-delta and C fibre input into the CNS may be perceived as pain.[31,40,41] A summary of these inputs is demonstrated in Figure 8.1. The list of potential pain sources is long and includes the cranium, periosteum, intra- and extracranial blood vessels, skin, muscles, sinuses, meninges, teeth and their surrounding structures. The eye is also a potential source of pain. The cornea and deeper structures such as the ciliary body and the iris are innervated by the trigeminal nerve and may become a source of deeper eye pain. The only structure which is not a source of nociceptive pain is the brain itself.[5,10,42]

Note, in Figure 8.1, the arrow pointing out from the nerve terminals and also the representation of a sympathetic terminal. The nervous system can contribute to inflammation. 'Backfiring' C fibres allow an efferent contribution from the peripheral nervous system to nociceptive pain. Substance P and other peptides are released from terminal boutons via an antidromic impulse (an impulse which travels in an efferent direction on an afferent nerve fibre). This occurs normally – the peptides stimulate tissue healing – but the process may become maladaptive with increased antidromic impulses arising from injury to the nervous system. Antidromic impulses may arise from the dorsal horn in the CNS[43–45] or sites of neuropathy in peripheral nerves.[46,47] Peptides are highly vasoactive and encourage enzyme activity and also the release of histamine from mast cells. The sympathetic efferent fibres are also known to secrete chemicals such as noradrenaline, which is involved in the inflammatory process.[31,37]

Nerve endings will also become sensitized from repeated noxious stimulation occurring from repeated inflammatory, mechanical or ischaemic states.[37,48] Classes of nociceptive endings which 'sleep' until awoken by inflammation will become active.[49] Local ischaemia may be another pain stimulus. Both low and high threshold nerve endings are sensitized and excited by hypoxia,[50] making tight muscles or scarred tissues candidates for ischaemic nociceptive pain which would clearly benefit from movement. These processes not only relate to the kind and intensity of the local pain, but they also combine to create a powerful afferent barrage into the central nervous system that is likely to adapt and respond in various ways.

Identification of nociceptive pain

Nociceptive pain should be an easy kind of pattern to identify, notwithstanding the complexity and specialization of nerve endings in the head. Often, the pain mechanisms are easier to identify than the source. Nociceptive pain frequently has a clear stimulus/response relationship, that is, pressure may evoke pain and then once pressure is off the pain eases, although in some inflammatory nociceptive pains the pain may be ongoing. It is usually acute and related to tissue injury. The pattern is often one of increased pain with movement and there is often a diurnal pattern where pain is worse in the morning. If the cervical spine is involved, patients may complain of stiffness in the morning.

As the injury or disease settles and the tissues become healthier, nociceptive pain should ease. Various treatments such as anti-inflammatory medication, ice, graded active and passive movements may speed up what should be a natural occurrence. The aim should be to do what you can to make the relevant tissues more healthy. It will also help recovery if any anxiety or fear created by the pain, related sensory phenomena and the painful event is decreased and diffused.

Any of the innervated tissues may refer pain. Superficial structures refer pain locally, for example a right frontal sinus infection can cause right forehead pain. Deeper structures have a less precise referral, for example an irritated trigeminal nerve root may result in facial pain.[51,52] The cervical spine and TMJ structures are major candidates for pain referral to the head. (See Chapters 2 and 3 for referral patterns to the head.)

Peripheral neurogenic pain

The second category of the input dominant pain mechanism is peripheral neurogenic pain. It has been argued for some years[53–55] that this is an underestimated pain mechanism. Peripheral neurogenic pain arises from processes in peripheral neural tissues, that is, tissues which lie outside the dorsal or medullary horns. Clinical syndrome examples are trigeminal or occipital neuralgia.

The axolemma of peripheral and cranial nerves are designed for impulse transmis-

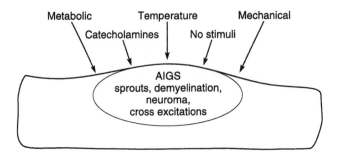

Figure 8.2 Stimuli which may activate an abnormal impulse generating site

sion, not generation. For pain to arise mid-axon, the number and sensitivity of ion channels in the axolemma at the injury site or elsewhere must alter. In addition, the kind of ion channels may change.[54] The injured or altered sites, if causing a sensory discharge, are known as abnormal impulse generating sites (AIGS). Pathological changes allowing ion channel pooling and sensitivity changes within an AIGS include demyelination and neuroma development. Alpha adrenoreceptor expression on injured axolemma may also occur post-injury,[56] thus allowing a contribution to depolarization from stress-induced circulating chemicals such as noradrenaline. (See Devor[54] for a review.)

Once an AIGS is set up, the stimuli leading to the perception of pain may be mechanical forces, catecholamines released during stress, or metabolic changes such as ischaemia. Some injury sites may fire spontaneously or in response to temperature increases[54] (see Figure 8.2 for a summary). In response to the neuropathy, neuronal function further along the nerve, especially in the dorsal root ganglion and in the CNS, may be altered, probably due to ion channel number and sensitivity changes[54,56] Note that if a nerve servicing a painful tissue is cut, it does not mean that pain is abolished. This dramatic alteration of input to the higher neurons may actually

increase pain since the cut ends of nerves can themselves become abnormal impulse generators,[4] in addition to neuroplastic changes in the CNS which may amplify input.

As stated above, a peripheral neuropathy may also contribute to an inflammatory nociceptive pain by creating antidromic impulses releasing neurotransmitters such as substance P and calcitonin gene related peptide (CGRP) which have a pro-inflammatory effect on target tissues.[57] For example, an injury or dysfunction in the trigeminal nerve or an alteration in its higher controls may be a major cause of migraine via inflammatory effects on intracranial blood vessels or any innervated tissue.[58,52,59] Some eye pains may have similar mechanisms.[60] Drugs such as sumatriptan block this neurogenic inflammation.

Many factors such as the health of the neural connective tissues, endoneurial fluid pressure, axonal transport systems and the quality of the vasa nervorum can influence impulse conduction.[61,62] The epineurium, perineurium and endoneurium of peripheral neural tissues are highly innervated and reactive connective tissues, and quite probable sources of symptoms in neuropathies.[53,63–65]

Perhaps most importantly for chronic pain management, a nerve injury, particularly a nerve root injury, continually injects abnormal trains of impulses and abnormal levels of transmitter chemicals into the central nervous system. This may have devastating effects on the subtly controlled balances of inhibition and excitation needed for normal sensory processing and even lead to morphological, perhaps irreversible, changes in synaptic connectivity. This is discussed further below.

Identification of peripheral neurogenic pain

Before discussing patterns, clinicians should be aware that some people sustain injuries such as nerve entrapment or nerve root compression and may never complain of pain.[66,67] In some patients, the pain may begin some days after injury,[54] probably due to a combination of the regulatory influences of the central nervous system and the slow development of an AIGS at the place of injury. Neural connective tissue injury or irritation should really be considered as a unique category of nociceptive pain which is perhaps responsible for some localized pains[63] much in the way a tendon or ligament may hurt.

The following features may help identify peripheral neurogenic pain. Symptoms (pain and/or paraesthesia) are within all or part of the innervation field of a nerve trunk or within the dermatome, myotome or sclerotome of a nerve root. The quality of symptoms may be influenced by the type of tissue innervated by the damaged fibres.[68] Thus, fibres that normally innervate muscle may give rise to deep aching or cramping pain, and fibres to skin may produce superficial burning, paraesthesia or stinging sensations. Tests that mechanically influence a nerve (such as a neurodynamic test), muscle contraction, or sustained postures that compress or stretch a reactive nerve may evoke a variety of pain

symptoms.[54] These responses may be a short burst of pain that ends before the stimulus is removed, symptoms remaining for the period the stimulus is present, or symptoms that continue after the physical stimulus has been removed. There may also be a slow build-up of symptoms during the application of the stimulus, subsiding slowly once the stimulus is removed. These features, particularly the stimulus after discharge, should be easily recognizable in nerve root irritation syndromes of the neck and perhaps of the trigeminal nerve.

Biologically-based management of peripheral neurogenic pain should include any possible way of dampening down AIGS activity. This may involve rest or graded movement of the nerves and their surrounding tissues, and attempts to increase blood flow to the nerve. It should also involve education about the disorder and its prognosis with the aim of lessening the likelihood of catecholamine contributions to depolarization and central sensitization. In addition, temperature-initiated activation may be managed by appropriate environmental modifications.

Central sensitization – pain related to altered CNS circuitry and processing

The medullary horn or cervicotrigeminal nucleus provides a variable response potential to input. Far more than a simple relay station, this small piece of neural tissue contains complex circuitry with a variety of neurons, neurotransmitters and receptors. This circuitry is controlled by excitatory and inhibitory influences from the brain, the periphery and spinal and segmental neurons.[4] While only a part of a much greater and more powerful CNS response system, recent research beginning with Woolf[69] and involving dorsal horn cells has provided an indication of the enormous plasticity of CNS circuitry,[70] in particular the potential of nociceptive enhancement.

Adult neurons will not replicate but they exhibit considerable neuroplasticity, and in particular their relationship to other neurons changes continually. The neuroplastic process includes time-dependent excitation or inhibition of neighbouring neurons, cell death and sprouting of new axons.

Inputs release neurotransmitters such as glutamate, aspartate and substance P into the synaptic cleft to bathe interneurons and second order neurons. These transmitters are excitatory and will sensitize the second order neurons by a process of ion channel opening or a longer lasting change in the second order neurons via channels which open for a longer period of time (G protein gated channels). There is a control system; after all, it would be of little use if all input hurt. Many of the interneurons are inhibitory and these are powerfully supplemented by controls which descend from higher areas, allowing inhibitory transmitters and modulators such as serotonin and the enkephalins to dampen synaptic activity. The above description is a normal response to input and once the afferent input ceases then the changes in the second and third order cells should dampen down and the system revert to its previous state, albeit leaving some synaptic memory of how it acted in response to that particular input.

A sensitive nervous system can be of great adaptive value to promote protective motor activity and healing behaviour, but sometimes (perhaps often, if the epidemiological data above are considered), this enhanced excitability state persists long after peripheral tissues have healed to the best of their abilities. If the input persists and there are poor descending controls, then some long-term morphological changes at the synaptic level may occur. This may involve local inhibitory neuron death,[33] new and inappropriate synapsing,[71] and cell membrane changes allowing cells that under normal conditions only respond to nociceptive inputs to respond to inputs that are innocuous.[72] Large-diameter primary afferent neurons may begin to express substance P,[73,74] something normally only associated with C fibre activity. In addition these cells respond far more, for longer, and increase their receptive field (area of tissue which can excite a neuron). Cells therefore change their response properties. While this dorsal horn sensitivity may be maintained by a 'trickle' of small-fibre afferent input from the periphery, it may persist even when the original injury has healed.[71,75] Inputs are not only physical. Inputs are also thoughts and feelings. Review the pain definition above. Conceptually, the dorsal horn is easier to grasp than higher centres, although similar processes of glutamate-inspired cell death, axon sprouting, neuropeptide concentration changes and receptive field alterations have been documented in CNS centres.[76–78] Pain states related to maladaptive central processing have been considered similar to memory processes by some, meaning that chronic pain may be very difficult to remove.[79–82]

Identification of a maladaptive central processing state

All patterns, including the ones listed above, are not pathognomic. The pattern suggested below provides a reasoned clinical categorization based on the best possible evidence to allow a management process. Remember that all pain states will have multimechanisms. It is the overall presentation which is important.

A frequent clue to the presence of maladaptive central sensitivity is when a patient's symptoms are ongoing after tissues have had time to heal, appreciating that tissues such as ligament take longer to go though inflammatory and remodelling phases than other tissues such as skin.

Therapists may consider the symptoms weird and wholly inappropriate to the history. There may be no familiar anatomical 'textbook' patterns to the symptoms. Evaluation reveals excessive sensitivity to inputs that would not normally provoke pain, yet the tissues under scrutiny seem to be healthy (secondary hyperalgesia). There is rarely a physical test that does not hurt in some way, and rarely a test where the patient reports an improvement in symptoms. Thus, everything may hurt, for example, ligament, muscle, joint and neurodynamic tests. In some instances, movements and activities can be non-painful at the time they are performed but produce a reactive latent response. Occasionally, grossly abnormal movement patterns, (which may be related to fear of pain or a need to demonstrate the pain) are displayed, other patients prefer to keep silent. Symptoms may be more intense under stressful circumstances and, similar to some peripheral neurogenic pain states, are often described as having 'a mind of their own'. Patients may provide histories of psychologically traumatic events that weaken their overall coping capacity and which might be significant to ongoing pain states. Some studies of populations of chronic pain sufferers have noted increased incidences of childhood physical and sexual abuse, abandonment, and emotional neglect and abuse.[83,84] Factors such as dislike of work[85] and heightened anxiety and frustration[86] are a few of the many features that can influence the patient's recovery, levels of distress and suffering.[87] Finally, responses to passive treatments are quite variable. A specific treatment may vastly improve symptoms on one occasion, yet the same treatment performed at another time may exacerbate the symptoms. Perhaps it is best to summarize the pattern as that group whose symptom complex was disbelieved in the past.

With this emerging information, many therapists, particularly manual therapists, may be questioning their worth. However, it should provide new treatment options. Many chronic pain sufferers can be taught to focus less on their pain and more on recovery of function once they have a better understanding of the pain mechanisms involved.[88,89] I would advocate focusing on a recovery process, where patients clearly understand their pain and where function is the goal, rather than a focus on pain relief and specific tissue therapy. In particular, with this CNS mechanism dominant, patients need to be aware that their pain level has been magnified by processes in the CNS rather than damaging processes in tissues. In this framework, tissues can be made healthier by whatever means are available. Manual therapists should not despair about the lack of moving parts in the head, other than the jaw; the movement limitations are likely to be more general or related to fitness level, rather than specific to a particular tissue.

Prolonged and maladaptive central sensitization is a big challenge for clinicians to integrate. It is a dangerous state for the patient. Therapists' doubt creeps in about the validity of the experience. This is compounded by the fact that there is no test, either imaging or biochemical, that can identify this subtle state of affairs. In this pain state, treatments such as unnecessary surgery, injection, and repeated and forceful manipulation are unwarranted, often leading to dashed hopes for a gullible patient in the presence of a convincing practitioner.[90] Pain evoked by physical tests may have little to do with the local tissues. It may simply be quite normal inputs which are wrongfully processed by the CNS to be perceived as noxious.

Output mechanisms

In response to input, the circumstances of input, our makeup, and the environment of injury or disease, there will be an 'output'. The CNS will give value to an input and this is reflected in a number of systems – the autonomic nervous system, the endocrine system, the motor system, the immune system and the descending pain control systems. The complexity of the processing involved in the value judgement is difficult to comprehend. The responses of some output systems are obvious, such as the motor system (e.g. spasm, altered movement patterns) and the sympathetic nervous system (e.g. sweating). Not so visible is the behaviour of the endocrine and the immune systems. There is a growing literature on the influence of mental stress on disease states via the sympathetic, neuroendocrine and immune system pathways.[91]

Autonomic and endocrine system responses

All physically or mentally registered inputs (including any treatments) will evoke a stress response. This is a primitive survival-driven response, well known as the 'flight or fight' response. (See Sapolsky[92] and any neurological text book for details.)

The sympathetic nervous system (SNS) has often been blamed for many pain states due to the apparent successful alleviation of symptoms following sympathetic block techniques.[93,94] However, the importance of the sympathetic nervous system may have been overemphasized. There are many patients who appear to have sympathetically maintained pain (SMP) symptoms that do not respond to sympathetic block techniques. Many ongoing pain states comprise multiple mechanisms, and all aspects of ongoing pain, particularly neuroplastic changes in the CNS, need consideration. Finally, the weight of modern evidence suggests that where a disorder has a component of SMP, it is not so much the fault of an abnormal sympathetic system but that abnormal sensitivity to *normal* sympathetic secretions occurs in injured nerves and peripheral nociceptor terminals,[95] as has been discussed earlier in this chapter.

Recent pain sciences investigations have challenged the dominance given to the SNS in the reflex sympathetic dystrophy (RSD) construction. This is useful because it challenges the focus of diagnosis on one element of a very complex and disabling pain state. It also encourages a re-examination of the role of the SNS in pain states generally. Clinicians are urged to review the current debate in pain sciences[95] and be aware that the reflex sympathetic dystrophy construction has now been labelled complex regional pain syndrome (CRPS).[96] This title encourages a broader look at the problem rather than a focus on the sympathetic nervous system.

Endocrine responses essentially revolve around the stress chemical cortisol. Sapolsky[92] is a worthwhile read here too; for more detail read Lovallo.[97] With input, particularly maintained stressful input, corticotrophin releasing factor (CRF) from the hypothalamus stimulates the anterior pituitary, releasing ACTH into the bloodstream and soon bathing the adrenal cortex. Glucocorticoids (cortisol) pour out into the circulation. Cortisol affects every major organ system in the body. Essentially it activates or excites body processes which are essential for immediate survival (e.g. enhanced memory and sensitivity), and it shuts down those processes which are not (e.g. reproduction, inflammatory processes). Short-term cortisol bursts are not harmful, however, long-term elevated levels may lead to depression, sleep disorders, neuronal death and weakened tissues.

The key message for clinicians is that no matter what they do or say to patients they will be influencing the stress system and therefore the sympathetic and the endocrine systems. Graduated strengthening, return of range of movement, increasing physical fitness and function and improving tissue health may be worthwhile manual therapy aims. However, decreasing catecholamine levels by easing anxiety, fear and frustration and using relaxation and other techniques may also be a vital aspect of management. When pain is chronic, the educative process may be more important for a beneficial outcome than actual passive physical manoeuvring. It is well worth explaining to the patient the relationship of negative/unhelpful thoughts and emotions to increased tissue sensitivity to catecholamines. Not only does this gives them an explanation for odd pain behaviours, but it also encourages them to use other strategies such as relaxation and meditative techniques and to utilize other clinicians involved in rehabilitation.[89] (For a psychological approach see Chapter 11.)

The other major output-related pain mechanism is via the motor system. The motor system responds to pain in various ways. Grossly there may be learnt postures and movements which the patient believes are best for his or her circumstances and these may have secondary ill-health effects on tissues such as the muscles and joints of the neck and on general fitness. The motor system's response to pain may be maladaptive if neuroplastic events have occurred in associated neural networks such as the somatosensory cortex[98] and/or dorsal/medullary horns. Injured muscle and ongoing inappropriate muscle activity may cause local pain, probably from ischaemia or mechanical influences on nociceptors, and be a source of noxious input into the CNS.[99] Conscious and subconscious muscle activity also occurs as a result of thoughts and feelings about injury, disease and their circumstances.[100]

Conclusion

Pain above the neck is common, recurrent, often idiopathic and frequently resistant to therapy. It does not necessarily relate to tissue damage or disability, and is individual-specific. This chapter calls for a greater exploration of the pain phenomenon, and in particular joins others in calling for attempts to make clinical diagnoses based on processes of pain.

Increasing scientific exploration into the pain phenomenon has meant that some patterns of head pain can be linked with known neurobiological processes, allowing better categorization and therapies which at least have evidence-based biological underpinnings.

Take pain on. It provides a common link with many medically related professions, including a precious common language. It stimulates research and it must direct therapy. As always, outcome studies are needed, but for the patients who cannot wait there is an overwhelming scientific revolution which powerfully indicates that we must begin to change and adapt therapy. These are exciting times in science.

We need to take this science to patients and make it exciting for them as well.

References

1 Melzack, R. and Wall, P. D. (1965). Pain mechanisms: a new theory. *Science.*, **150**, 971–979.

2 Crook, J., Rideout E. and Browne G. (1984). The prevalence of pain in a general population. *Pain*, **37**, 215–222.

3 Magni, G., Caldieron, C. and Rigatti-Luchini, S. *et al.* (1990). Chronic musculoskeletal pain and depressive symptoms in the general population: an analysis of the first national health and nutrition examination survey data. *Pain*, **43**, 299–307.

4 Melzack, R. and Wall, P. D. (1996). *The Challenge of Pain*, 3rd edn. Penguin.

5 Wall, P. D. and Melzack, R. (1994). *Textbook of Pain*. Churchill Livingstone.

6 Morris, D. (1991). *The Culture of Pain*. University of California Press.

7 Delvecchio-Good, M., Brodwin, P. E., Good, B. J. and Kleinman A. (1992). *Pain as Human Experience*. University of California Press.

8 Merskey, H. and Bogduk N. (1994). *Classification of Chronic Pain*, 2nd edn. IASP Press.

9 Chapman, R. C., Oka, S. and Jacobson, R. C. (1997). Phasic pupil dilation response to noxious stimulation in humans. In: *Proceedings of the 8th World Congress on Pain* (T. S. Jensen, J. A. Turner and Z. Wiesenfeld, eds), pp. 449–458. IASP Press.

10 Lance, J. W. (1993). *Mechanisms and Management of Headache*, 5th edn. Butterworth-Heinemann.

11 Darof, R. B. (1988). Classification and diagnostic criteria for headache disorders, cranial neuralgias and facial pain. *Cephalagia*, **8**, 1–96.

12 Diamond, S. and Diamond, M. L. (1994). Differential diagnosis of headache pain. In: *Handbook of Pain Management*, 3rd edn (C. D. Tollinson *et al.* eds), pp. 239–252. Williams and Wilkins.

13 Schoenen, J. and Maertens de Noordhout, A. (1994). Headache. In: *Textbook of Pain*, 3rd edn (P. D. Wall and R. Melzack, eds), pp. 495–522. Churchill Livingstone.

14 Sharav, Y. (1994). Orofacial pain. In: *Textbook of Pain*, 3rd edn (P. D. Wall and R. Melzack, eds), pp. 563–582. Churchill Livingstone.

15 Kanner, R. M. (1996). Headache and facial pain. In: *Pain Management: Theory and Practice* (R. K. Portenoy and R. M. Kanner, eds), pp. 51–79. F.A. Davis.

16 Butler, D. S. (1998) Integrating pain awareness into physiotherapy – wise action for the future. In: *Topical Issues in Pain* (L. S. Gifford, ed), pp. 1–26. NOI Press.

17 Gifford, L. S. (1998). Pain, the tissues and the nervous system: A conceptual model. *Physiotherapy*, **84**(1), 27–36.

18 Gifford, L. S. and Butler D. S. (1997). The integration of pain sciences into clinical practice. *J. Hand Ther.*, **10**, 86–95.

19 Devor, M. (1996). Pain mechanisms and pain syndromes. In: *Pain – An Updated Review* (J. N. Campbell, ed), pp. 103–112. IASP Press.

20 Sidall, P. J. and Cousins, M. J. (1997). Spinal update: spinal pain mechanisms. *Spine*, **22**, 98–101.

21 Woolf, C. J., Bennett, G. J., Doherty, M. *et al.* (1998). Towards a mechanism-based classification of pain. *Pain*, **77**, 227–229.

22 Melzack, R. and Casey, L. (1968). Sensory, motivational and central control determinants of pain: a new conceptual model. In: *The Skin Senses* (D. Kenshalo, ed), pp. 423–443. Charles C Thomas.

23 Melzack, R. and Katz, J. (1994). Pain measurement in people in pain. In: *Textbook of Pain*, 3rd edn (P. D. Wall and R. Melzack, eds), pp. 337–356. Churchill Livingstone.

24 Chapman, C. R. (1995). The affective dimension of pain: a model. In: *Pain and the Brain* (B. Bromm and J.E. Desmedt, eds), pp. 283–302. Raven Press: Advances in Pain Research and Therapy; vol 22.

25 Ziegler, D. K., Hassanein, R. S. and Couch J. R. (1977). Characteristics of life headache histories in a non-clinic population. *Neurol.*, **27**, 265–269.

26 Diehr, P., Wood, R. W., Barr, V. *et al.* (1981). Acute headaches: presenting symptoms and diagnostic rules to identify patients with tension and migraine headache. *J. Chron. Dis.*, **34**, 147–158.

27 Hopkins, A. (1989). Lessons for neurologists from the United Kingdom third national morbidity survey. *J. Neurol. Neurosurg. Psych.*, **52**, 430–433.

28 Hopkins, A., Menken, M. and De Friese, G. A. (1989). A record of patient encounters in neurological practice in the United Kingdom. *J Neurol. Neurosurg. Psych.*, **52**, 436–438.

29 Backonja, M. M. (1996). Primary somatosensory cortex and pain perception. Yes sir, your pain is in your head (part 1). *Pain Forum*, **5**, 171–180.

30 Woolf, C. J. (1991). Generation of acute pain: central mechanisms. *Br. Med. Bull.*, **47**, 523–533.

31 Meyer, R. A., Campbell, J. N. and Raja, S. N. (1994). Peripheral neural mechanisms of nociception. In: *Textbook of Pain*, 3rd edn (P. D. Wall and R. Melzack, eds), pp. 13–44. Churchill Livingstone.

32 Moriwaki, K. and Yuge, O. (1999). Topographical features of cutaneous hypoesthetic and hyperesthetic abnormalities in chronic pain. *Pain*, **81**, 1–6.

33 Dubner, R. (1988). Neuronal plasticity and pain following peripheral tissue inflammation or nerve injury. In: *VIth World Congress on Pain* (M. R. Bond, J. E. Charlton and C. J. Woolf, eds), pp. 263–276. Elsevier.

34 Cohen, M. L. (1995). The clinical challenge of secondary hyperalgesia. In: *Moving in on Pain* (M. O. Shacklock, ed), pp. 21–26. Butterworth-Heinemann.

35 Lewis, T. (1942). *Pain*. Macmillan.

36 Portenoy, R. K. (1996). Basic mechanisms. In: *Pain Management: Theory and Practice* (R. K. Portenoy and R. M. Kanner, eds), pp. 19–39. F. A. Davis.

37 Levine, J. and Taiwo, Y. (1994). Inflammatory pain In: *Textbook of Pain*, 3rd edn (P. D. Wall and R. Melzack, eds), pp. 45–56. Churchill Livingstone.

38 Wall, P. D. (1993). The mechanisms of fibromyalgia: a critical essay. In: *Progress in Fibromyalgia and Myofascial Pain* (H. M. Voeroy and H. Merskey, eds). Elsevier.

39 Woolf, H. G. (1963). *Headache and Other Head Pain.* Oxford University Press.

40 Treede, R. D., Meyer, R. A., Raja, S. N. *et al.* (1992). Peripheral and central mechanisms of cutaneous hyperalgesia. *Prog. Neurobiol.*, **38**, 397–421.

41 Dickenson, A. H. (1996). Pharmacology of pain transmission and control. In: *Pain – An Updated Review* (J. N. Campbell, ed.), pp. 113–122. IASP Press.

42 Oleson, J., Tfelt-Hansen, P. and Welch, K. M. A. (1993). *The Headaches.* Raven Press.

43 Levine, J. D., Coderre, T. J. and Basbaum, A. I. (1988). The peripheral nervous system and the inflammatory process. In: *Vth World Congress on Pain* (R. Dubner, G. F. Gebhart and M. R. Bond, eds), pp. 37–43. Elsevier Science.

44 Sluka, K. A. and Rees, H. (1997). The neuronal response to pain. *Phys. Theory Pract.*, **13**, 3–22.

45 Sluka, K. A., Willis, W. D. and Westlund, K. N. (1995). The role of dorsal root reflexes in neurogenic inflammation. *Pain Forum*, **4**, 141–149.

46 Wall, P. D. and Devor, M. (1983). Sensory afferent impulses originate from dorsal root ganglia and chronically injured axons: a physiological base for the radicular pain of nerve root compression. *Pain*, **17**, 321–339.

47 Chahl, L. and Ladd, R. (1976). Local oedema and general excitation of cutaneous sensory receptors produced by electrical stimulation of the saphenous nerve in the rat. *Pain*, **2**, 25–34.

48 Schmidt, R. F., Schaible, K. M., Heppelmann, B. *et al.* (1996). Silent and active nociceptors: structure, functions and clincial implications. In: *7th World Congress on Pain* (G. F. Gebhart, D. L. Hammond and T. S. Jensen, eds), pp. 213–250. IASP Press.

49 McMahon, S. B. and Koltzenburg, M. (1994). Silent afferents and visceral pain. In: *Progress in Pain Research and Management* (H. L. Fields and J. C. Liebeskind, eds), pp. 11–30. IASP Press.

50 Kieschke, J., Mense, S. and Prabhakar, N. R. (1988). Influence of adrenaline and hypoxia on rat muscle receptors in vitro. *Prog. Brain Res.*, **74**, 91–97.

51 Ray, B. S. and Woolf, H. G. (1940). Experimental studies on headache: pain sensitive structures of the head and their significance in headache. *Arch. Surg.*, **41**, 813–856.

52 Giammarco, R., Edmeads, J. and Dodick, D. (1998). *Critical Decisions in Headache Management.* Decker, B. C.

53 Sunderland, S. (1978). *Nerves and Nerve Injuries*, 3rd edn. Churchill Livingstone.

54 Devor, M. (1994). The pathophysiology of damaged peripheral nerves. In: *Textbook of Pain*, 3rd edn (P. D. Wall and R. Melzack, eds), pp. 79–100. Churchill Livingstone.

55 Loeser, J. D. (1985). Pain due to nerve injury. *Spine*, **10**, 232–235.

56 McLachlan, E. M., Janig, W., Devor, M. *et al.* (1993). Peripheral nerve injury triggers noadrenergic sprouting within dorsal root ganglia. *Nature*, **363**, 534–536.

57 Hasue, M. (1993). Pain and the nerve root. An interdisciplinary approach. *Spine*, **18**, 2053–2058.

58 Moskowitz, M. A. (1993). The trigeminovascular system. In: *The Headaches* (J. Olesen, P. Tfelt-Hansen and K. M. A. Welch, eds), pp. 57–68. Raven Press.

59 Moskowitz, M. A. (1984). The neurobiology of vascular head pain. *Ann. Neurol.*, **16**, 157–168.

60 Bill, A., Stjernschantz, J., Mandahl, A. *et al.* (1979). Substance P: release on trigeminal nerve stimulation, effects in the eye. *Acta Phys. Scand.*, **106**, 371–373.

61 Lundborg, G. (1988). *Nerve Injury and Repair.* Churchill Livingstone.

62 Lundborg, G. and Dahlin, L. B. (1996). Anatomy, function and pathophysiology of peripheral nerves and nerve compression. *Hand Clinics.*, **12**, 185–193.

63 Asbury, A. K. and Fields, H. L. (1984). Pain due to peripheral nerve damage: an hypothesis. *Neurol.*, **34**, 1587–1590.

64 Zochodne, D. W. (1992). Epineurial peptides: a role in neuropathic pain? *Can. J. Neurol. Sci.*, **20**, 69–72.

65 Hromada, J. (1963). On the nerve supply of the connective tissue of some peripheral nervous system components. *Acta Anat.*, **55**, 343–351.

66 Neary, D. and Ochoa, R. W. (1975). Sub-clinical entrapment neuropathy in man. *J. Neurol. Sci.*, **24**, 283–298.

67 Boden, S. D., Davis, D., Dina, T. S. *et al.* (1990). Abnormal magnetic-resonance scans of the lumbar spine in asymptomatic subjects: a prospective investigation. *J. Bone Joint Surg.*, **72A**, 403–408.

68 Devor, M. and Rappaport, Z. H. (1990). Pain and the physiology of damaged nerve. In: *Pain Syndromes in Neurology* (H. L. Fields, ed), pp. 47–84. Butterworth Heinemann.

69 Woolf, C. J. (1983). Evidence for a central component of post-injury pain hypersensitivity. *Nature*, **306**, 686–688.

70 Coderre, R. J., Katz, J., Vaccarino, A. L. and Melzack, R. (1993). Contribution of central neuroplasticity to pathological pain: review of clinical and experimental evidence. *Pain*, **52**, 259–285.

71 Shortland, P. and Woolf, C. J. (1993). Chronic peripheral nerve section results in a rearrangement of the central axonal arborizations of axotomized A beta primary afferent neurones in the rat spinal cord. *J. Comp. Neurol.*, **330**, 65–82.

72 Cook, A. J., Woolf, C. J., Wall, P. D. and McMahon,

S. B. (1987). Expansion of cutaneous receptive fields of dorsal horn neurones following C-primary afferent fibre inputs. *Nature*, **325**, 151–153.

73 Neumann, S., Doubell, T. P., Leslie, T. and Woolf, C. J. (1996). Inflammatory pain hypersensitivity mediated by phenotypic switch in myelinated primary sensory neurones. *Nature*, **384**, 360–364.

74 Noguchi, K., Kawai, Y., Fukuoka, T. *et al.* (1995). Substance P induced by peripheral nerve injury in primary afferent sensory neurons and its effect on dorsal column nucleus neurons. *J. Neurosci.*, **15**, 7633–7643.

75 Woolf, C. J. and Doubell, T. P. (1994). The pathophysiology of chronic pain - increasd sensitivity to low threshold A beta fibre inputs. *Curr. Opin. Neurobiol.*, **4**, 525–534.

76 Kandel, E. R., Schwartz, J. H. and Jessell, T. M. (1995). *Essentials of Neural Science and Behaviour.* Appleton & Lange.

77 McGaugh, J. L., Weinberger, N. M. and Lynch, G. (1995). *Brain and Memory: Modulation and Mediation of Neuroplasticity.* Oxford University Press.

78 Thomas, R. J. (1995). Excitatory amino acids in health and disease. *J. Am. Geriatric Soc.*, **43**, 1279–1289.

79 Basbaum, A. I. (1996). Memories of pain. *Sci. Med.*, **3**, 22–31.

80 Katz, J. and Melzack, R. (1990). Pain 'memories' in phantom limbs: review and clinical observations. *Pain*, **43**, 319–336.

81 Lenz, A. F., Tasker, R. R., Dostrovsky, J. O. *et al.* (1988). Abnormal single-unit activity and response to stimulation in the presumed ventrocaudal nucleus of patinets with central pain. In: *Pain Research and Clinical Management* (R. Dubner, G. F. Gebhart and M. R. Bond, eds), pp. 157–164. Elsevier.

82 Gifford, L. S. (1997). Pain. In: *Rehabilitation of Movement* (J. Pitt-Brooke, H. Reid, J. Lockwood and K. Kerr, eds), pp. 196–234. W.B. Saunders.

83 Schofferman, J., Anderson, D., Hines, R. *et al.* (1993). Childhood psychological trauma and chronic refractory low back pain. *Clin. J. Pain*, **9**, 260–265.

84 Linton, S. J., Larden, M. and Gillow, A. (1996). Sexual abuse and chronic musculoskeletal pain: prevalence and psychological factors. *Clin. J. Pain*, **12**, 215–221.

85 Bigos, S. J., Battie, M. C., Spengler, D. M. *et al.* (1992). A longitudinal, prospective study of industrial back injury reporting. *Clin. Orthop. Rel. Res.*, **279**, 21–34.

86 Indahl, A., Velund, L., Reikeraas, O. (1995). Good prognosis for low back pain when left untampered: a randomized clinical trial. *Spine*, **20**, 473–477.

87 Skevington, S. M. (1995). *Psychology of Pain.* John Wiley.

88 Bradley, L. A. (1996). Cognitive–behavioural therapy for chronic pain. In: *Psychological Approaches to Pain Management* (R. J. Gatchel and D. C. Turk, eds), pp. 131–147. The Guildford Press.

89 Turk, D. C., Meichenbaum, D. and Genet, M. (1983). *Pain and Behavioural Medicine. A Cognitive–Behavioural Perspective.* The Guildford Press.

90 Loeser, J. D. and Sullivan, M. (1995). Disability in the chronic low back pain patient may be iatrogenic. *Pain Forum*, **4**, 114–121.

91 Ader, R., Felton, O. L. and Cohen, W. (1991). *Psychoneuroimmunology*, 2nd edn. Academic Press.

92 Sapolsky, R. M. (1994). *Why Zebras Don't Get Ulcers.* Freeman.

93 Wallin, B. G., Torebjork, E. and Hallin, R. G. (1976). Preliminary observations on the pathophysiology of hyperalgesia in the causalgic pain pattern. In: *Sensory Functions of the Skin in Primates* (Y. Zotterman, ed), pp. Pergamon Press.

94 Bonica, J. J. (1990). Causalgia and other reflex sympathetic dystrophies. In: *The Management of Pain*, 2nd edn (J. J. Bonica, ed.). Lea & Feabiger.

95 Janig, W. (1996). The puzzle of 'reflex sympathetic dystrophy': Mechanisms, hypotheses, open questions. In: *Reflex Sympathetic Dystrophy: a Reappraisal* (W. Janig and M. Stantin-Hicks, eds). IASP Press.

96 Stanton-Hicks, M., Janig, W., Hassenbusch, S. *et al.* (1995). Reflex sympathetic dystrophy: changine concepts and taxonomy. *Pain*, **63**, 127–133.

97 Lovallo, W. R. (1997). *Stress and Health.* Sage publications.

98 Byl, N. N. and Melnick, M. (1997). The neural consequences of repetition: clincial implications of a learning hypothesis. *J. Hand Ther.*, **10**, 160–174.

99 Ohrbach, R. and McCall, W. D. (1996). The stress–hyperactivity pain theory of myogenic pain. Proposal for a revised theory. *Pain Forum*, **5**, 51–66.

100 Flor, H. and Turk, D. C. (1996). Integrating central and peripheral mechanisms in chronic muscular pain. An initial step on a long road. *Pain Forum*, **5**, 74–76.

9

The influence of posture and alteration of function upon the craniocervical and craniofacial regions

L. Bryden and D. Fitzgerald

Introduction

When examining patients presenting with signs and symptoms of craniocervical and craniomandibular dysfunction, the examination should involve assessment of posture and muscle function. The purpose of this chapter is to examine the relationship between alterations in posture and musculoskeletal function of the upper quadrant in relation to persistent neck, head and facial pain states. Much debate exists regarding the degree of variation in posture and muscle function which is of clinical significance. It is often unclear whether postural changes occur as a result of altered function or are implicated as a cause of altered function. Optimal posture is classically described by Kendall and Kendall,[1] although it is clear that few of us meet all the criteria described for optimal posture. While it must be acknowledged that the quantification of 'normal' musculoskeletal function still remains largely speculative at this stage, our focus will relate to management issues which confront the clinician on a daily basis. Despite the paucity of normative data relating to musculoskeletal function we can draw from many fields of basic science such as comparative anatomy, biomechanics, and physiology to establish a basis of optimal function. The issue then becomes one of quantifying the significance of suboptimal posture and function in relation to clinical presentations.

The application of these principles dictates that rehabilitation specialists utilize a clinical framework which tends to be more holistic in nature rather than purely focusing on a local source of a patient's pain.

Influences on muscle function

The evolutionary changes displayed in the musculoskeletal system reflect structural adaptations to functional requirements over a prolonged period. These changes give us some insight into potential mechanisms for musculoskeletal dysfunction which may occur during activities of daily living but over a considerably shorter time scale. The alterations which occurred in the change from quadruped to bipedalism are reflected in many aspects of upper quadrant anatomy. The relative mass of the head has reduced from 10% of body weight in primates to 5.4% of body weight in humans.[2] The redistribution of mass allows the centre of gravity of the head to be distributed more directly through the axial column, requiring less counterbalancing from the associated cervical musculature. This is reflected in a more symmetrical distribution of muscle mass throughout the neck in humans, in comparison to the predominantly posterior musculature in quadrupeds and primates.

The upper limb also shows significant alterations as a consequence of change in function from predominantly weight bearing to predominantly prehensile. These changes not only relate to changes in bone mass and range of movement but also to a reduction in muscle mass of scapular stabilizers (trapezius, levator scapulae and rhomboids) and propulsive upper limb muscles such as pectoralis major and latissimus dorsi. Given that the upper limb is largely suspended from the axial skeleton and head by suspensory muscles as well as the articulation with the clavicle, the functional interdependence of the cervical spine and upper limb can readily be appreciated.

The following discussion will focus on the anatomical basis for cervicogenic head and neck pain; identifying the possible clinical consequences of postural variations in the upper quadrant in relation to the presentation of symptoms in the head and neck; the principles underlying the functional examination of the musculoskeletal system; the functional anatomy of the upper quadrant; and the principles involved in addressing faulty posture and altered muscle function.

The anatomical basis for cervicogenic head and neck pain

Upper cervical joint dysfunction (occiput to C3) has long been recognized as a potential source of head and neck pain.[3–6]

Clinically interrelated segmental dysfunction in lower cervical and upper thoracic segments is also often noted and can change head and facial symptoms when treated manually or following surgical intervention. Muscle spasm in the upper cervical segments has been shown to contribute directly to pain referral patterns in the head and face[7,8] and, in practical terms, usually coexists with myofascial and articular dysfunction. Dural sensitivity is also a significant contributor to head and neck pain.[9] A neuroanatomical link between the cervical spine and cranium is formed by the trigeminal nucleus (often referred to as the trigeminocervical nucleus[4]), and is of particular significance when considering possible mechanisms of pain in the region of the head and neck. It reaches from the pons in the brainstem to the level of the third or fourth cervical spinal segment. Because of this position it receives afferent inputs not only from the trigeminal nerve, but also from the dorsal nerve roots of C1 to C3, the facial nerve, the glossopharyngeal nerve, and the vagus nerve. It is therefore possible that an increase in afferent impulses originating from pain receptors in the upper cervical joints may produce symptoms in areas which are not giving rise to these impulses, providing a mechanism where changes in the cervical spine joints may precipitate symptoms in the face, which in turn may lead to postural adaption of an antalgic nature and contribute to secondary dysfunction.

The interaction of peripheral and central mechanisms in chronic pain states is a source of much debate within contemporary literature.[10] Undoubtedly peripheral tissue irritation can cause central hypersensitivity which perpetuates long beyond normal tissue healing time.

(For further information please refer to Chapter 8.)

Posture

There are many theories as to why an individual may develop poor postural alignment. Habitual sustained postures related to occupation and lifestyle may contribute to long-term postural changes, and it seems reasonable that the degree of physical activity taken by an individual might also be influential in determining postural alignment. There is also the possibility of genetic influences. Disregarding the mechanism by which poor postural alignment occurs, the important clinical issue is the functional consequence of these changes. Data is available which implicates a forward head posture in association with cervical dysfunction.[11–13] Weakness of deep cervical flexor muscles (longus colli) in patients with cervical pain has also been described.[14,15] Importantly, the severity of weakness and diminished endurance appear to be related to the degree of forward head posture.[13] Changes in thoracic curvature with age have been well documented[16–18] and shown to influence the range of cervical motion. Additionally, previous studies have suggested that head posture is an aetiological factor in the development of temporomandibular dysfunction,[12,13,19–23] though a causal relationship between posture and temporomandibular dysfunction has not been established.[19,24]

Given these findings it would appear rational to improve postural alignment in situations where the malalignment can be shown (through systematic examination) to affect the symptomatic region.

Measurement of posture

There is surprisingly little in the literature on both normal values for and external measurement of head posture. Several methods of measuring head and neck posture are described in the literature, though many of these are of little practical value in the clinical situation. Some examples follow.

Braun and Amundsen[25] describe a computer-assisted slide digitizing system called postural analysis digitizing system (PADS), which allows determination of angular relationships in the head, neck, and shoulders.

Profile photographs have also been employed to measure posture, using a set lens-to-subject distance, and markers on the subject to allow positions to be measured.[26] Zonnenberg et al.[27] used photographs taken from frontal, dorsal and lateral positions with surface markers on anatomical landmarks, and with a screen of 10-cm squares positioned behind the patient. This enabled them to plot coordinates from the anatomical landmarks to evaluate postural changes. A further value of photographs is that patients are also able to visualize their faulty posture, which may give better incentive for improvement.

Hanten et al.[28] measured forward head posture by marking the skin over the zygomatic arch, 3 cm below the corner of the eye, and then measuring the perpendicular distance of this mark from a wall.

In a previous study by Bryden and Power,[29] a spondylometer was used to measure cervical posture. The mobile arm of the spondylometer has an attachment for a measuring bar that holds a series of probes which slide back and forward in the bar to allow alignment against the contour of the head, neck, and upper thoracic spine. The measuring bar is removable and allows a tracing to be taken onto graph paper from the tips of the needles. This method of measuring posture has the advantage of being reasonably quick and easy to use in the clinical situation.

Braune and Fischer[30] used plumb lines in standing, while Kendall and Kendall[1] developed a method of measuring posture which reached a compromise between the line of gravity and the exact centres of the joints. The points of reference given for the ideal posture are in a line falling slightly in front of the ankle joint; slightly anterior to the midline through the knee; through the greater trochanter of the femur; approximately midway through the trunk; through the shoulder joint; and through the lobe of the ear.

Rocabado[31] described the ideal posture of the head as placing the centre of gravity 'of the head' slightly anterior to the cervical spine, and terms this the 'orthostatic position of the head and neck'. Here a tangent line is drawn from the back of the head passing through the apex of the thoracic curve, the average distance from this line to the mid-cervical spine is 6 cm, with higher measurements indicating a greater degree of forward head posture.

In practice most clinicians will visually evaluate posture with reference to anatomical landmarks (as described by Kendall and Kendall[1]), as more precise measurement is only usually required as part of research data. As mentioned earlier, photographic records provide good visual evidence of postural changes and can be combined with a variety of measurement techniques.

It is clear that posture is no simple thing to measure, that there is a wide variation of postural types, and that it is difficult to give normal values for posture. A further consideration is that all the types of postural measurement descibed here relate to the measurement of posture in the static situation, and the measurement of 'dynamic posture' is an area that will require more sophisticated analysis.

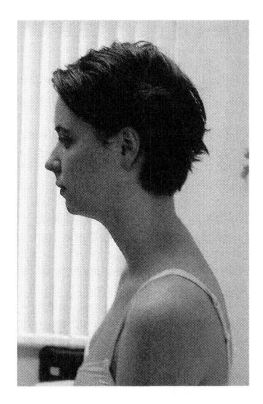

Figure 9.1 A female subject with forward head posture

Head Posture

Kapandji[32] describes the balance of the head on the neck as follows:

The centre of gravity of the head lies just anterior to the occipital condyles, and as a mechanical arrangement the head would tend to tip forward if there were not some force to hold it erect. This force is provided by the posterior cervical muscles. These muscles need to not only oppose the force of gravity which tends to pull the head forward but also to resist the tension in the muscles of mastication and the supra and infra hyoid muscles during functional movements of the head and neck such as eating, swallowing and speaking.

Of interest is a study by Vig *et al.*[33] who found when they artificially changed the centre of mass of the skull, that there was a wide variation in the postural adaptations made by the subjects.

The most commonly observed faulty posture in the clinical situation is that of forward head posture. It is seen in patients with all types of clinical presentations and may be implicated as a source or result of the presenting signs and symptoms. Forward head posture is said to exist when the head rests anterior to the anatomical points of reference as described by Kendall and Kendall (Figure 9.1).

The changes in forward head posture involve extension at CO–1 and C1–2 levels, a decrease in the mid-cervical lordosis and an increase in the upper thoracic kyphosis. Protraction and elevation of the scapula accompanied by apparent internal rotation of the humerus follow.[34]

There may also be alteration in the rest position of the mandible, upper thoracic respiration with subsequent hyperactivity of the accessory muscles of respiration, mouth breathing, and a loss of rest position of the tongue. The changed mechanics of this posture may lead to excessive compressive forces on the cervical apophyseal joints and posterior part of the vertebral bodies, while anterior structures such as the muscles of neck flexion and the infrahyoid muscles may undergo stretching and subsequent lengthening and weakness, with elevation of the hyoid bone. The suprahyoid muscles are thought to become shortened, as are the suboccipital muscles due to this alteration in head posture[31] (Figure 9.2).

The effects of head posture on craniomandibular function

Mandibular position

Many studies link changes in cervical posture to changes in mandibular position.[31,35–38] Forward movement of the head (forward head posture) in relation to the

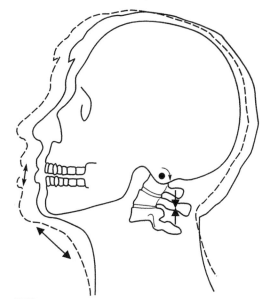

KEY

––– Outline soft tissue head in forward head posture

● Fulcrum of movement

↕ Angle in upper cervical spine decreases posteriorly in forward head posture

↘ Increase in tension in anterior soft tissue structures in forward head posture

↕ Increase in vertical dimension of occlusion in forward head posture

Figure 9.2 The effects of forward head posture on craniomandibular relationships

thorax increases the elastic tension that the supra- and infrahyoid muscles place upon their thoracic attachments. This in turn places a pull in a downward and backward direction on the mandible.[31]

The effect of this is a change in the relationship of the mandibular condyle to the temporal fossa, which is then likely to produce a change in temporomandibular joint mechanics. This in turn may have an effect on masticatory muscle function, cervical muscle function and tongue position.

Mandibular position is influenced by movement at the craniovertebral level with or without involvement of the middle and lower cervical spine. If the head is flexed at the CO–1 and C1–2 levels, the mandible will move in an upward and forward direction with a consequent decrease in the interocclusal distance (the distance between the lower border of the upper incisors and the upper border of the lower incisors). Conversely, craniovertebral extension will result in an increase in the interocclusal distance.[39,40]

Changing mandibular position alone by use of a mouth-opening device[38] has also been seen to result in craniovertebral extension. Two theories as to why this may occur are proposed. When the mandible is lowered passively the hyoid muscles relax, allowing the hyoid bone to drop back and thereby reducing the pharyngeal airway. In order to open the airway the head is extended, thereby tightening the hyoid muscles and pulling the hyoid bone forwards again. This of course occurs at a subconscious level of activation.[38] A further suggestion[41] is that the mouth-opening device provokes a proprioceptive response in the periodontal ligaments and that this is projected to the spinal nucleus of the trigeminal nerve, causing contraction of the posterior cervical muscles in an attempt to reduce occlusal forces.

Forward head posture has been shown to correlate directly with an increase in the vertical dimension of occlusion of the mouth (VDO). This is thought to be as a result of increased tension in the soft tissues which attach to the mandible, thereby pulling the mandible downwards and backward.[22,34]

The rest position of the mandible

The rest position of the mandible in the upright posture is defined as that in which all stomatognathic structures are in a balanced but not necessarily non-pathological condition.[34] This position is also referred to as the UPPM – the upright postural position of the mandible.[42] In this position there is some activity in the masticatory muscles.[43] The normal value for the space between the lower border of the upper incisors and the upper border of the lower incisors in the mandibular rest position is between 2 and 5 mm. This is known as the freeway space.

It is clear that mandibular rest position will vary in an individual and certainly between individuals, but it is considered important that a resting position can be achieved which reduces muscle activity to a minimum, allowing rest and repair in the associated structures. Failure to achieve a rest position is thought to be a significant contributory factor in craniomandibular pain/dysfunction syndrome. Many studies have examined the effects of changing head posture on hyoid bone position. As the hyoid bone provides attachment for muscles, fascia and ligaments of the cervical spine, cranium, mandible and scapula, its position is of interest as an indicator of changing craniomandibular relationships. Several studies support the view that the hyoid bone is a good indicator of mandibular position, finding that the hyoid bone moves in a consistent manner in response to anteroposterior movement of the mandible.[44–46] Others have suggested that the hyoid bone has a more constant relationship to the cervical spine than to the mandible.[47–50] The general consensus is that changes in hyoid bone position are coordinated with changes in both mandibular position and craniocervical posture.

Muscle activity

Some studies have employed electromyography to measure activity in muscles during altered mandibular or head posture.[34,51,52] A study using rats as subjects has shown that the tonic neck reflex influences the tone of the jaw muscles.[53] A later study by the same authors[54] examined the effect of voluntary alteration of head posture on the jaw musculature and its relationship to occlusal interference in man. It was found that certain head movements influenced electromyographic (EMG) activity: for example, head flexion was found to increase tone in the digastric muscle, while extension of the head increased the tone in temporalis bilaterally.

Winnberg *et al.*[36] employed electromyography and videofluorographic techniques to quantify the effects of altered head posture on the interplay of masseter and suprahyoid muscle activity, lip–mandibular movements, and the working angle of the suprahyoid muscles, the results confirming that a change in head posture has influences on masseter and suprahyoid activity and upon excursion distance of the hyoid bone during the open–close–clench cycle. The duration of increased activity in the masseter and suprahyoid muscles and distance of excursion of the hyoid bone was seen to vary when head posture was altered from flexion to neutral to extension.

Forsberg,[55] in a study of 30 normal adults, used EMG to determine postural activity in the neck and masticatory muscles in positions of head flexion and extension. Activity in the posterior cervical muscles decreased when the head was extended and increased during flexion. Activity in sternocleidomastoid muscle increased at 20° of extension and was unchanged during flexion. Masseter activity increased between 10–20° of extension of the head and again showed no change during flexion. He also proposed that compensatory muscle function caused by altered head posture may be one of the determinants of craniofacial morphology.

Hellsing and Hagberg[52] found that maximum bite force was higher in an extended head posture compared to natural head posture in association with a change in position of the hyoid bone, which increased its distance from the mandible and moved closer to the anterior pharyngeal wall, possibly reflecting a change in muscle balance between the elevators and depressors of the mandible.

There is general agreement among authors that flexion of the head on the cervical spine generally decreases masticatory muscle activity and that extension of the head increases masticatory muscle activity.[54,55] The logical extension of this finding is that if the rest position of the mandible is altered by changes in head posture, then the path of closure of the mandible will also be altered.[35]

Perry[56] states that prolonged retraction of the mandible due to spasm in temporalis causes a reflex contraction of the posterior cervical muscles due to offsetting the balance between the masseter and temporalis and the suprahyoid muscles.

Frumker and Kyle[57] found that positive feedback exists between the cervical spine posture and the state of excitation of the mandibular musculature. They suggest that a forward head posture and cervical dysfunction elicit afferent discharges from the mechanoreceptors in the cervical spine which ascend to the fusimotor neurons in the motor pools of mandibular muscles.

Clarke and Wyke[58] studied the contributions of temporomandibular articular mechanoreceptors to the control of mandibular position. They found that afferent discharges from these receptors make a continuous contribution to the reflex control of the masticatory muscles both at rest and during movement. Furthermore, if these discharges were changed by dysfunction in any group of receptors the reflex activity of the mandibular muscles was altered in response. Klineberg *et al.*[59] studied the morphology of these receptors and made the point that clinical electromyographic analysis of masticatory muscle changes is often difficult to interpret because of the variety of reflex influences which combine to control motor unit activity. Mechanoreceptors located in masticatory muscles and their tendons, TMJ capsules, mandibular and maxillary periosteum and periodontal membranes all provide afferent discharges to motor neuron pools in the central nervous system and in practice it may be difficult to determine from which precise source abnormal muscle activity is derived.[59]

The literature recognizes the existence of a relationship between the cervical spine and head posture, and the position of the mandible, although opinions differ as to whether this relationship is based upon mechanical factors, muscle activity, neural links, or a combination of these factors.

Further consquences of altered head posture

The relevance of occlusion

Occlusion is often cited as a significant contributor to temporomandibular dysfunction. Levy[60] expressed the view that most temporomandibular or associated myofascial dysfunctions stem from dental malocclusion and that management should be by modifying the occlusal position.

The occlusal position describes the relationship of the upper and lower teeth when all the teeth are fully interdigitated. The position will depend upon the presence/absence/shape and position of the teeth. It is a transitional position at the end of empty mouth closure. The occlusal position will have an effect upon the rest position of the mandible via afferent input to the central nervous system from the periodontal ligaments, which provide information regarding the position and quality of the load. This enables the masticatory musculature to adjust its activity to avoid overloading of the teeth and temporomandibular joints. The periodontal ligaments are affected by occlusal contact and so if, for example, there is premature tooth contact in one area, there is activation of a feedback loop from receptors in the periodontal ligaments to the masticatory musculature to avoid the premature contact in order to minimize loading of the teeth and/or the temporomandibular joints.[61]

This positioning away from premature contact is associated with an increase in the level of masticatory muscle activity.[55] Additionally, the vertical dimension of occlusion (VDO) will affect cervical spine and head posture. The VDO is measured from the base of the nose to the base of the chin when the teeth are fully interdigitated. By maintaining an increase in VDO[38] by means of a mouth-opening device, head extension was seen to occur; this is supported by Vig *et al.*[62]

Extending the head at the craniovertebral junction will lead to altered initial occlusal contact from that experienced in the neutral head position. Similarly, flexing the head will change initial contacts again. There is however no change in the position of maximum intercuspation.[63]

Opinions vary considerably as to the relevance of occlusion in temporomandibular dysfunction. A summary of epidemiological and patient study data by Gray *et al.*[64] reported that occlussion was variable across all subgroups.

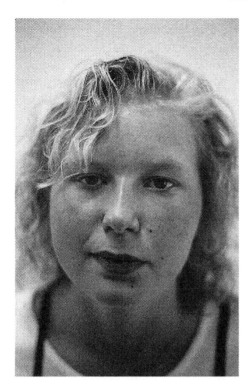

Figure 9.3 An example of altered craniofacial morphology in a female subject, showing asymmetry in the lower two-thirds of the face

Nasal airflow

Obstruction of the nasal airway causes decreased air flow through the nasal cavity. As a result, tongue position will change to allow more room for air to flow between it and the palate. The tongue moves forward and the mandible is depressed (mouth breathing). In addition, upper cervical extension occurs to facilitate the increased air flow.[62]

Craniofacial morphology

Head posture has been shown to have a relationship with craniofacial morphology.[65–67] An example of altered craniofacial morphology is shown in Figure 9.3. Extension of the head in relation to the cervical spine has been correlated with large anterior and small posterior facial heights, small anteroposterior craniofacial dimensions, large inclination of the mandible to the anterior cranial base and to the nasal plate, facial retrognathism, a large cranial base angle and a small nasopharyngeal space. Subjects with an increase in adenoid development in the nasopharynx exhibited a forward and downward tongue position and an extended head posture, apparently in an attempt to increase the airway.[66,68] For further clinical implications see Chapters 2 and 7.

In summary there exists a large body of work supporting a relationship between cervical spine and head posture, and craniomandibular function. It is important for the clinician to be aware of this relationship when planning treatment programmes for patients with signs and symptoms of dysfunction in the head and neck.

The following section discusses the factors which contribute to the control of posture and muscle function, and how this control may become disrupted.

Biomechanical aspects of functional movement

A theoretical framework to explain the mechanisms of spinal segmental stability has been proposed[69] and has attracted considerable interest in the field of rehabilitation. It provides a theoretical framework for evaluating the stability of the cervical spine and challenges some of the conventional wisdom regarding spinal instability.

The concept integrates multiple factors which may contribute to spinal segmental control, and thus provides a basis for specific application of therapies to the dysfunctional component. The theoretical framework integrates the osseoligamentous, muscular and neural regulation mechanisms of segmental control. This framework is outlined in Figure 9.4.

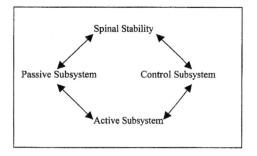

Figure 9.4 Theoretical framework for evaluating the stability of the cervical spine (Adapted from Panjabi 1992[69])

The passive subsystem refers to the osseoligamentous structures, which have been discussed in detail. The active subsystem refers to muscle biomechanics in the control of spinal segments and is discussed below. The control subsystem refers to the proprioception, coordination and neural regulation of muscle function. Impaired muscle contribution to segmental control may be due to impairment in force-generating capacity of the relevant muscles (muscle fibre incompetence) or inappropriate neural regulation of muscle function.

In attempting to understand the relative functions of specific muscles, subdivision into global and local muscle systems has been proposed.[70] The relevant characteristics of global and local muscles are outlined below.

Characteristics of local (stability) muscles

- Deep, relatively small, integral with passive structure, i.e. capsule
- Positioned close to joint axis

- Monoarticular
- Dominant compressive (stabilizing) force component
- Multipennate/oblique fibre orientation
- Tonic activation (continuous) in weight bearing and joint motion
- Slow fibre dominant or ratio favouring endurance function (type I)
- Most vulnerable to disuse atrophy
- Tendency to lengthen
- Tendency to inhibition and stretch weakness (preferential disuse)
- Fatigue resistant.

Characteristics of global (mobility) muscles

- Relatively superficial
- More distant from joint axis
- Dominant movement force component (long leverage)
- Biarticular
- Fast fibre dominant (type IIa,b)
- Fatiguable
- Least vulnerable to disuse atrophy
- Tendency to shorten
- Tendency to hyperactivity (preferential recruitment/dominance).

In the lumbar spine, dysfunction of global muscles is associated with increased rigidity[71–73] and increased segmental compression.[74,75] These concepts remain speculative in relation to the cervical spine, but are attracting increasing attention in the field of rehabilitation.

Mechanisms of functional disturbance

With the exclusion of systemic disease processes, functional disturbance of the cervical spine and upper limb can be broadly grouped into either primary traumatic mechanisms or secondary acquired mechanisms. The most common mechanism of traumatic onset is motor vehicle accidents involving a flexion/extension mechanism of injury. The mechanics of forces involved will determine the tissues traumatized and the extent of damage, which will in turn dictate the degree of reversibility. There is mounting evidence that current radiological investigations do not detect significant irreversible damage which may perpetuate chronic pain in this region.[5,6]

In conjunction with the local inflammatory response, an alteration in motor output occurs in order to minimize irritation of sensitized tissues. In effect this may produce hyperactivity in some muscles regions and inhibition in others, with a net result of relative immobilization of the sensitized structures. Studies in the field of pain science have shown that inflammatory reactions enhance the flexion withdrawal reflex, lower the threshold at which this reflex is initiated and prolong the duration of the reflex,[76,77] and that these alterations in synergies may be perpetuated long after the pain has resolved.[78] This would appear to correlate with the clinical observations of painful hyperactivity in muscles of the head/neck region.

Alternatively, acquired changes in upper quadrant function may result as a consequence of maladaptation to previous trauma, postural loading as a result of occupation or habitual usage, or alterations in muscle recruitment due to physical training. A high incidence of muscle hypertonicity has been noted with postural abnormalities,[7] and a high incidence of postural abnormalities in association with pain.[79] These alterations in function may cause primary myofascial pain, secondary painful articular dysfunction or neural irritation. For example, many weight-training regimens perpetuate muscle hyperactivity by creating hypertrophy of pectoralis major, upper trapezius and deltoid, causing postural malalignment of the upper quadrant. Conversely, postural malalignment may also be a consequence of decreased use, with postural muscles showing a higher propensity for disuse atrophy. Of course the role of emotion and higher centres cannot be neglected, as the so-called 'flight or fight' response induces both postural and muscle adaptations that may become habitual in the long term. It is important to recognize this symptom pattern and instigate multidisciplinary management with this patient population. Clinical presentations typically display an increase in symptoms in relation to stress, inconsistent response to manual techniques, and the perpetuation of sensations of stiffness when potential structural causes have been eliminated.

Functional anatomy of the upper quadrant

The cervical articulations

The cervical spine is divided into two functional units; the upper complex (occiput, C1, C2), which contributes about one-third of the flexion extension and half the axial rotation of the cervical spine, and the remaining six vertebrae from C3 to T1. The large range of motion available in the cervical spine is achieved at the expense of stability – a feature common to the upper quadrant in general. There are a number of features which contribute to both the structural and functional stability of the cervical spine. The osseoligamentous stability is achieved through the specific morphology of the region, which differs from other parts of the spine. The vertebral body, intervertebral disc, uncovertebral joints and the zygapophyseal (facet) joints are equally weight bearing. The facet joint orientation of 30°–60° to the coronal plane offers low torsional protection to the intervertebral disc but achieves a relatively large range of motion. In flexion there is progressively diminishing facet contact (5 mm^2 common surface area), creating a stepped appearance and dictating an important contribution from the posterior musculature and ligaments.

The ligamentous structures (zygapophyseal joint capsules, supraspinous and interspinous ligaments, ligamentum flavum and ligamentum nuchae) contribute to limiting the extremes of motion but are unlikely to provide major tension through range, given the relatively large excursions required. This brief description of functional biomechanics alludes to an important potential role of muscle activation to control motion and stabilize the region. Some data are emerging in support of this hypothesis and will be considered in the following sections.

Cervical muscle anatomy

The muscular anatomy of the cervical spine should be viewed in relation to the region of primary mechanical effect. The multilayered configuration dictates that the most superficial muscles act upon all regions crossed, and the effects of these stresses depend on the synergic function of deeper muscles. Thus we can consider short intersegmental muscles, polysegmental muscles with cervical attachment, polysegmental muscles with cranial attachment and polysegmental muscles with scapular attachment.

Anterior cervical muscles from superficial to deep

- Sternocleidomastoid

- Scalenus anterior
- Scalenus medius
- Scalenus posterior
- Longus colli
- Longus capitis
- Sternohyoid, omohyoid and digastric.

Posterior cervical muscles from superficial to deep

- Trapezius
- Levator scapulae (layer one)
- Splenius capitus
- Splenius cervicis (layer two)
- Semispinalis capitus
- Semispinalis cervicis
- Longissimus thoracis (layer three)
- Iliocostalis
- Multifidus
- Rectus capitis posterior major
- Rectus capitis posterior minor (suboccipital muscles layer four)
- Obliquis capitis superior
- Obliquis capitis inferior.

The muscles of mastication

The muscles of mastication can be divided into two main groups – the mandibular elevators and the mandibular depressors (Figure 9.5). The following description of the various muscle actions is brief, and the reader is referred to detailed anatomy texts for further information.

Temporalis – the primary function of this muscle is mandibular elevation. The posterior fibres are important for retrusion and lateral deviation of the mandible to the ipsilateral side.

Masseter – its primary action is elevation of the mandible and clenching of the jaws. It also acts to retrude the mandible from full protrusion.

Medial pterygoid – acts with masseter as

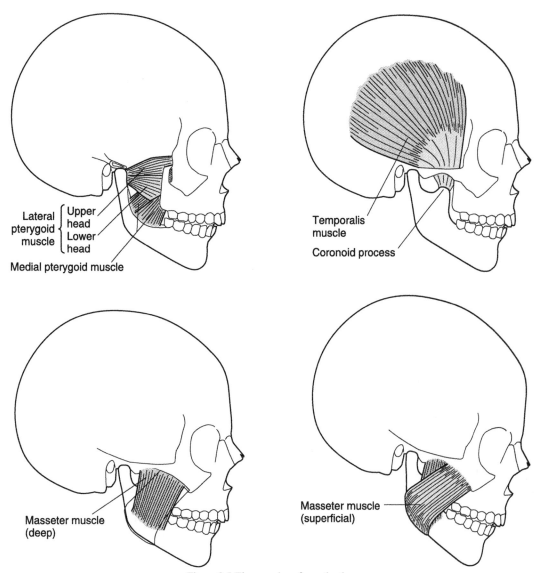

Figure 9.5 The muscles of mastication

a sling to suspend the angle of the mandible. When acting bilaterally the muscles help to elevate the mandible with masseter and temporalis. Unilaterally the medial pterygoid deviates the mandible toward the opposite side.

Lateral pterygoid – the two divisions of the lateral pterygoid are functionally and anatomically two separate and reciprocating muscles. The inferior head exerts a forward and downward pull on the mandible, i.e. opening the mouth. It protrudes the mandible and, when acting unilaterally, it deviates the mandible to the opposite side. Arguments exist as to whether the superior lateral pterygoid is inactive during the opening phase of the mandible and acts to rotate the disc anteriorly on the condyle during closing,[80] or whether it pulls the disc anteriorly during opening of the mouth.[81]

The suprahyoid muscles

The muscles attached from the mandible to the hyoid bone are referred to as suprahyoid muscles.

The muscles included in this group are the geniohyoids, the digastrics, the mylohyoids and the stylohyoids. Both the geniohyoids and the digastrics act to depress the mandible, while the hyoid bone is stabilized by the infrahyoid muscles. Acting together the digastrics assist in mandibular retrusion and, when the mandible is fixed, elevate the hyoid bone. Mylohyoid acts to stabilize the tongue or to elevate it during swallowing, and stylohyoid draws the tongue upwards and backwards during swallowing.

The infrahyoid muscles

The sternohyoid, omohyoid, sternothyroid and thyrohyoid muscles cover the front and much of the sides of the larynx, trachea, and thyroid gland. They represent a continuation in the cervical spine of the straplike rectus abdominus muscle. The continuation of fibre orientation and deep fascia provides an intermuscular continuum from the mandible to the symphysis pubis.

As a group, the infrahyoid muscles depress the larynx and hyoid bone. Together with the suprahyoid muscles they fix the hyoid bone, providing a firm base on which the tongue and mandible can be moved. These muscles are innervated by fibres from upper cervical nerves.

Recognizing this configuration allows us to consider in more detail specific muscle function in relation to its mechanics as well as its synergic functions. Given that it is not possible completely to isolate individual muscle contraction, we can devise tests which give useful information regarding postural function, particularly in relation to poor head–neck alignment. In general terms these causes may be quantified as either mechanical restrictive disorders or muscular control disorders. Gross mechanical disorders may present as obvious restrictions in range of motion but if confined to single motion segments will require specific manual examination.[82] This degree of examination specificity is not the rule in general medical practice, and dictates a more holistic overview of functional assessment[83] in conjunction with clinical expertise.

Testing muscle strength

Assessing muscle strength relevant to postural control requires modification of standard resistance tests. Several clinical approaches have been advocated for assessing muscle control in the cervical spine,[84–87] which attempt to quantify synergic muscle function and segmental control and are described below. It should be remembered that the upper limb is virtually suspended from the cervicothoracic region and dysfunction of the upper limb may have direct consequences upon the head/neck complex. The concepts of dysfunction are based upon the following tenets.

Joint stability is enhanced by co-contraction of agonist and antagonist muscles in close proximity to the joint.[88] Afferent feedback modifies gamma motorneuron discharge.[89] Gamma input modifies alpha motorneuron control of tonic, slow twitch muscle fibres.[89] Some muscles have a tendency to become overactive (upper trapezius, levator scapulae, sternocleidomastoid, scalenes, and pectorals,[84] the suboccipital extensors,[31] masseter and the suprahyoids[36]), while others have a tendency to become inhibited (deep cervical flexors, mid- and lower trapezius,[82] infrahyoid muscles[31]).

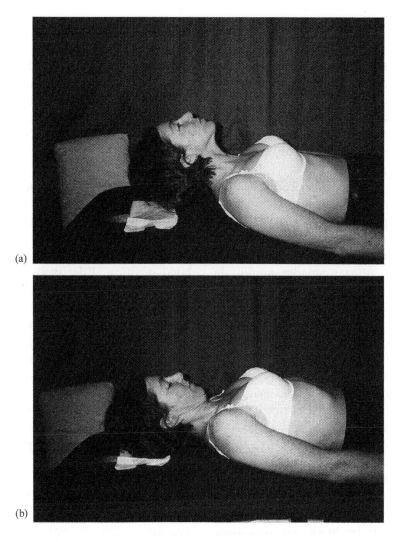

(a)

(b)

Figure 9.6 (a) Assessment of deep neck flexor function. Note the protrusion of the chin indicative of some overactivity. **(b)** Activation of deep neck flexors producing corrected cervical flexion

Dysfunction of these stabilizing systems may predispose to overload of spinal structures.

Rehabilitation of the spinal complex should address automatic coordination of muscle activity to control posture as well as addressing torque-producing capability.[82]

It can be seen from the above accounts that standard muscle resistance tests will not yield the relevant information regarding function. Assessment of postural stabi-

lity is dependent upon targeting the relevant muscles, loading at the appropriate intensity and observing for muscle substitution.

Testing deep neck flexor function

This test is performed in supine. The subject is asked to raise the head from the supporting surface and progressively move through flexion towards the sternum.[15,83,88–91] Observation of the mandible determines whether the movement is carried out predominantly by spinal segmental flexion (producing a smooth arch of movement) or whether the chin pokes forwards at initiation of lifting. Relative poking of the chin indicates weakness of the deep neck flexors, allowing upper cervical extension by gravity. It can also be associated with overactivity of sternocleidomastoid, which in this position is an upper cervical extensor by virtue of its alignment relative to the axis of motion. Modification of this test protocol[82] utilizes smaller amplitude movements without full lifting of the head to accommodate subjects initially unable to support the weight of the head. Specific biofeedback devices have been designed for this purpose.[82] Observation should also be made for a tendency to shoulder protraction and flexion of the trunk, which is associated with mass flexor muscle recruitment as opposed to isolated cervical muscle activation. It is not uncommon in clinical practice for patients to present with secondary cervical strain following abdominal strengthening exercises as a result of this mass muscle recruitment pattern. Observation should also be made for rotational deviations, which indicate an asymmetry in anterior muscle control unless articular restrictions are dictating an altered movement pattern (Figure 9.6).

Testing deep neck extensors[92]

The purpose of this test is to ascertain the synergic interaction of the cervical extensor muscles. Trapezius and levator scapulae (the most superficial and powerful of the cervical extensors) can contribute to excessive upper cervical extension associated with a head-forward position. The mid- and lower cervical lordosis is often compromised or lost and is associated with relative flexion and anterior translation of the cervical segments. The rationale of testing and exercise prescription is therefore to correct this postural compromise. The test is carried out with the subject in a prone position resting on the elbows (sometimes called sphinx position). The head is allowed to drop forwards, hanging under gravity, and the subject is asked to draw in the chin, thereby producing upper cervical flexion. While maintaining upper cervical flexion, the mid- and lower cervical spine is brought into an extended/posteriorly translated position. Effectively this manoeuvre reduces the potential of the multisegmental superficial cervical extensors to be overdominant in the movement synergy. The clinical assumption therefore is that muscles such as splenius cervicis, semispinalis cervicis, iliocostalis and multifidus are the predominant muscles recruited in this motion pattern. Observation should be made for potential substitutions, indicated by elevation of shoulder girdles, increased activity in the interscapular muscles, a loss of upper cervical flexion throughout the manoeuvre or deviations from the sagittal plane (Figure 9.7). Of course these testing protocols can be turned directly into treatment techniques.

The information gained from these two tests yields information regarding the ability to maintain head–neck and neck–thorax alignment. As previously discussed, the typical head-forward posture is associated with relative stretching of the deep neck flexors and mid-cervical extensors. By virtue of the length–tension relationship, these muscle may display inner range weakness when aligned in neutral anatomical postures. For this reason the attainment of anatomical alignment often requires a structured, progressive postural exercise regimen, with optimal alignment being the

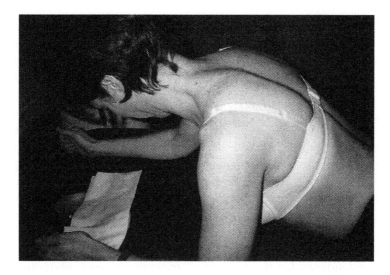

Figure 9.7 Combined activation of scapula stabilizers and neck extensors

end-stage goal. Instructions to stand up straight or throw the shoulders back are idealistic instructions rather than practical rehabilitation interventions.

Testing upper quadrant function[86,93,94]

Test 1. Cervical stability with arm elevation

The objective of this test is to evaluate the effect of upper limb motion on the cervical spine. In general, the head and neck should remain relatively stable while the arm is being elevated through flexion. Deviation of the head with this movement pattern implies that the effort of lifting the upper limb is producing potentially harmful stresses in the cervical spine. This could occur for a number of reasons, such as primary weakness of the cervical stabilizing muscles, overactivity of the scapular muscles (particularly upper trapezius and levator scapulae), or mechanical compromise of upper limb motion inducing compensatory cervical movement. The test is best per-

formed in sitting and the subject is asked slowly to lift the arm forwards through flexion into full elevation. The examiner stands in front and observes the head position throughout this movement pattern. The test is repeated on the opposite side. In a typical faulty pattern the cervical spine side flexes to the arm under test, coupled with either ipsilateral or contralateral rotation depending on the dominant muscle activity. Alternatively, the head and upper cervical spine may be observed to poke forwards at the cervicothoracic junction, particularly when a large, fixed cervicothoracic kyphosis is evident on examination. When dysfunction is less marked or not visible, it is worthwhile palpating the spinous processes of the cervical spine during this test. Sometimes a vertebral segment can be felt to move relative to its associated segments, implying a local segmental muscle incompetence. If cervical muscle testing reveals incompetence, then the rational of exercise prescription is to target this area primarily. If examination of the upper quadrant reveals either a loss of flexibility in the shoulder complex or impaired scapular muscle control, then this should be addressed as a primary cause.

Test 2. Testing scapular control

Assessing the pattern of scapular motion during arm elevation can yield useful information regarding the synergic function of scapular muscles.[83,92,94] With the subject in a seated position the observer stands behind. The subject is asked to elevate each arm alternately while the observer monitors the contour of the upper trapezius and any tendency for the scapula to migrate superiorly. Biomechanically the function of the scapula is to rotate the glenoid upwards during arm elevation, and this is accomplished primarily by scapular protraction and upward rotation producing movement of the inferior angle around the chest wall. This is achieved by a force couple generated by upper and lower fibres of trapezius and serratus anterior, while the middle trapezius and rhomboids act to stabilize the scapulae on the thorax. A tendency for superior scapula migration during this movement pattern implies that the upper trapezius is more dominant in the synergy. Whether the cause is primary trapezius hyperactivity or weakness/inhibition of lower trapezius/serratus anterior, the therapeutic goal is to reduce or diminish the tendency for superior scapula migration. This can be done by the therapist either applying a downward force on the scapula as the motion occurs in order to give feedback or by prescribing specific scapula stabilization exercises (described below).

Test 3. Scapular stability assessment

The simplest position to test scapular control is in prone with the hands by the sides. The scapula is manually placed into a neutral anatomical position on the thorax by the therapist and instruction is given to maintain this position under voluntary control. Observation is made to ensure a downward and medial movement of the scapula attributable to lower trapezius, together with scapula apposition on the thorax attributable to serratus anterior. This initial test position constitutes relatively low scapular load and altering the position of the upper limb by removing the support from the bed and progressively moving through abduction into elevation challenges the scapular stabilizers to a greater extent. As the level of load increases it is important to observe for substitution, typically hyperactivity of upper trapezius, which if it occurs will have an extensor effect upon the upper cervical spine.

Postural re-education

The clinical tests outlined thus far provide useful information about the functional interaction of the craniomandibular, craniocervical and shoulder complexes. Specific testing procedures have been outlined which attempt to quantify the mechanical capacity of the most significant postural muscles. The rationale of therapeutic intervention is then to target these muscles in isolation, improve their force-generating capacity, and reintegrate this capacity into postural control. To fulfil this requirement postural re-education exercise must replicate the demands of daily living specific to the individual. The typical head-forward posture which has been discussed is often part of a generalized postural syndrome in which the alignment against gravity is inefficient.[92]

Three basic postural variations from

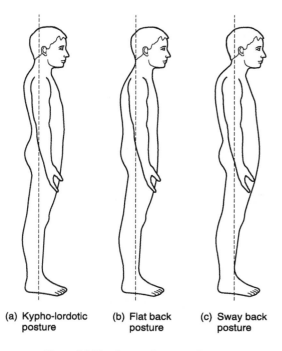

(a) Kypho-lordotic posture   (b) Flat back posture   (c) Sway back posture

Figure 9.8 The three main postural types

ideal alignment have been described[87] and the clinician should be aware that the correction of poor head and neck posture will often require a global, systematic approach. The postural variations described can be considered as kyphosis/lordosis, flat-back and sway-back, as indicated in Figure 9.8.

One of the first important goals is to create kinaesthetic awareness of optimal postural alignment. In practice this means the use of both verbal and visual feedback in the form of mirrors, tactile stimulation by the therapist, or varying forms of EMG biofeedback. Verbal instruction to 'stand up straight' is usually an inadequate stimulus in isolation to achieve postural realignment. In fact, such instruction often produces muscle hyperactivity as subjects attempt to attain a military-type posture which is sustained no longer than the period of observation.

It is important to recognize that optimal alignment will not feel 'normal' for a patient if it is not their habitual posture. If changes in alignment can be shown to reduce or alleviate symptoms, or reduce palpable tension in hyperactive muscles, for example in the neck and jaw, then this will improve the likelihood of compliance.

Preliminary postural exercises to address forward head position and therefore support an optimal craniomandibular relationship (minimizing downward and backward forces on the mandible) can be performed in supine using a chin-tuck exercise as described for assessment of deep neck flexors. Most importantly, any tendency to protract the chin should be corrected as this is indicative of superficial neck flexor dominance (as previously described) and will negate the effect of specific postural exercises. Scapular control at low load can also be encouraged by aligning the scapula against the supporting surface, thus opposing a tendency to scapular protraction. Mid-cervical extensor function can be initially improved from a prone position resting on elbows, as described for cervical extensor assessment, with the subject retracting the neck while maintaining a chin-tuck position. Simultaneous activation of scapular stabilizers can be achieved by encouraging scapular retraction and depression with relative increased load by virtue of elbow weight bearing. This can be further progressed by sliding each arm forward alternately while maintaining scapular position and preventing displacement of the trunk. This enhances trunk, scapular and neck stability simultaneously at a reasonable level of load prior to activity in upright. Progression to sitting or standing can then be made, depending on the specific functional deficits (Figure 9.9).

Postural alignment can be guided by therapist facilitation and visual and verbal feedback. All the previously described

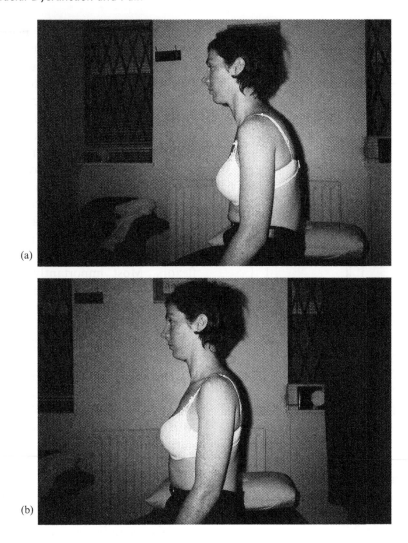

Figure 9.9 Postural alignment. (**a**) Suboptimal alignment, increased thoracic kyphosis and head and neck protraction. (**b**) Postural realignment. Restoration of cervical lordosis and reduced thoracic kyphosis

exercises can be performed in the upright position, and progression can be made using external resistance such as elastic tubing, hand weights or pulley systems. The cardinal rule is the maintenance of alignment with the progression of load.

Postural stability can be challenged to a greater extent by reducing the base of support or making it unstable. Typically this will involve the use of large (65-cm diameter) therapeutic gym balls, wobble boards or any other apparatus which challenges postural stability in this manner. There are many philosophies of movement re-education which have largely remained outside the medical spectrum but have useful clinical applications. Systems such as Alexander technique, Feldenkrais, Rolphing, Pilates, Yoga and Tai Chi[95–98] have common elements which attempt to

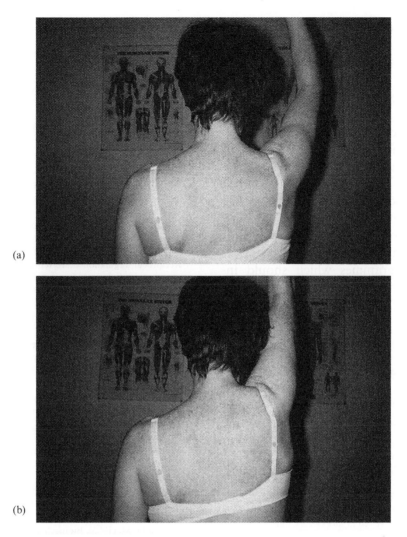

(a)

(b)

Figure. 9.10 (a) Assessment of scapula control with arm elevation. Scapula motion should primarily be that of rotation indicating good muscle coordination. **(b)** Assessment of scapula control indicated by elevation of scapula as a result of upper trapezius overactivity

enhance kinaesthetic and postural awareness. Zinc oxide tape can also be used as proprioceptive reinforcement. This is particularly useful in the thoracic spine and scapular region. Maintenance of good posture is likely to require maintenance exercise in conjunction with vigilance in situations of potential compromise (VDU operation, reading). Efficient locomotor system function requires prophylactic intervention, as do all biological systems, and awareness of optimal posture forms an important element of musculoskeletal function.

Summary

It is important for clinicians managing patients with head and neck pain to be aware of the influence of posture upon this region. The potential effects of altered posture, in particular forward head posture and its possible effect on temporomandibular joint mechanics, have been discussed and strategies for assesment and management have been suggested. Various aetiological factors have been proposed for the development of temporomandibular dysfunction, including occlusion, life stresses, and postural influences. The debate continues and it seems likely that all these factors are possible contributors to the development of symptoms. Clinicians must consider all possible sources of symptoms in their examination and plan appropriate treatment programmes which should include addressing any postural contribution to the patients' problems.

References

1 Kendall, H. O. and Kendall, F. P. (1968). Developing and maintaining good posture. *Phys. Ther.*, **48**, 319–336.

2 Rightmire, G. P. (1993). *The Evolution of Homo Erectus.* Cambridge University Press.

3 Williams, P..L., Warwick, R., Dyson, M, and Bannister, L. (1989). *Gray's Anatomy*, 37th edn, Churchill Livingstone.

4 Bogduk, N. (1986). Cervical causes of headache and dizziness. In: *Modern Manual Therapy of the Vertebral Column* (G. Grieve ed.), 289–302. Churchill-Livingstone.

5 Barnsley, L., Bogduk, N. and Lord, S. (1994). Whiplash injury. *Pain*, **58**, 283–307.

6 Bogduk, N. and Aprill, C. (1993). On the nature of neck pain, discography and cervical zygapophyseal joint blocks. *Pain*, **54**, 213–217.

7 Travell J. G. and Simons, D. G. (1983). *Myofacial Pain and Dysfunction: the Trigger Point Manual, the Upper Extremities.* Williams and Wilkins.

8 Bogduk, N. and Simons, D. G. (1993). Neck pain: joint pain or trigger points: In: *Progress in Fibromyalgia and Myofascial Pain* (H. Vaeroy and H. Merskey, eds), pp. 267–273. Elsevier.

9 Butler, D. S. (1991). *Mobilisation of the Nervous System.* Churchill-Livingstone.

10 Woolf, C. J. and Manion, R. J. (1999). Neuropathic pain: aetiology, symptoms, mechanisms and management. *Lancet*, **353**, 1959–2058.

11 Sakuta, M. and Sakuta, Y. (1989). Drooping head syndrome: the significance of neck posture and neck instability as a cause of muscle contraction headache. *Cephalgia*, **9** (suppl. 10), 19.

12 Braun, B. (1991). Postural differences between asymptomatic men and women and craniofacial pain patterns. *Arch. Phys. Med. Rehab.*, **72**, 653.

13 Watson, D. and Trott, P. (1993). An investigation of natural head posture and upper cervical flexor muscle performance. *Cephalgia*, **13**, 272.

14 Krout, R. M. and Anderson, T. P. (1966). Role of anterior cervical muscles in production of neck pain. *Arch. Phys. Med. Rehab.*, **69**, 603.

15 Silverman, J., Rodriquez, A. and Agre, J. (1991). Quantitative cervical flexor strength in healthy subjects and in subjects with mechanical neck pain. *Arch. Phys. Med. Rehab.*, **72**. 679.

16 Loebel, W. Y. (1967). Measurement of spinal posture and range of motion. *An. Phys. Med.*, **9**, 103–110.

17 Stangara, P., DeMauroy, J. C., Dran, G. *et al.* (1982). Reciprocal angulation of vertebral bodies in a sagittal plane: approach to references for the evaluation of kyphosis and lordosis. *Spine*, **7**, 335–342.

18 O'Gorman, H. and Jull, G. (1987). Thoracic kyphosis and mobility: the effect of age. *Physiother. Prac.*, **3**, 154–162.

19 Darlow, L. A., Pesco, J. and Greenberg, M. S. (1987). The relationship of posture to myofascial pain dysfunction syndrome. *JADA*, **114**, 73–75.

20 Clarke, G. T., Green, E. M., Doran, M. R. and Flack, V. F. (1987). Craniocervical dysfunction levels in a patient sample from a temporomandibular joint clinic. *JADA*, **115**, 251–256.

21 Huggare, J. A. and Raustia, A. M. (1992). Head posture and cervicovertebral and craniofacial morphology in patients with craniomandibular dysfunction *Cranio*, **10**, 173–177, discussion 178–179.

22 Darling, D., Kraus, S. and Glasheen-Wray, M. (1984). Relationship of head posture and the rest position of the mandible. *J. Pros. Dent.*, **52**, III.

23 Rocabado, M. (1983). Biomechanical relationship of the cranial, cervical, and hyoid regions. *Phys. Ther.*, **1**, 62–66.

24 Lee, W. Y., Okeson J. P. and Lindroth, J. (1995). The relationship between forward head posture and temporomandibular disorders. *J. Orofacial Pain*, **9**, 161–167.

25 Braun, B. L. and Amundsen, L. R. (1989). Quantitative assessment of head and shoulder posture, *Arch. Phys. Med. Rehabil.*, **70**, 322–329.

26 Young, J. D. (1988). Head posture measurement. *J. Pediatr. Ophthalmol. Strabismus*, **25**, 86–89.

27 Zonnenberg, A. J., Van Maanen C. J., Oostendoorp, R. A. and Elvers, J. W. (1996). Body posture photographs as a diagnostic aid for musculoskeletal disorders related to temporomandibular disorders (TMD). *J. Craniomandibular Pract.* **14**, 225–232.

28 Hanten, W. P., Lucio, R. M., Russell, J. L. and Brunt, D. (1991). Assessment of total head excursion and resting head posture. *Arch. Phys. Med. Rehabil.*, **72**, 877–880.

29 Bryden, L. and Power, A. (1992). An investigation into the inter-relationship between clinical measurement of cervical posture and X-ray measurement of cervical lordosis and hyoid bone position. *Manip. Physiother.*, **24**, 18-22.

30 Braune, W. and Fischer, O. (1889). Uber den Schwerpunkt des menschlichen Korpers mit Rucksicht auf die Ausrustung des deutschen Infanteristen. *Abhdlg D Kg Sach Wissenschaften*, **26**, 561, as cited in Sahrmann, S. A. (1988). Adult posturing. In: *TMJ Disorders. Management of the Craniomandibular Complex. Clinics in Physical Therapy* (S. L. Kraus, ed.). Churchill Livingstone.

31 Rocabado, M. (1981). *Diagnosis and Treatment of Abnormal Craniocervical and Craniomandibular Mechanics*. Rocabado Institute.

32 Kapandji, I. A. (1974). *The Physiology of the Joints – Volume 3. The Trunk and the Vertebral Column*, p. 217. Churchill Livingstone.

33 Vig, P., Rink, J. and Shoufety, K. (1983). Adaptation of head posture in response to relocating the centre of mass: a pilot study. *Am. J. Orthod.*, **83**, 138–42.

34 Ayub, E., Glasheen-Wray, M. B. and Kraus, S. L. (1984). Head posture: a case study on the effects of the rest position of the mandible. *J. Orthop. Sports Phys. Ther.*, **5**, 179.

35 Mohl, N. (1976). Head posture and its role in occlusion. *NY Dent. J.*, **42**, 17–23.

36 Winnberg, A., Pancherz, H. and Westesson, P. (1988). Head posture and hyo-mandibular function in man. A synchronized electromyographic and videofluorographic study of the open–close–clench cycle. *Am. J. Orthod. Dentofacial Orthoped.*, **94**, 393–404.

37 Passero, P. L., Wyman, B. S., Bell, J. W. *et al.* (1985). Temporomandibular joint dysfunction syndrome: a clinical report. *Phys. Ther.*, **65**, 1203–1207.

38 Daly, P., Preston, C. B. and Evans, W. G. (1982). Postural response of the head to bite opening in adult males. *Am. J. Orthod.*, **82**, 157–60.

39 Preiskel, H. W. (1965). Some observations on the postural position of the mandible. *J. Prosth. Dent.*, **15**, 625–633.

40 Urbanowicz, M. (1991). Alteration of vertical dimension and its effect on head and neck posture. *Cranio*, **9**, 174–179.

41 Abrahams, V. C. and Richmond, F. J. R. (1977). Motor roll of the spinal projections of the trigeminal system. In: *Pain in the Trigeminal Region* (D. J. Anderson and B. Mathews, eds). Elsevier.

42 Rugh J. D. and Drago C. J. (1981). Vertical dimension: a study of clinical rest position and jaw muscle activity. *J. Prosth. Dent.*, **45**, 670.

43 Garnick, J. and Ramfjord, S. P. (1962). Rest position. An electromyographic and clinical investigation. *J. Prosth. Dent.*, **12**, 895.

44 Kuroda, Nunota, E., Hanada, K., Ito, G. and Shilsaski, Y. (1966). A roentgenocephalometric study on the position of the hyoid bone. *Bull. Tokyo Med. Dent. Univ.*, **13**, 228.

45 Nagai, M., Kudo, A., Matsuno, I. *et al.* (1989). Hyoid bone position and airway accompanied with influence of head posture (Abs). *Nippon. Kyosei. Shika. Gakkai. Zasshi*, **48**, 214–225.

46 Ingervall, B., Carlsson, G. E. and Helkimo, M. (1970). Change in location of hyoid bone with mandibular positions. *Acta Odontol. Scand*, **28**, 337.

47 Carsloo, S. and Leijon, G. (1960). A radiographic study of the position of the hyo-caryngeal complex in relation to the skull and cervical column in man. *Trans. R. Schools Dent. Stockh. Umea*, **5**, 13.

48 Takaji, Y., Gamble, J. W., Proffitt, W. R. and Christiansen, R. L. (1967). Postural change of the hyoid bone following osteotomy of the mandible. *Oral Surg. Oral Med. Oral Pathol.*, **23**, 688–692, as cited in Tallgren, A. and Solow, B. (1987). Hyoid bone position, facial morphology and head posture in adults. *Eur. J. Orthod.*, **9**, 1–8.

49 Fromm, B. and Lundberg, M. (1970). Postural behavior of the hyoid bone in normal occlusion before and after surgical correction of mandibular protrusion. *Swed. Dent. J.*, **63**, 425–433 as cited in Tallgren, A. and Solow, B. (1987). Hyoid bone position, facial morphology and head posture in adults. *Eur. J. Orthod.*, **9**, 1–8.

50 Tallgren, A. and Solow, B. (1987). Hyoid bone position, facial morphology and head posture in adults. *Eur. J. Orthod.*, **9**, 1–8.

51 Zuniga, C., Miralles, R., Mena, B. *et al.* (1995). Influence of varation in jaw posture on sternocleidomastoid and trapezius electromyographic activity. *J. Craniomandibular Pract.*, **13**, 157–162.

52 Hellsing, E. and Hagberg, C., (1990) Changes in maximum bite force related to extension of the head. *Euro. J. Orthod.*, **12**, 148–153.

53 Funakoshi, M. and Amano, N. (1973). Effects of the tonic neck reflex on the jaw muscles of the rat. *J. Dent. Res.*, **52**, 668–673.

54 Funakoshi, M., Fujita, H. and Takehana, S. (1976). Relationship between occlusal interference and jaw muscle activities in response to changes in head position. *J. Dent. Res.*, **55**, 684–690.

55 Forsberg, C. M., Hellsing, E., Linder-Aronson, S. and Sheik Holesham, A. (1985). Postural muscle activity of the neck muscles in relation to extension and flexion of the head. *Eur. J. Ortho.*, **7**, 177–184.

56 Perry, H. T. (1956). Facial, cranial and cervical pain associated with dysfunctions of the occlusion and articulations of the teeth. *Angle Orthod.*, **26**, 121–128.

57 Frumker, S. C. and Kyle, M. A. (1985). The dentist's contribution to rehabilitation of cervical posture and function: orthopaedic and neurological considerations in the treatment of craniomandibular disorders. *Basal Facts*, **9**, 105–109.

58 Clarke, R. K. F. and Wyke, B. D. (1974). Contributions of temporomandibular mechanoreceptors to the control of mandibular posture: an experimental study. *J. Dent.*, **2**, 121.

59 Klineberg, J., Greenfield, B. E. and Wyke, B. D. (1970). Contributions to the reflex control of mastication from mechanoreceptors in the TMJ capsule. *Dent. Pract. Dent. Rec.*, **21**, 73.

60 Levy, P. H. (1981). Physiological response to dental malocclusion and misplaced mandibular posture: the keys to temporomandibular joint and associated neuromuscular disorders. *Basal Facts*, **4**, 103–122.

61 Eberle, W. R. (1951). A study of centric relation as recorded in a supine position. *J. Am. Dent. Assoc.*, **42**, 15, cited Kraus (1994).

62 Vig, P., Showfety, K. and Philips, C. (1980). Experimental manipulation of head posture. *Am. J. Orthod.*, **77**, 258–268.

63 Kraus, S. L. (1994). Temporomandibular disorders, 2nd edn. *Clinics in Physical Therapy*, pp. 325–412. Churchill Livingstone.

64 Gray, R. J. M., Davies, S. J. and Quayle, A. H. (1995). *Temporomandibular Disorders: a Clinical Approach*, pp. 1–7. BDA Publication.

65 Wenzel, A., Hojensgaard, E. and Henriksen, J. M. (1985). Craniofacial morphology and head posture in children with asthma and perennial rhinitis. *Eur. J. Orthod.*, **7**, 83–92.

66 Solow, B. and Tallgren, A. (1976). Head posture and craniofacial morphology. *Am. J. Phys. Anthrop.*, **4**, 417–436.

67 Rocabado, M. and Iglash, Z. A. (1991). *Musculoskeletal Approach to Maxillofacial Pain*. J. B. Lipincott Co.

68 Ricketts, R. M. (1968). Respiratory obstruction syndrome. *Am. J. Orthod.*, **54**, 495–507 cited in Solow, B. and Tallgren, A. (1976). Head posture and craniofacial morphology. *Am. J. Phys. Anthrop.*, **4**, 417–436.

69 Panjabi, M. M. (1992). The stabilising system of the spine. 1: Function, dysfunction, adaptation and enhancement. *J. Spinal Disord.*, **5**, 383–389.

70 Bergmark, A. (1989). Stability of the lumbar spine. A study in mechanical engineering. *Acta Orthopaed. Scand.*, **230** (suppl.), 20–24.

71 Hides, J. A., Richardson, C. A. and Jull, G. A. (1996). Multifidus muscle recovery is not automatic following resolution of acute first episode low back pain. *Spine*. **21**, 2763–2769.

72 O'Sullivan, P. B. and Twomey, L. T. (1994). Evaluation of specific stabilising exercise in the treatment of chronic low back pain with radiological diagnosis of spondylosis or spondylolisthesis. *Thesis*, Curtin University of Technology, Western Australia.

73 O'Sullivan, P. B., Twomey, L. T. and Allison, G. T. (1997). Evaluation of specific stabilising exercise in the treatment of chronic low back pain with radiological diagnosis of spondylosis or spondylolisthesis. *Spine*, **22**, 2959–2967.

74 Lavander, S. A., Mirka, G. A., Schoenmarklin, R. W., *et al.* (1989). The effects of preview and task symmetry on trunk muscle response to sudden loading. *Hum. Factors*, **31**, 101–115.

75 Mirka, G. A. and Marras, W. S. (1993). A stochastic model of trunk muscle coactivation during trunk bending. *Spine*, **18**, 1396–1409.

76 Woolf, C. J (1984). Long term alterations in the excitability of the flexion reflex produced by peripheral tissue injury in the chronic decerebrate rat. *Pain*, **18**, 325–343.

77 Woolf, C. J. and McMahon, S. B. (1985). Injury-induced plasticity in the flexor reflex in chronic decerebrate rats. *Neuroscience*, **16**, 395–404.

78 Steinmetz, J. E. Beggs, A. L., Lupica, C. R. and Patterson, M. M. (1983). Effects of local anaesthesia on persistence of peripherally induced postural asymmetries in rats. *Behav. Neurosci.*, **97**, 62–67.

79 Griegel, P., Larson, K., Mueller, K. and Oatis, C. (1992). Incidence of common postural abnormalities in the cervical, shoulder, and thoracic regions and their association with pain in two age groups of healthy subjects. *Phys. Ther.*, **72**, 425–430.

80 Bourbon, B. M. (1988). Anatomy and biomechanics of the TMJ. In: *TMJ Disorders. Management of the Craniomandibular Complex. Clinics in Physical Therapy* (S. L. Kraus, ed.). Churchill Livingstone.

81 McDevitt, W. E. (1989). *Functional Anatomy of the Masticatory System*. Wright Butterworth & Co. Ltd.

82 Jull, G. (1998). *Physical Therapy of the Cervical and Thoracic Spine*, 2nd edn, pp. 262–273. Churchill Livingstone.

83 Lewitt, K. (1991). *Manipulative Therapy in Rehabilitation of the Locomotor System*, 2nd edn. Butterworth-Heinemann.

84 Janda, V. (1988). Muscles and cervicogenic pain syndromes. In: *Physical Therapy of the Cervical and Thoracic Spine*, pp. 153. Churchill Livingstone.

85 Jull, G. (1994). Headaches of cervical origin. In: *Physical Therapy of the Cervical and Thoracic Spine*, pp. 271–274. Churchill Livingstone.

86 Sahrmann, S. (1990). *Diagnosis and Treatment of Muscle Imbalances Associated with Regional Pain Syndromes.* (Course notes) Washington University, School of Medicine, Physical Therapy Department.

87 Kendall, F. P., McCreary, E. K. and Provance, P. G. (1993). *Muscles: Testing and Function*, 4th edn. Williams and Wilkins.

88 Anderson, G. and Winters, J. (1990). Role of muscle in postural tasks: spinal loading and postural stability. In: *Multiple Muscle Systems* (J. Winters and S. Y. Woo, eds), pp. 375–395. Springer-Verlag.

89 Johansson, H. and Sojka, P. (1991). Pathophysiological mechanisms involved in genesis and spread of muscular tension in occupational muscle pain and in chronic musculoskeletal pain syndromes: a hypothesis. *Med. Hypoth. Physiother. Pract.*, **3**. 154–162.

90 Beeton, K. and Jull, G. (1994). Effectiveness of manipulative physiotherapy in the management of cervicogenic headache. *Physiotherapy*, **80**, 417–422.

91 Watson, D. and Trott, P. (1991). Cervical headache: an investigation of natural head posture and upper cervical flexor muscle performance. In: *Manipulative Phy-*

siotherapists Association of Australia 7th Biennial Conference, pp. 19–24. Manipulative Physiotherapists Association of Australia.

92 Janda, V. (1983). *Muscle Testing and Function*. Butterworth-Heinemann.

93 Poppen, N. K. and Walker, P. S. (1976). Normal and abnormal motion of the shoulder. *J. Bone Joint Surg.*, **58A**, 175.

94 Culham, E. and Peat, M. (1993). Functional anatomy of the shoulder complex. *J. Orthopaed. Sports Physiother.*, **18**, 342–350.

95 Feldenkrais, M. (1984). *The Master Moves*. Meta Publications.

96 Bond, M. (1993). *Rolfing Movement Integration*. Healing Art Press.

97 McMillan, A. Proteau, L. Lebe, R.-M. (1998). The effect of Pilates-based training on dancers' dynamic posture. *J. Dance Med. Sci.*, **2**(3).

98 Gelb, M. (1987). *Body Learning – An Introduction to the Alexander Technique*. Arum Press.

10

Clinical reasoning – a basis for examination and treatment in the cranial region

M. Jones and H. J. M. von Piekartz

Clinical reasoning refers to the thought processes and decision making associated with a clinician's examination and management of a patient or client. Clinical reasoning is intentional, goal-oriented thinking applied in a clinical context. In the past, clinicians were expected to acquire skilled clinical reasoning through the course of their education and clinical practice. The science and skill of clinical reasoning was not overtly taught. Even today resistance still exists among some educators and clinicians, who believe their own clinical reasoning ability and success in the clinic vindicates their view that formal attention to the reasoning process and reasoning strategies is unnecessary. A common argument, highlighted by Nickerson,[1] is that 'All of us compare, classify, order, estimate, extrapolate, interpolate, form hypotheses, weigh evidence, draw conclusions, devise arguments, judge relevance, use analogies, and engage in numerous activities that are typically classified as thinking', despite never having had formal instruction in critical thinking or clinical reasoning. But this is not to say that we do these things well in all circumstances or that we could

not learn to do them better. That is, it is not enough simply to recognize a clinical situation you have encountered in the past and apply a solution that has worked before. Rather, clinicians must acquire and apply critical and creative thinking skills in order to validate their clinical beliefs, develop improved understanding of human pain and dysfunction and increase the effectiveness and efficiency of patient management. There is now an increasing international acceptance across the health professions that clinical reasoning is the foundation of clinical practice and in order to optimize patient outcomes and promote clinicians' lifelong learning, health science students and clinicians must understand the key aspects of clinical reasoning including an awareness of their own reasoning strengths and weaknesses.[2]

This chapter provides a brief overview of clinical reasoning processes, with particular attention to key aspects influencing clinicians' ability to reason well, and an introduction of reasoning strategies used by clinicians across the health professions. A transcript of a patient interview with craniofacial pain is presented along with a

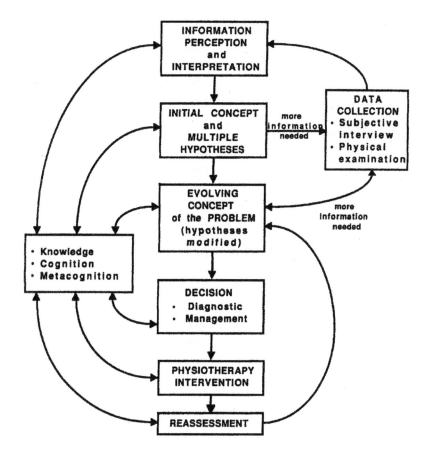

Figure 10.1 The clinical reasoning process (adapted from Barrows and Tamblyn, 1980)

comparison of the clinical reasoning of six clinicians from different health professions. While the full depth of the clinicians' reasoning is unlikely to have emerged in this exercise, and the reasoning of any one clinician should not be seen to represent a whole profession, it does highlight common errors in clinical reasoning, the importance of recognizing one's own limitations and the need for greater collaboration across the health professions. All clinicians in each profession are vulnerable to being locked into their own clinical patterns. The safeguard to such narrow reasoning is to ensure clinicians understand their reasoning and the errors to avoid while promoting an open yet critical and reflective thinking style.[3] In this way clinicians will be less likely to accept unquestioningly unsubstantiated theory or the latest popular view. Instead, skilled clinical reasoning combined with creative lateral thinking will encourage clinicians continually to challenge their existing beliefs, clinical patterns and associated management strategies and in the process expand the breadth and depth of their understanding of patients' problems.

Clinical reasoning can broadly be portrayed as a hypothetico-deductive process where patient data elicit the consideration of hypotheses, which are in turn tested through further data collection. It is a cyclic process that commences with the initial information obtained about the patient (Figure 10.1). For example, in a rehabilitation setting this may be a referral, case notes, observation of the patient in the waiting room, as well as opening introductions and inquiries with the patient and/or family. This preliminary information will elicit a range of impressions or working interpretations. While typically not thought of as such, these can be considered hypotheses in that clinicians' initial thoughts should guide their further inquiries, with clinical decisions being made on the weight of supporting and negating evidence.

The thinking involved in this generation of hypotheses includes a combination of specific data interpretations or inductions (also called forward reasoning or pattern recognition) and the synthesis of multiple clues or deductions (also called backward reasoning). While diagnostic hypotheses are most easily recognized, other categories of hypotheses have also been proposed, including.[4,5]

- dysfunction
- pathobiological mechanisms
- source of the symptoms (often equated with diagnosis)
- contributing factors
- prognosis
- management.

Initial hypotheses tend to be quite broad, such as 'appears to be a back or hip problem', or 'the way he is coping with his stress and frustration suggests a potential central pain mechanism with maladaptive or dysfunctional coping strategies'. As further clarifying information is obtained, the clinician's evolving understanding of the patient's problem leads to a refinement of hypotheses considered. By the end of the patient interview the clinician should have acquired sufficient understanding of the patient and the patient's problem to be able to tailor the physical examination to test specifically those hypotheses which emerged from the interview. By taking time to search for clues of physical dysfunction and, equally importantly, how the patient's problems are affecting him personally, including his understanding of and feelings about his problem, the clinician can then interpret the physical findings in the broader context of how the patient's life has been affected by the problem, or his pain experience. This hypothesis-oriented approach should then continue through the ongoing patient management, where the success or failure of different treatment strategies contribute to the clinician's evolving understanding of the patient's problem.

As illustrated by the box to the left in Figure 10.1, their cognition, metacognition and knowledge largely influence the overall success of clinicians' reasoning. In this context, cognition refers to purposeful thinking, which occurs at multiple levels. To start, the clinician must perceive a piece of information as being relevant, a point where novices often make their first mistake in simply not recognizing key information. Next, each piece of information must be interpreted and then the collective clues acquired throughout the examination must be synthesized in the context of that patient's unique presentation. Hypotheses which emerge from this synthesis of information must then be tested against further information collected through the patient interview, physical examination and ongoing management.

While conceptually quite simple, thorough reasoning can be very difficult and is fraught with errors. Errors of reasoning can occur through any stage of the reasoning process, including errors of perception, interpretation, inquiry, synthesis, goal setting, planning and self-monitoring.[3] The most common errors are an overemphasis on findings which support an existing hypothesis, misinterpreting non-contributory information as confirming an existing hypothesis, ignoring findings which did not support a favoured hypothesis, and incorrect interpretations related to inappropriately applied inductive and deductive logic.[3,6–10]. Many clinicians, however, will be unaware of the thinking processes they use when examining and treating a patient, and hence errors may well go unnoticed.

The most common error is an over focus on a favourite hypothesis. This of course is an inherent limitation of pattern recognition – that is, when you try to put things into discrete boxes, the boxes themselves become the focus of your attention and it is difficult to see any patterns outside those boxes. Care is needed to avoid a preoccupation with one diagnosis, one structure or one system at the expense of the others, as this will be reflected in the management. That is, if all you have is a hammer, everything looks like a nail.

Metacognition refers to clinicians' awareness of their own thinking, that is their ability to monitor or think about their thinking.[2] This advanced thinking skill, characteristic of experts across all professions,[11] enables clinicians to recognize the need for further clarifying information, carefully to scrutinize the reliability and validity of information obtained and, importantly, to recognize limitations in their own knowledge base and clinical skills.[12,13] Through metacognition, critical thinkers pay attention to the context in which their ideas and actions are generated and thereby develop an awareness of the assumptions under which they, and others, think and act.[14] This reflective scepticism ensures that theories and protocols are not taken for granted simply because they have existed unchanged for a period of time or have been presented by a source of authority.

Knowledge is a third key factor influencing clinicians' reasoning. Errors of interpretation and synthesis may be related less to the clinician's limited amount of medical or clinical knowledge than one might think, and more to the clinician's inadequate organization of that knowledge limiting the ability to retrieve relevant knowledge already stored in memory.[15–17] The hypothesis categories proposed by Jones[18] and expanded on by Gifford and Butler[5] provide a useful framework for organizing knowledge in the neuro-orthopaedic area. These hypothesis categories, discussed in more detail in Chapter 8, require clinicians to recognize common patterns of dysfunction, pain mechanisms, pathology, healing, contributing factors, and risk to management and prognosis. To hypothesize and reach decisions across this wide range of clinical concerns requires a good biomedical knowledge base linked to its clinical significance, with attention to psychological (cognitive, affective and behavioural), social, cultural, environmental and physical cues extracted from the patient's story and physical examination.

In addition to the interrelated aspects of cognition, metacognition and knowledge organization, expert clinicians also appear to possess reasoning strategies (e.g. diagnostic reasoning, narrative reasoning, interactive reasoning, collaborative reasoning, predictive reasoning, and ethical reasoning) which they employ to assist their understanding and management of patients and their problems. Reasoning strategies are lines of inquiry, styles of dialogue or a specific focus of thinking which clinicians adopt in particular clinical situations. The nature and use of these strategies or styles of reasoning have been previously

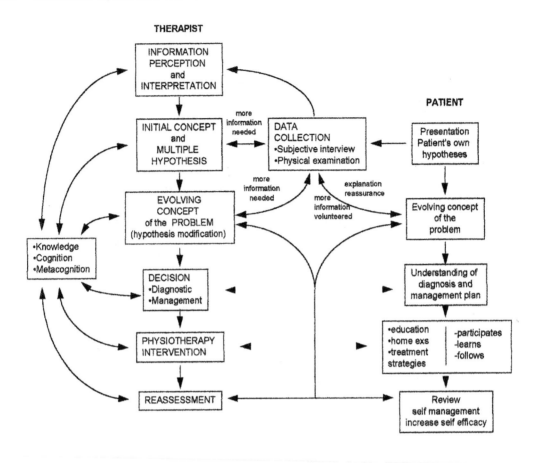

Figure 10.2 Cooperative decision making between patient and therapist (Jones[18])

described in the occupational therapy and nursing literature,[19–20] and more recently our own research has documented their use among expert physiotherapists.[22]

Diagnostic reasoning is that reasoning aimed to reveal the patient's dysfunction and the underlying pain mechanisms, structures at fault, pathophysiology and factors contributing to the development and maintenance of the dysfunction. While diagnostic reasoning is the most familiar reasoning strategy, in clinical practice it is intermixed with other strategies to establish patient rapport, educate and promote patient self-efficacy and responsibility.

Interactive reasoning occurs when dialo-gue in the form of social exchange is used purposely to enhance or facilitate the assessment/management process. This may be in terms of putting a patient at ease, establishing rapport, engaging the confidence of a patient and directly finding out more about the patient's context (work, family, belief systems) or may be conversa-tion about matters in the life of the patient and/or the clinician that indirectly achieves the above. Such socializing during a patient encounter, while not always the case, provides an effective means of better understanding the context in which the patient's problem(s) exist, while creating a relationship of interest and trust which is essential to promote change successfully in patient attitude, behaviour and responsibility, as is frequently required. While all clinicians interact with their patients, not everyone engages in interactive reasoning.

Narrative reasoning describes the use of stories regarding past or present patients that are told by the clinician to the patient for the purpose of explaining/educating, reassuring and building rapport. The use of a 'story', or commonly an account of a patient who had a similar situation, is frequently used to make a point. Such real life scenarios bring credibility to the advice or explanation which they are used to support, and can be strategically employed by clinicians to strengthen their message.

Collaborative reasoning refers to the shared decision making that ideally occurs between clinician and patient. Here the patient's opinions and not just information about the problem are actively sought and utilized. The concept of collaborative reasoning is illustrated in Figure 10.2. Where Figure 10.1 portrayed the clinician's reasoning, Figure 10.2 attempts to highlight that patients will also go through a thinking process regarding their problem. That is, patients arrive for their assessment with their own ideas about their problem, usually based on either previous personal experiences or the opinions of family members or other health professionals. When the encounter with the health clinician is one-sided, with patients simply being passive providers of information and passive recipients of treatment, their initial understanding of their problem either goes unchanged or is further confused by yet another opinion. Similarly, without good understanding of the management and opportunity to contribute to management decisions, patients are less likely to accept responsibility for their part in the recovery and their self-efficacy is at

risk. In contrast, collaborative reasoning, with shared decision making between clinician and patient, promotes patients' evolving understanding of their problem and shared responsibility for the management, with greater patient self efficacy and increased likelihood of compliance.

Predictive reasoning is that part of the clinician's thinking directed to estimating patient responses to treatment and likely outcomes of management based on information obtained through the patient interview, physical examination and response to management interventions.

Ethical/pragmatic reasoning alludes to those less recognized but frequently made decisions regarding moral, political and economic dilemmas which clinicians regularly confront. For example, deciding how long to continue treatment when progress is slow or making judgements on the treatment of other health professionals requires careful consideration of the available data and the implications of the decision reached.

Teaching as reasoning occurs when clinicians consciously use advice, instruction and guidance for the purpose of promoting change in patient understanding, feelings and behaviour.

Underpinning all dimensions of clinical reasoning is the ability of clinicians to recognize relevant cues (e.g. behavioural, psychological, social, cultural, environmental, etc.) and their relationship to other cues, and to test or verify these clinical patterns through further examination and management. This again highlights the hypothetico-deductive nature of the clinical reasoning process. How well clinicians learn from the results of their decisions depends on the thoroughness of their deliberations and the time and attention given to their conscious reflection.

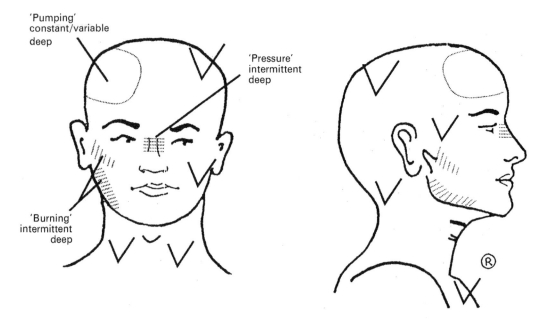

'Pumping'
constant/variable
deep

'Pressure'
intermittent
deep

'Burning'
intermittent
deep

Figure 10.3 Body chart

Patient case–initial subjective examination of a patient with long-term craniofacial pain

Interview

Patient personal profile: 29-year-old male. Married with no children. Employed full time as a bank operator with 80% of work involving computer activities. He has some medical background as he started nursing education but did not complete it. His hobbies include soccer (plays 1 hour per week) and biking (rides 2 hours per week).

Section 1 – Patient interview regarding type and area of symptoms patient is experiencing (See body chart, Figure 10.3 for area of symptoms)

Physiotherapist: Please can you tell me what, at this moment, is your main problem?

Patient: Yes, my main problem at this moment is a headache in this part of my head (see Figure 10.3). I feel a burning pain on my cheek and a kind of pressure in the upper part of my nose. The headache especially occurs when I'm very busy.

Physiotherapist: Which of those three symptoms, the headache, the burning feeling in your cheek or the pressure in your nose, is your main problem?

Patient: At this moment I think my headache is my main problem.

Physiotherapist: Can you please describe your headache?

Patient: Yes, it feels like my heartbeat is in my head. It's kind of beating.

Physiotherapist: Is it constantly there, or does it come and go?

Patient: Well, I have a headache every day but sometimes it's worse than others.

Physiotherapist: Are there any times when your headache is completely gone?

Patient: Yes, but recently it's been more frequent.

Physiotherapist: OK, and the pain in your

cheek, what kind of pain is that?

Patient: It's a kind of burning pain. It's just like a sunburn-pain, only not of my skin but within my cheek.

Physiotherapist: So, you feel this burning pain more inside your cheek?

Patient: Yes, it's not the skin, which burns, but what is underneath it.

Physiotherapist: Is that pain only in this area of your cheek (see Figure 10.3), or does it spread?

Patient: Yes, it's only in this area.

Physiotherapist: OK, and the pain over your nose, can you explain the kind of pain you feel there?

Patient: Well, it's not really a pain, it's more a kind of pressure feeling in my nose.

Physiotherapist: OK, and is that pressure there all the time or does it come and go?

Patient: The pressure is constant but increases when I bend over.

Physiotherapist: So, when you move your head or body forward the pressure increases?

Patient: Yes, especially when I write or work on the computer.

Physiotherapist: So, your beating headache is your main problem. The burning in your cheek is your next concern and the pressure in your nose is the least problem of the three?

Patient: Yes, that's right.

Physiotherapist: Now, just to be certain I'm aware of all symptoms, do you have any discomfort or sensations of any kind in your jaw, left cheek or the rest of your head (indicating each area on the patient while asking)?

Patient: No, just those areas I've mentioned.

Physiotherapist: How about your neck, upper back, shoulders and arms (also indicating each area on patient)?

Patient: No, those areas are OK as well.

Physiotherapist: And in your throat, any problems there?

Patient: Well, sometimes I suffer a dry throat but that is mainly caused by the hot weather.

Question 1. What are your thoughts about the patient's information?

Orthodontist: At this stage I would be considering an occlusal, sinus or tooth problem. There is also the suggestion of a stress-related problem.

Dentist: Probably a right sinusitis.

Physiotherapist: Good witness – he describes the qualities of his symptoms very well.

Neurologist: Atypical facial pain, could be a tension headache.

House doctor: There are a number of problems that need to be considered here including trigeminal neuralgia; prolapsed cervical disc; traumatic problem; multiple sinusitis; and visual disturbances.

Psychologist: My first impression is that he has a matter-of-fact like way of expressing his complaints.

Question 2. What further information would you like at this stage?

Orthodontist: I would want to assess pressure on nerves in the right infraorbital region and also ask the patient to tilt his head forward and down to find hints of a sinus problem.

Dentist: I would like more information about what appears to be a classic sinusitis pattern.

Physiotherapist: I would like to know about the relationship between the different symptoms and whether any features of sympathetic nervous system involvement are present.

Neurologist: Patient history.

House doctor: How long did he have the complaints? Details of the onset? Any visual complaints? Is the pain related to position or movement?

Psychologist: I would like to know more personal data such as his work and marital history, and begin to explore his thoughts and feelings about his problems.

Question 3. What sources do you think are implicated?

Orthodontist: Muscle, nerves, sinus, occlusion, and teeth.

Dentist: Sinus frontalis, sinus maxillaris, and sinus ethomoidalis.

Physiotherapist: Headache: the quality of the headache (pumping like a heart beat) leads me to consider the sympathetic nervous system more than cervical spine. Burning pain in cheek: nervous system (e.g. maxillaris nerve, trigeminal nerve). Pressure feeling in nose: sinuses, cranium, TMJ, cervical spine.

Neurologist: Muscle, psychological, blood vessels.

House doctor: Neurogenic.

Psychologist: He indicates that his complaints are being increased by certain stress situations such as being very busy at work; other potential sources of stress in the workplace and the family system will also need to be explored.

Question 4. What factors do you think could be contributing to maintaining this man's problem?

Orthodontist: Inadequate stress management; occlusal problem; pulpitis (*i.e. orofacial pain due to pulpal inflammation*).

Dentist: Expansion of a rhinitis, dental problem or sinusitis.

Physiotherapist: This patient describes his complaints perfectly which can reflect a personality which strives for perfectionism, and as such influence his ability to cope with his problem. He also associated his headache with being very busy at work, which may be an indication that stress is a contributing factor.

Neurologist: His congenital narcissism (*i.e. dysfunctional self-love*).

House doctor: The cervical spine and perhaps the patient's personality.

Psychologist: There is an early indication that stress may be a contributing factor.

Question 5. What would you examine and what are your thoughts about treatment at this moment?

Orthodontist: Teeth, occlusion, muscles, TMJ, life situation. As for treatment, at this stage I would consider a referral to an ENT specialist.

Dentist: X-ray sinuses, dental and nasal examination. Treatment considered at this stage: medication, sinus flushing.

Physiotherapist: All potential local somatic (e.g. TMJ, craniofacial tissues, local muscles and teeth) and neurogenic structures (e.g. function and neurodynamics of trigeminal nerve) will need to be assessed as well as any structures capable of referring symptoms to this area, such as the upper cervical spine. The occlusal/dental examination may require referral to an orthodontist or dentist. If stress proves to be a relevant factor then he may also benefit from an examination with a psychologist. With my cervical spine examination I will need to be aware of sympathetic reactions, especially during cervical movements such as flexion, extension and lateral flexion due to the potential influence these movements can have on the cervical ganglia. With respect to treatment, it's really too soon to say. If there proves to be physical dysfunction in the craniofacial or cervical structures then manual therapy may be helpful, but if stress turns out to be a significant component then other hands-off strategies will need to be employed.

Neurologist: X-rays (anterior, posterior). Treatment considerations include antibiotics and possibly a neuroleptic medication (*i.e. antipsychotic action principally affecting psychomotor activity*).

House doctor: No change in thoughts from previous section.

Psychologist: I would examine the patient's consciousness of any pain behaviours and coping strategies. As for treatment, I'm not sure at this stage.

Section 2 – Subjective examination/ patient interview regarding behaviour of patient's symptoms

Physiotherapist: You said your symptoms come and go, what do you think brings them on?

Patient: Well, when I'm busy at work or when I am working under mental pressure, my headache increases. Bending over writing seems to particularly aggravate the headache and pressure feeling.

Physiotherapist: What about the burning pain in your cheek and the pressure feeling in your nose, do they occur then as well?

Patient: No, it always starts with my headache and then within a few moments the pressure in my nose increases.

Physiotherapist: And how about the burning pain in your cheek?

Patient: Well, the burning is present all day but when I get busy, it increases too.

Physiotherapist: Does that mean the burning feeling is provoked by different activities than your headache and the pressure in your nose?

Patient: Yes.

Physiotherapist: Is it totally different situations?

Patient: Not totally different. Where the headache and pressure in my nose fluctuate with the mental stress I suffer, with no headache or pressure when I relax, the burning in my cheek is always present and increases when I'm really busy.

Physiotherapist: Are there any more things that provoke your symptoms?

Patient: Well, it's not only with writing, the pain also increases when I pick something up from the floor and things like that. In general you can say that when I bend forward with my head the headache and pressure feeling increase.

Physiotherapist: How is it when you drive a car?

Patient: Well, if I am not too tired I have no problems driving a car, but when I am getting tired the headache and nose pressure increase.

Physiotherapist: So, the combination of tiredness and driving the car provokes those symptoms?

Patient: Yes.

Physiotherapist: Are there any other things in your daily life that provoke any of your symptoms?

Patient: Yes, for example playing sports like soccer or athletics. In general when I increase my activities, all the pains increase with it.

Physiotherapist: What do you think it is about playing sport that aggravates your symptoms.

Patient: I'm not sure.

Physiotherapist: Do you think it has anything to do with movements of your neck or arms or maybe the jarring associated with running?

Patient: I don't know, it seems like it has to do with the overall effort of playing. Although general movements of my head do seem to affect the headache and pressure, this is only after some 20 minutes of playing sport.

Physiotherapist: What about other times when you exercise without impact such as your bike riding, would that aggravate your symptoms?

Patient: I don't know for sure as I haven't ridden my bike since the surgery.

Physiotherapist: Are there any activities that influence the burning pain in your cheek?

Patient: No, maybe slight rotations of my head, but I'm not really sure about this.

Physiotherapist: Would you say the three symptoms seem to influence each other, that is if one increases the other two follow within a few moments?

Patient: Yes, they always go together. The only difference is that the pain in my cheek is always present at a low level whereas my headache and the pressure in my nose sometimes disappear.

Physiotherapist: Can you describe the pattern of your symptoms from when you go to bed, when you first wake and then how they vary through the day?

Patient: Well, at night getting to sleep is difficult, especially when I have had a busy day because then I usually have more pain than when I've had a lazy day. During the morning when I get up I usually have very few complaints. It's typical that when I increase my activities the symptoms increase as well. And then I will try and reduce them by lying down.

Physiotherapist: So does lying down or resting decrease your symptoms?

Patient: Oh, I always feel better when I lie down.

Physiotherapist: Can you compare the intensity of your pain in the morning and in the afternoons?

Patient: In general, in the morning I've got less pain than in the afternoon.

Physiotherapist: So your pain has a cumulative pattern?

Patient: Yes that's right.

Physiotherapist: If you rest during the day then, would you have less pain than if you didn't get the chance to rest?

Patient: Yes.

Physiotherapist: How about your concentration and your memory, have they been affected?

Patient: I have got problems with my concentration, especially when I'm very busy at work it's hard for me to keep focused on what I do. And about my memory, I know I forget more than before my operation.

Physiotherapist: Do you mean you can't remember past events (*i.e. long-term memory*)?

Patient: No, that's OK. It's just that sometimes when I'm talking I get a bit confused and forget what I was saying.

Physiotherapist: Have you had any problems with brushing your teeth or with biting and chewing?

Patient: No I don't have any problems with cleaning teeth or eating.

Physiotherapist: Earlier you said your symptoms ease when you lie down, are there any other things you can do to ease any of your symptoms?

Patient: No, not that I can think of.

Physiotherapist: Have you ever tried squeezing your skull? Some people find that affects their symptoms.

Patient: Yes, I forgot about that. But when I have a headache and I squeeze my skull like this (bilateral pressure with palms of both hands), the headache does decrease.

Physiotherapist: How long do you need to squeeze your skull for the headache to decrease?

Patient: Well, it's hard to say how many minutes it takes. I just squeeze my skull 'til the pain is gone.

Physiotherapist: And how about your concentration?

Patient: I don't know if the squeezing

influences that.

Physiotherapist: What about the other symptoms, are they affected by squeezing your skull?

Patient: Yes, everything decreases, the headache, the burning pain in my cheek and the pressure in my nose as well.

Physiotherapist: And have you found that is the only place where the squeezing will ease your symptoms?

Patient: Well, when I put pressure on my nose like this (index finger and thumb on the cranial part of the nose), it also decreases the nose pressure and headache somewhat, although not as much as the relief I get from pressure on my skull.

Question 1. What are your thoughts about this additional information regarding the behaviour of the patient's symptoms?

Orthodontist: I need more information about the nose region to understand this problem.

Dentist: Sinus frontalis/sinus maxillaris problem.

Physiotherapist: Since all areas of pain are provoked by what the patient refers to as 'mental stress', this suggests either a common central pain mechanism exists for all three symptoms or possibly this stress occurs in conjunction with poor posture and associated increased muscle tension predisposing to cervical and/or cranio-facial somatic and neurogenic dysfunction. He does present with a typical 'postural' pattern where his symptoms are better in the morning, increase through the day and appear related to his tiredness. Therefore posture, muscle tone, length and control will all need to be carefully assessed in the physical examination.

Neurologist: With this new information I would now consider a referral to an ear,

nose and throat specialist.

House doctor: Neurotic patient? I'm surprised at the detailed information this patient has provided. I don't see these kind of patients.

Psychologist: No change to my previous thinking.

Question 2. What further information would you like at this stage?

Orthodontist: In addition to my answer from the previous section, I would like to have radiography results of the sinus maxillaris from the ENT examination.

Dentist: History.

Physiotherapist: Yes, given what he has already said about his mental pressure, over the next couple of appointments I will try to find out more about his general lifestyle, the effect his problem has on it and in particular his understanding and feelings about all this. I would also like to know the specialist's diagnosis.

Neurologist: History of his symptoms and therapy until now.

House doctor: History of his problem.

Psychologist: What coping strategies does he have. Also, how does he perceive his complaints, I mean his emotional appraisal of the aforementioned complaints?

Question 3. What sources do you think are implicated?

Orthodontist: Muscles, sinuses, teeth and occlusion (in the sense of parafunctional habits such as clenching and their effect on the symptoms).

Dentist: Sinus frontalis, sinus maxillaris, and sinus ethomoidalis.

Physiotherapist: Since mechanical pressure on his head gives him relief and rotation and bending affect his symptoms, this would fit with a nociceptive or peripheral neurogenic problem:

- nociceptive: cranium – nasofrontal, dura, cranial blood vessels, TMJ, upper cervical spine
- peripheral neurogenic: trigeminal nerve (maxillaris nerve), intracranial.
- sympathetic nervous system (hypothalamus is bedded in sella tursica of sphenoid bone and can be affected by cranial dysfunction with hormonal/neurotransmitter links to the central and sympathetic nervous system)
- affective: stress, fear.

Neurologist: Olfactory bulb disturbance.
House doctor: Neurogenic.
Psychologist: Patient's further reference to 'mental pressure' and 'mental stress' highlights the likely role this is having in his problem.

Question 4. What are your thoughts about prognosis so far?

Orthodontist: If not an isolated sinus problem, help could come from splint therapy, physiotherapy and stress management.
Dentist: Good.
Physiotherapist: The potential affective stress-related component is a relatively negative prognostic indicator. Also, the skull and associated tissues, if involved, may require a longer time to heal.
Neurologist: Good prognosis.
House doctor: Not clear, need more information.
Psychologist: I would need more information to comment on prognosis.

Question 5. What factors do you think could be contributing to maintaining this man's problem?

Orthodontist: In addition to my previous

thoughts I would now also consider an ENT problem.
Dentist: Chronic sinus inflammation.
Physiotherapist: Increased muscle tone and/or insufficient muscle control are potential contributing factors to increased cervical and craniofacial dysfunction. Stress and other psychosocial factors may also be contributing factors either via central pain mechanisms or through their potential effects on the muscular, immune and neuroendocrine systems.
Neurologist: No change to previous thoughts.
House doctor: No change to previous thoughts.
Psychologist: No change to previous thoughts that stress is the most likely contributing factor.

Question 6. Given the information you now have, what do you feel needs to be examined and what are your thoughts on treatment at this stage?

Orthodontist: No change to previous thoughts.
Dentist: X-ray and examination by ENT specialist. Treatment of antibiotics and flushing of sinuses.
Physiotherapist: No new structures have been implicated for assessment by this additional information. However, TMJ dysfunction is now considered less likely since there are no apparent masticatory problems, although the TMJ will still need to be examined for confirmation. The cranium itself (i.e. craniofacial tissues and sinuses), local muscles, cervical spine and neural tissues (function and neurodynamics) must be examined, with consequent reassessment of all symptoms. There is now further support for potential cognitive/affective dysfunction which highlights

that, in addition to any physical measures that may be used in treatment, a broader overall pain management approach will be required where explanation, patient education and stress management feature strongly.

Neurologist: No change to previous thoughts regarding assessment or management.

House doctor: Thoughts unchanged.

Psychologist: Thoughts unchanged.

In screening questioning regarding general health and other questions that may alert the clinician to the need for caution, the following information was obtained:

- General health (e.g. heart, lungs, any form of arthritis, diabetes, neurological conditions, etc.) – no apparent present or past disorders.
- Spinal cord or central nervous system involvement (bilateral pins and needles and/or gait disturbance) – no apparent disorder.
- VBI dysfunction (dizziness, dysarthria, dysphagia, diplopia, drop attacks, nausea) – no apparent disorder.
- Medications – presently on antibiotics, 300 mg of difantoine (anti-convulsant – standard medication following cranial surgery) a day and paracetamol for pain as needed. Has never required blood thinners or any form of steroids.
- Medical investigations include X-ray (no apparent disorder) and nasofrontal CT scan (revealed 1.8 cm cyst pressing on frontal lobe). Blood/rheumatalogical tests negative.
- Familial factors – no relevant family history.

Subjective examination/patient interview regarding history of patient's symptoms

Physiotherapist: Can you tell me when these problems started?

Patient: Well, 3 months ago I had brain surgery.

Physiotherapist: Why?

Patient: I had an abscess in my brain.

Physiotherapist: Do you know exactly where it was?

Patient: It was in the frontal part of the right half of my brain.

Physiotherapist: Do you know what caused the abscess?

Patient: I had a chronic cold or sinusitis for the past 5 years. As I understand it, since I never had the sinusitis treated with antibiotics, the bacteria dug a hole in my skull and moved into my brain.

Physiotherapist: Before the operation, having the sinusitis, did you ever have any of the symptoms you have now?

Patient: No.

Physiotherapist: When did you decide to see a doctor?

Patient: Well that was about 4 months ago. The doctor told me to see an ENT specialist and a neurologist.

Physiotherapist: What was the diagnosis after the consultation with the specialists?

Patient: The ENT specialist put me on antibiotics and the neurologist ordered a CT scan.

Physiotherapist: Do you know what the CT scan showed?

Patient: Yes, it showed there was a big cyst of 2 by 3 cm in my brain that attracted a lot of fluid. Therefore there was a lot of pressure on the right half of my brain.

Physiotherapist: At what moment did these symptoms begin, or did you suffer any other complaints?

Patient: At that time I had a headache

during my periods of sinusitis.

Physiotherapist: Was that the same headache as you have now?

Patient: No, it was a different headache. The headache I suffered then was on both sides of my head just above my eyebrows, although when I went into the hospital I wasn't having any headaches at the time, only a really stuffy nose and blocked sinuses. Oh, I suppose I should also mention I was also having some sort of change in character.

Physiotherapist: In what way did your character change?

Patient: I became aggressive and egotistic. I told everybody that I could do everything on my own and I didn't need any help from anyone. When somebody tried to help me with something I behaved very aggressively and violently. That is something I usually wouldn't do and therefore my friends started to think that there was something wrong with my brain.

Physiotherapist: What did the doctors do after they saw the results of the CT scan?

Patient: At first they treated me with antibiotics by infusion. This didn't work because within 2 weeks three more abscesses developed on my brain. They then decided to operate to take out the big abscess.

Physiotherapist: Did they operate through your skull or was it a laser surgery?

Patient: They had to go through my skull.

Physiotherapist: Can you show me where and how?

Patient: Yes, they drilled four holes in my skull right here..., here..., here..., and here in a square shape like this (see Figure 10.3). After they had sawed from hole to hole they took this piece of my skull out and went into my brain to take the big abscess out. When they got the abscess out, they put the piece of skull back and stitched my skin again.

Physiotherapist: You have a scar here on your nose as well, what caused that?

Patient: That scar is from an operation on my nose, a so-called septum correction.

Physiotherapist: Was that done at the same time as the abscess surgery?

Patient: Yes, they did them both together.

Physiotherapist: Wow, they did a lot.

Patient: Yes, they sure did.

Physiotherapist: OK, and what else did they do? You had surgery in this region as well (indicates medial, cranial side of the right orbit)?

Patient: Yes, during my nose operation they cleared the ethmoids on both sides of my nose too.

Physiotherapist: How was it with you after the operation? When did these symptoms start?

Patient: About a couple of weeks after the operation. I went home and the headache slowly started. First on a very low level but it became stronger with time.

Physiotherapist: So the headache started after the operation? Can you also say which of the following three started first? Was it your headache, the pressure in your nose or the burning pain in your cheek?

Patient: At first there was the headache, after that came the burning pain in my cheek but I'm not sure when the pressure in my nose started.

Physiotherapist: Now your complaints have been present for about two and a half months. Can you tell if there is any change in the level of your symptoms?

Patient: Well, the level fluctuates a bit through the day with my work but overall week to week it is staying the same.

Physiotherapist: So it's not getting worse?

Patient: No.

Physiotherapist: How about the change to your character you mentioned, has that improved at all?

Patient: Well, my wife and friends say I'm

not as aggressive but I still get agitated very easily and my wife thinks my personality is different than before all this started.

Physiotherapist: And your colds and sinusitis, are they better than before?

Patient: Yes, before my surgery when I suffered a cold it would take at least 2 weeks to go, now they're less severe and settle in just a couple of days.

Past history

Other than the chronic sinusitis problem he has no past history of spinal, TMJ or dental/orthodontic problems. Specific screening for congenital/developmental/behavioural factors that may influence cranial and orofacial development (e.g. normality of birth, congenital disorders, previous trauma, mouth breather, thumb sucker, etc.) reveals no relevant history.

Questions 1. What are your thoughts about this new information regarding the history of the patient's problem?

Orthodontist: Concerning my field, if there is even a minor occlusal problem a splint could help to decrease the burning pain in the region of the right zygomatic bone and assist in the overall stress management.

Dentist: Chronic frontal sinusitis and postoperative neuralgia.

Physiotherapist: Sources and pain mechanisms become clearer now with this additional information regarding the onset of his symptoms. His initial problems (i.e. sinusitis, a different sort of headache and changes in character) appear to have commenced as a combination of a chronic sinus infection and a central neurogenic disorder of the brain itself. While the character changes may be the direct result of the brain abscess, cognitive/affective

influences associated with the stress and frustration he now reports are also likely to be contributing to his symptoms. The postoperative problems (current headaches, nasal pressure, burning sensation and continued character changes) appear to be an iatrogenic combination of nociceptive and neurogenic involvement secondary to the cranial and sinus-nasal surgery with swelling-induced cranial hypomobility, muscle tension/poor control and possible cervical dysfunction.

Neurologist: Diagnosis changed to cerebral disorder, possibly a lobus frontalis pathology.

House doctor: Strange that pressure in his face relieves the complaints. Did he have a sinusitis, meningitis or encephalitis?

Psychologist: Character changes such as he describes are not uncommon with some frontal pathologies, I would like to see the surgeon's report. It is encouraging anyway that he is aware of these changes and comfortable to report them. I would want to explore these much further, especially the circumstances they manifest, the reactions of his wife and work colleagues and how he is presently coping with these changes.

Question 2. What further information would you like at this stage?

Orthodontist: Data concerning my field such as past history regarding the patient's occlusion and teeth. Will also need a thorough physical examination of the occlusion and teeth including functional analysis of the occlusion, inspection of the teeth and panoramic radiograph of the teeth.

Dentist: I would now want to conduct a physical assessment.

Physiotherapist: Information about morphological changes of the cranium and intracranial tissue such as blood vessels, dura and the brain. I would also like further information regarding the cause of his burning pain and his personality changes. I will discuss his character changes with him more over the next few appointments but a psychologist referral may be appropriate.

Neurologist: I would like to know more about the ENT specialist's examination and findings.

House doctor: I would like to know more about the neurosurgeon's assessment.

Psychologist: Dealing process (assimilation) with the surgery? Analysing his frustrated behaviour. Emotional strength – what stronger and weaker aspects of himself (relevant skill, capacities) can he bring forward? Also, lifespan areas: are there marital problems? More information is needed about the aforementioned stress at work. Does he fear something? Motivation and resistance: what are his motivating powers? In what way can his motivation (to better his situation) be improved and what resistance can be identified? What about his ability to set realistic goals?

Question 3. What sources do you think are implicated?

Orthodontist: Predominantly neurogenic in origin but muscles, occlusal and dental factors could amplify the central problem.

Dentist: The pressure pain in the nose region and the burning pain in sinus maxillaris region implicate involvement of the sinuses (i.e. frontalis, ethomoidalis, maxillaris and zygomaticum bone).

Physiotherapist: In addition to previous thoughts this latest information particularly implicates intracranial tissue (e.g. intracranial dura), craniofacial tissues and nervous system dysfunction (e.g. central

nervous system and trigeminal nerve).

Neurologist: Compression phenomenon of the olfactory tract and bulb within the basal forebrain as implicated by the personality changes.

House doctor: Neurogenic.

Psychologist: Organic but also psychosocial.

Question 4. What are your thoughts on prognosis now?

Orthodontist: I would expect all his symptoms to improve although he may well have continued sinus problems. Physiotherapy and an occlusal splint could help and improve his prognosis.

Dentist: No idea because of the onset of these complaints after the surgery.

Physiotherapist: The long history of morphological changes and the personality changes are both negative prognostic indicators although the hint of improvement in his character is encouraging. These will now need to be considered in light of his physical examination findings.

Neurologist: Good. Personality changes are somewhat better after the operation.

House doctor: The continued presence of post-operative symptoms is a negative indicator of prognosis.

Psychologist: While he needs further psychosocial assessment to determine his emotional strength and weakness, at this stage I would still say the prognosis is good.

Question 5. Have your thoughts regarding factors contributing to maintaining this man's problem changed at this stage?

Orthodontist: An inadequate muscular balance may be a factor. Also, this patient appears to need pain in his life. This would suggest central pain mechanisms are likely to be contributing to maintaining his pain.

Dentist: New infection of the sinuses, stress.

Physiotherapist: Personality changes and possibly the cognitive dysfunction as well as muscle control factors mentioned previously.

Neurologist: His mental changes so far.

House doctor: Post-encephalitis pattern. I would like to know what the neurosurgeon thinks.

Psychologist: He appears to have received an inadequate explanation of his problems thus far, which may well be contributing to his stress. Of course, it may also be that with his changes in personality and memory, an appropriate explanation was provided which he has not recalled.

Question 6. What would you examine and what are your thoughts now regarding management?

Orthodontist: Muscles, occlusion, teeth.

Dentist: Refer to ENT specialist, neurologist and physiotherapist. I would be hopeful that he would get a reduction of pain from manual therapy.

Physiotherapist: Hands on assessment and management: passive movement assessment and treatment as indicated of the cranium (e.g. nasofrontal palate); nervous system assessment and treatment via trigeminal nerve neurodynamic testing/mobilization as indicated; hands off assessment and management via further explanation of the sources and contributing factors to his symptoms with particular attention to the relationship between his feelings and pain (e.g. the effects of stress, anger, etc. chemically on levels of pain). Referral to psychologist or psychiatrist for assistance with coping strategies as needed.

Neurologist: Examinations that should be considered include an EEG and an MRI. Management should include anti-swelling medications and antibiotics.

House doctor: Treatment by a house doctor not useful in this phase. Consideration should be given to consultation with psychologist and return to neurosurgeon.

Psychologist: Psychosocial assessment (e.g. his emotional strength and weakness).

After the whole subjective examination

Question 1. What are your thoughts about how the patient's life has been affected by his problem?

Orthodontist: Maybe he has developed his physical problems as part of a special coping mechanism for his frustration. Hopefully now after his surgery, and with appropriate education and management, he will be able to reach a new turning point with a better understanding of his problems and more healthy feelings.

Dentist: Patient has chronic pain during effort and is obstructed by his short-term memory problem and his actual symptoms.

Physiotherapist: My feelings so far are that his personality changes and concentration disturbance affect him more than his facial pain. There is probably still an ongoing form of frustration together with ongoing nociceptive and peripheral neurogenic input. More information about his acceptance and social behaviour is needed in the next appointments.

Neurologist: Not really. He has made improvement since surgery. If his character changes are still present after a time, psychological consult would be advised.

House doctor: Patient seems strong yet hampered by his problem. My question is, how far is it really hampering him?

Psychologist: There is still much I would want to know in order to understand how this patient's life has been affected. For example:

1 Categorizing the stress factors. What factors increase the complaints and what stress factors (and possible problems) play an important part in life? How does he cope with stress factors and problems.
2 The meaning/impact of the complaint. What are his thoughts, feelings, emotions with respect to his complaints?
3 The function of the complaint. What habits, rituals or complaint circles are involved? What about the presence of secondary gain from these complaints?
4 (Self)-management of complaints. Does he feel responsible for his behaviour? What skills does he have to cope effectively with his complaints and what skills does he perceive are lacking?

Question 2. What are your thoughts about how the patient is feeling about the problem and how he is coping with the problem? Does this influence your thoughts regarding the pain mechanisms, which may be maladaptive?

Orthodontist: Patient is developing coping mechanisms by himself and appears quite prepared to receive help. In my view he is doing that very well, open and clear.

Dentist: Positive.

Physiotherapist: While this patient's craniofacial symptoms are likely to have both a nociceptive and peripheral neurogenic basis, his apparent psychological changes are also likely to have contributed to his pain presentation. There may already be a degree of centrally maintained pain, or at least his character changes present a risk of the pain mechanisms shifting into a central state, making them considerably more difficult to resolve.

Neurologist: The patient seems pre-occupied with his pre-surgery physical dysfunction or character changes which may be contributing to his present pain.

House doctor: He does not appear to be coping well at all.

Psychologist: Stress situation, dissatisfaction etc. about the surgery plays an important role that will influence his pain behaviour.

Summary of key findings from physiotherapy physical examination

Due to limitations in space, only key features of the physical examination are highlighted here. Other examinations not recorded can be presumed negative.

Symptoms present at the time of the physical examination included his headache (H) at an intensity of 4/10, his nose pressure (N) at an intensity of 4/10 and his burning cheek pain (B) with an intensity of 1/10.

Inspection: Slight lateral flexion of the head on neck to the right. This asymmetry was easily corrected and produced no change to any of his symptoms.

Assessment of patient's functional work position

In a simulated typing position with the head and neck in relative flexion (types looking at his hands), bilateral pressure to his skull simulating the squeezing that he reported eased his symptoms and produces an immediate decrease in the headache and nose pressure. Both symptoms return to the same level on release of the pressure. In contrast, when this functional position is maintained and various components of the position are systematically altered (e.g. positional changes to head on neck, neck on thorax, thoracic flexion/extension, lumbar flexion/extension, arms, knee extension and clenching teeth), there is no change to any symptoms.

Neurological examination (conduction tests)

- Lower motor neuron tests. No apparent disorder.
- Cranial nerve tests. No apparent disorder.
- Upper motor neuron tests. No apparent disorder.

Cervical physiological movements

Flexion
- Full flexion – normal range of movement with pulling sensation and upper to mid-cervical pain, right greater than left
- Upper cervical flexion – normal range of movement with sharp local upper cervical pain, right greater than left (not something he had felt before)

Extension
- Full extension – normal range of movement and symptom free
- Upper cervical extension – normal range of movement with sharp local upper cervical pain, right greater than left

Lateral flexion
- Full lateral flexion left and right – normal range of movement and symptom free

Rotation
- Normal range of movement and symptom free.

Soft tissue assessment

Standing and simulated work/typing posture
- Apparent shortening or increased tone of scapular elevators, glenohumeral internal rotators, scapular protractors, upper cervical extensors and mandibular elevators
- Apparent increased length of scapular depressors and retractors, glenohumeral external rotators and upper cervical flexors

Supine and prone
- Able to relax with encouragement, revealing normal tone and length of all muscle groups. Patient least aware and greatest difficulty relaxing upper cervical extensors and mandibular elevators.

Passive physiological intervertebral movements (cervical spine)

Occiput/C1
- Extension stiff bilaterally
- Flexion stiff bilaterally
- Lateral flexion right stiff compared to left
- Rotation right stiff compared to left.

Passive accessory intervertebral movements (cervical spine)

Unilateral postero-anterior movement over the right C1/C2 zygapophyseal joint
- stiff with sharp local pain (same as reproduced with upper cervical movements)

Unilateral postero-anterior movement over the right C2/C3 zygapophyseal joint
- stiff with local pain.

Neurodynamics: (√√means normal range and symptom free)

Right upper limb tension test 1

- Glenohumeral abduction√√, plus forearm supination√√, plus wrist and finger extension√√, plus glenohumeral lateral rotation√√, plus elbow extension – restricted 20° with pulling sensation through whole arm and an increase in headache and nose pressure to 6/10. Release of wrist and finger extension decreases all symptoms

Left upper limb tension test 1

- Normal range (full elbow extension) with only slight pulling in cubital fossa

Mandibular neurodynamic test

- Full cervical flexion – full range with a pulling sensation and upper to mid-cervical pain, right greater than left. When left cervical lateral flexion is added, the lateral flexion is restricted 50% eliciting a sharp local upper cervical pain and the patient's burning sensation in the cheek. Depression (opening) of the mandible and left mandibular lateral excursion added to this position elicit an increase in symptoms (headache increased to 4/10, nose pressure to 6/10 and burning in the cheek to 8/10) with a 50% reduction in the depression and lateral excursion movements compared to the same movements tested in neutral. When sensitizing movements to the right arm are added to the mandibular neurodynamic test, the combination of shoulder girdle depression and glenohumeral abduction further increase all symptoms

Slump test

- Full cervical flexion – full range with a pulling sensation and upper to mid-cervical pain, right greater than left.

When right knee extension is added to this position, the extension is restricted 20° and the movement elicits an additional pulling sensation in the right mandibular region, which is eased with the release of knee extension. In comparison, left knee extension is also restricted 20°, however, with this movement there is only the cervical pulling/pain and a pulling felt in the posterior knee region.

Passive accessory cranial movements

Occipital-frontal compression

- Headache and nasal pressure decrease

Left occiput–sphenoid junction

- Transverse movement to the right of the sphenoid – stiff compared to same movement on the right with increase in patient's headache
- Rotation to the right around a sagittal axis – normal movement with decrease in headache and nasal pressure
- Rotation to the left around a sagittal axis – normal movement with increase in headache and nasal pressure

Right occiput–sphenoid junction

- All movements normal range and no effect on symptoms

Occipital suture movements

- Normal mobility and no change to symptoms with any movements

Nasofrontal suture junction

- Longitudinal caudad – normal mobility with increase in nasal pressure
- Transverse to the left – restricted with decrease in nasal pressure and slight increase in burning sensation
- Postero-anterior pressure – normal mobility with increase in headache and nasal pressure but no change to burning sensation

Palate
- General bilateral distraction of maxillary bones – normal mobility with increase in nasal pressure and extreme increase (8/10) in burning sensation
- Longitudinal directed cranially of hard palate cephalad/cranial on the left maxilla – normal mobility with increase in headache and nasal pressure
- Longitudinal directed cranially of hard palate cephalad/cranial on right maxilla – normal mobility with increase in headache and nasal pressure and marked increase (9/10) in burning sensation.

Maxillofacial assessment

Temporomandibular joint mobility
- Normal range of movement in all directions except longitudinal directed caudally, slight restriction on the right TMJ producing a pulling discomfort in the right mandibular region. When the longitudinal was maintained and cervical flexion was added, the mandibular area pulling spread into the area in which the patient reports feeling the burning pain

Palpation
- Tender in area of temporalis, medial pterygoid, masseter and suprahyoid muscles

Resisted tests
- All normal

Occlusion
- No obvious occlusal dysfunction but marked wearing from bruxing apparent

Breathing pattern
- Mouth breather with hyperactivity of suprahyoids, scalenes, sternocleidomastoid and upper cervical extensors.

Reassessment following physical examination:
- Headache intensity 3/10, nasal pressure 4/10, burning sensation 4/10
- Inhalation improved with increased opening of right nostril
- Upper cervical flexion and extension still produced sharp local pain but less intense
- Neurodynamics: Right ULLT 1 – elbow extension now only limited 10° with same pulling through whole arm, but headache only 2/10
- Mandibular neurodynamic test – left lateral excursion still restricted 50%, but headache now 4/10, nasal pressure 4/10 and burning only 2/10.

First treatment:
Left occiput–sphenoid junction
- Transverse mobilization pressure to the right of the sphenoid for 2 minutes at a grade IV⁻ without increasing symptoms.
- Symptoms and signs unchanged
Technique repeated stronger (grade IV) and for 5 minutes.
- All symptoms decreased to 1/10
- Upper cervical flexion and extension unchanged
- ULTT 1 unchanged
- Mandibular neurodynamic test – left lateral excursion range improved with no increase to symptoms
- Transverse mobilization of left occiput–sphenoid junction less stiff with only slight increase to headache (2/10).

Conclusion: Support for a nociceptive component to the patient's symptoms with dysfunction apparent in cranial tissue mobility, upper cervical spine, upper quadrant muscle tone and upper quadrant neurodynamics. Ongoing assessment will need to explore further the patient's pain experience (i.e. his understanding, feelings and coping strategies for the effect these problems are having on his life), his awareness of posture, movement patterns, muscle tone and breathing pattern, and his overall muscle control including his lower quadrants. This initial decrease of symptoms following the physical examination and further improvement following cranial mobilization is encouraging and suggests further treatment to this area should be tried, with systematic inclusion of treatment to the other key signs. The patient was given a clear explanation of the clinician's assessment, including how his stress and frustration could be contributing to his symptoms. Early incorporation of self-management is considered essential for this patient.

Further management

There was ongoing discussion regarding the effect the patient's problems were having on his life and his feelings about these problems. Numerous issues were raised in these discussions, including: his fears about having a tumour in his head; his frustrations with the health profession until now; his frustrations with his character changes, including how he is addressing this and what other avenues are available for help in this area (e.g. consultation with a psychologist); his medications and what they were for; the physical dysfunction found in the physiotherapy examination and the purpose of the various treatment techniques; the concept of chronic pain and the importance of him sharing responsibility in the management. These discussions were aimed at understanding more fully this patient's pain experience and assisting in reducing any cognitive/affective components to his pain.

Ongoing manual therapy consisted of the systematic treatment and reassessment of cranial and facial tissue mobilization, upper cervical mobilization, cranial nervous tissue mobilization and postural awareness/re-education. Treatments were used to evaluate further and improve any nociceptive dysfunction in the respective tissues. The most significant improvements were obtained with techniques aimed to improve sphenoid and palate tissue mobility and mandibular and maxillary neurodynamic mobility and sensitivity.

Progress

This patient received a total of six treatments over a period of 1 month. The headache had decreased about 25% and the nasal pressure and burning sensation 50% by the third treatment. By this time the patient had become quite proficient at self craniofacial and neural mobilization, and was working on his postural correction and muscle relaxation techniques throughout his work day. He attributed most improvement to the nasofrontal palate manual therapy, simple respiratory techniques and self-mobilization. The headaches improved further when cranial nervous tissue mobilization techniques were added, and after six treatments the nose pressure and burning in his cheek had completely resolved and his headaches were significantly improved in intensity and frequency, now only being present once or twice a week when he was very busy and stressed at work. While he felt there was slight improvement in his character changes over this time, he was still aware of easily becoming agitated, continued memory problems and difficulty managing the stress at work. He had initially been reluctant to seek any additional assistance with these problems; however, the improvement he made with physiotherapy appeared to encourage him and at his last appointment he agreed to a referral to a psychologist.

Analysis of clinicians' reasoning

It is important to appreciate that the clinicians in this activity were shown a videotape of the patient examination conducted by a physiotherapist and then asked to answer the specific questions. This meant that clinicians were not allowed to follow the line of questioning they may have preferred to take and could not necessarily get answers to questions they would have asked, although they were given the opportunity to nominate additional information they would like to have.

This exercise highlights the importance of skilled clinical reasoning with thorough hypothesis generation and testing, care to avoid premature conclusions, metacognitive awareness of your own reasoning and limitations, and better multidisciplinary collaboration.

The first impression one gets in reading through this case study is the obvious difference in hypotheses considered by the respective clinicians. This should not be surprising, as research to date has repeatedly shown that the quality of our hypothesis generation is closely related to our organization of knowledge.[17,23–32] Each profession has its own unique knowledge base which, unfortunately, is sometimes so esoteric and poorly understood by the other professions that collaboration across professions is lacking and patients all too often suffer the consequences of mixed and confusing information. Nevertheless, by looking at this problem from their own perspectives these clinicians frequently made the classic error of reasoning – focusing only on their favourite hypotheses. This is a reasoning error which even experts have been shown to make,[3,6,10] with the risk being that hypotheses not mentioned may then not be tested for in subsequent inquiries or treatments. For example, while all clinicians considered from one to four different possible sources for the patient's headache, none clearly attempted to discriminate between the common types of headache, such as tension, migraine with aura, migraine without aura, cluster, headache associated with craniomandibular dysfunction, dural, neurogenic, chronic paroxysmal hemicrania, hemicrania continua and cervical,[33,34] despite being given the opportunity to nominate further information they would like to have.

An intracranial source was never even considered until the patient reported the history of his brain abscess, and subjective differentiating features such as the temporal pattern, presence of side shift and premonitory symptoms were never requested. When the breadth of hypothesis generation is limited and inquiries are not used to try to discriminate among the different possibilities, the risk of incorrect diagnosis and management increases. In some cases this error of reasoning is likely related to the clinician's insufficient organization of knowledge, where for others, well familiar with the common patterns of headache, it is more an error of incomplete hypothesis generation and lack of thoroughness.

Despite this general lack of thoroughness, most clinicians did demonstrate their use of hypothesis testing in their reasoning through their requests for further clarifying information. It would have been even more interesting had the clinicians been requested to justify their hypotheses. This can be a useful reflective exercise to reveal your own biases, as clinicians will commonly only identify the supporting evidence without consideration to any negating evidence or those features which may not fit with their favourite hypothesis. For example, in response to the third question following section 2 (p. 199), the physiotherapist rightly highlights supporting evidence of 'mechanical' features which incriminate a nociceptive or peripheral neurogenic source. While clinicians in this exercise were not requested to identify negating evidence, this can be another very useful exercise to improve your reasoning. For example, in this situation it is important to weigh up what appears to be mechanical factors, such as the increase in headache with forward bending or head movements and relief with squeezing of the skull, against what may be seen as less clearly mechanical factors, including the effect of tiredness, mental pressure and general effort. By directing attention to both supporting and negating evidence, clinicians can alert themselves to what may prove to be overlapping clinical patterns or subcategories of patterns they had not previously recognized.

Another inquiry strategy, which is useful to reduce the risk of missing key information, is to screen for common problems or associated symptoms and typical aggravating and easing factors. While each profession will have its own screening questions related to the clinical patterns they must be able to recognize, all clinicians should be familiar with screening questions pertaining to general health and safety (e.g. review of systems, unexplained weight loss, vertebrobasilar insufficiency, spinal cord, medications, investigations etc.), and questions which will alert them to risk factors, or 'yellow flags' for long-term disability and work loss. Some examples of yellow flags include attitudes and beliefs about pain – such as pain is harmful, emotions such as fear of increased pain and depression, behaviours such as total activity avoidance, compensation issues, family responses such as over-protection, work requirements and employer support.[35]

On several occasions through this case study, judgements were made which seemed premature. For example, while most clinicians appeared to recognize the potential relevance of the patient's stress, frustration and character changes, the use of labels such as 'congenital narcissism', 'neurotic patient' or statements that the patient 'needs pain in his life' can be risky if these statements are made as conclusions as opposed to hypotheses. Insufficient knowledge in a particular area (e.g. psychology) can lead to hypotheses or even conclusions being made on insufficient information. While all clinicians will have areas where their knowledge will be lacking, the best safeguard to this unavoidable limitation is to have good metacognitive skills. In this case, metacognition of what you know and what you do not know is essential. It will assist you to avoid premature and unfounded conclusions and importantly will encourage your further acquisition of such knowledge and prompt your consultation with other health professionals. Such metacognitive awareness was evident in the clinicians' reasoning through this case each time they identified the need for referral to another professional, and where one clinician openly acknowledged not seeing these kinds of patients.

As you would expect from an initial patient examination, diagnostic reasoning was the dominant reasoning strategy underlying the physiotherapist's line of questioning and also evident in the clinicians' responses. This is in part due to the nature of the questions posed to the clinicians, which were diagnostically oriented towards sources and contributing factors, but is also consistent with the diagnostic emphasis of medical reasoning in general.[36] Interactive reasoning, which can range from apparent socializing to build rapport to specific questions regarding the effect the problem is having on the patient's life, including the patient's understanding and feelings about the problem, would have been more apparent through the subsequent management as evidenced by the physiotherapist's report regarding ongoing discussions of this nature. Nevertheless, the clinicians' responses to the final two questions regarding the effect on the patient's life and his feelings and ability to cope clearly illustrate they were thinking along these lines.

Similarly, narrative reasoning and teaching as reasoning could be expected to be used more during treatment sessions where for example, education was clearly a key component of the physiotherapist's management.

Collaborative reasoning, or shared decision making between clinician and patient, is essential to engender patient responsibility in rehabilitation. Had the physiotherapist pushed the patient into a psychological consult before he was ready, the likely benefit would have been diminished. Rather, by discussing this issue with the patient but waiting until the patient could see for himself the potential benefits, a shared decision was reached, increasing the likelihood of success.

This particular case was especially useful in that it highlights the value of a multidisciplinary approach which patients with ongoing pain states often need. The reasoning of any of these clinicians on their own would clearly not be as complete as their collective thoughts. Similarly, the mixed messages a patient would receive had they visited each clinician separately highlights the importance of adopting a common language for explaining pain to patients. Clinicians must continually strive to improve their organization of knowledge to at least be aware of clinical patterns recognized by their colleagues in other health professions. This in turn will promote

greater health-care collaboration between patient and the respective health providers.

This case also nicely demonstrates the importance of being alert to yellow flags in the clinical presentation, which should warn the clinician of the patient's risk of long-term disability and work loss. This requires a basic understanding of pain science, including the clinical patterns of not only common musculoskeletal syndromes, but also of pain mechanisms and strategies for altering management according to the balance of those mechanisms. A predominantly mechanical, nociceptive disorder such as dysfunction of the craniofacial tissues, upper cervical spine, TMJ, or teeth will respond to appropriate mechanical corrective measures. On the other hand, when an element of central pain is present or if it becomes dominant, then such traditional hands-on treatment is not only ineffective but may well contribute to the maintenance of the patient's pain. In this case study there was clearly a component of nociceptive dysfunction which was helped by manual treatments. However, the patient also appeared to have a component of central cognitive/affective dysfunction which, despite the improvement in the physical dysfunction, was still present and may well be contributing to the residual headaches as well as the continued affective and behavioural changes. Education and self-management were instigated from the start with this patient, which are essential for him to understand and accept responsibility for his recovery. This, combined with thorough reasoning, including attention to those aspects of his problem which had not changed sufficiently and a metacognitive awareness of his own limitations in addressing cognitive/affective dysfunction, led the physiotherapist eventually to succeed in encouraging this patient to seek further help.

Lastly this case study illustrates the need for all clinicians to be prepared to recognize their biases and challenge their assumptions. We all need occasionally to reformulate our representation of how we perceive a problem, and open discussion or comparison of reasoning, as attempted with this case study, is one way of prompting ourselves to consider alternative views.

References

1 Nickerson, R. S. (1987). Why teach thinking? In: *Teaching Thinking Skills: Theory and Practice* (J. B. Baron and R. J. Sternberg, eds), pp. 27–37. W.H. Freeman and Company.

2 Higgs, J. and Jones, M. (1995). Clinical reasoning. In: *Clinical Reasoning in the Health Professions* (J. Higgs and M. Jones, eds), pp. 3–23. Butterworth-Heinemann.

3 Jones, M. (1992). Clinical reasoning in manual therapy. *Phys. Ther.*, **72**, 875–884.

4 Jones, M., Jensen, G. and Rothstein, J. (1995). Clinical reasoning in physical therapy. In: *Clinical Reasoning in the Health Professions* (J. Higgs and M. Jones, eds), pp. 72–87. Butterworth-Heinemann.

5 Gifford, L. S. and Butler, D. (1997). The integration of pain sciences into clinical practice. *J. Hand Ther.*, **10**, 86–95.

6 Elstein, A. S., Shulman, L. S. and Sprafka, S. S. (1978). *Medical Problem Solving: an Analysis of Clinical Reasoning.* Harvard University Press.

7 Lesgold, A., Rubinson, H., Feltovich, P. *et al.* (1988). Expertise in a complex skill: diagnosing x-ray pictures. In: *The Nature of Expertise* (M. T. J. Chi, R. Glaser and M. Farr, eds), pp. 311–342. Lawrence Erlbaum Associates Inc.

8 Feltovich, P. J., Johnson, P. E., Moller, J. H. and Swanson, D. B. (1984). LCS: the role and development of medical knowledge in diagnostic expertise. In: *Readings in Medical Artificial Intelligence: The First Decade* (H. G. Schmidt and M. L. DeVolder, eds), pp. 275–319. Addison-Wesley.

9 Voytovich, A. E., Rippey, R. M. and Suffredini, A. (1985). Premature conclusions in diagnostic reasoning. *J. Med. Educ.*, **60**, 302–307.

10 Ramsden, E. L. (1985). Basis for clinical decision making: perception of the patient, the therapist's role, and responsibility. In: *Clinical Decision Making in Physical Therapy* (S. J. Wolf, ed.), pp. 25–60. F.A. Davis.

11 Glaser, R. and Chi, M. T. H. (1988). Overview. In: *The Nature of Expertise* (M. T. J. Chi, R. Glaser and M. Farr, eds), pp. xv–xxviii. Lawrence Erlbaum Associates Inc.

12 Flavell, J. (1979). Metacognition and cognitive monitor-ing: a new area of cognitive-developmental inquiry. *Am. Psychol.*, **34**, 906–911.

13 Nickerson, R. S., Perkins, D. N. and Smith, E. E. (1985). *The Teaching of Thinking.* Lawrence Erlbaum Associates Inc.

14 Mezirow, J. (1990). *Fostering Critical Reflection in Adulthood: a Guide to Transformative and Emancipatory Learning.* Jossey-Bass Publishers.

15 Bordage, G. and Allen, T. (1982). The etiology of diagnostic errors: process or content? An exploratory study. In: *Proceedings of the 21st Annual Conference of Research in Medical Education*, pp. 171–176. American Association of Medical Colleges.

16 Bordage, G. and Zacks, R. (1984). The structure of medical knowledge in the memories of medical students and general clinicians: categories and prototypes. *Med. Educ.*, **18**, 406–416

17 Bordage, G., Grant, J. and Marsden, P. (1990). Quantitative assessment of 'diagnostic' ability. *Med. Educ.*, **24**, 413–425.

18 Jones, M. (1995). Clinical reasoning and pain. *Man. Ther.*, **1**, 17–24.

19 Mattingly, C. (1991). What is clinical reasoning? *Am. J. Occ. Ther.*, **45**, 979–986.

20 Mattingly, C. and Fleming, M. H. (1994). *Clinical Reasoning: Forms of Inquiry in a Therapeutic Practice.* F.A. Davis.

21 Benner, P. (1991). The role of experience, narrative, and community in skilled ethical comportment. *Adv. Nursing Sci.*, December, 1–21.

22 Edwards, I., Jones, M. Carr, J. and Jensen, G. M. (1998). Clinical reasoning in three different fields of physiotherapy – a qualitative study. In: *Proceedings, Fifth International Congress, Australian Physiotherapy Association*, Hobart, Tasmania, May 11–15.

23 Barrows, H. S., Norman, G. R., Neufeld, V. R. and Feightner, J. W. (1982). The clinical reasoning of randomly selected physicians in general medical practice. *Clin. Invest. Med.*, **5**, 49–55.

24 Norman, G. R., Tugwell, P. and Feightner, J. W. (1982). A comparison of resident performance on real and simulated patients. *J. Med. Educ.*, **57**, 708–715.

25 Patel, V. L. and Groen, G. J. (1986). Knowledge-based solution strategies in medical reasoning. *J. Cogn. Sci.*, **10**, 91–108.

26 Patel, V. L. and Groen, G. J. (1991). The general and specific nature of medical expertise: a critical look. In: *Toward a General Theory of Expertise: Prospects and Limits* (A. Ericsson and J. Smith, eds), pp. 93–125. Cambridge University Press.

27 Grant, J. and Marsden, P. (1987). The structure of memorized knowledge in students and therapists: an explanation for 'diagnostic' expertise. *Med. Educ.*, **21**, 92–98.

28 Grant, J. and Marsden, P. (1988). Primary knowledge, medical education and consultant expertise. *Med. Educ.*, **22**, 171–172.

29 Bordage, G. and Lemieux, R. (1991). Semantic struc-

tures and 'diagnostic' thinking of experts and novices. *Acad. Med.*, **66**, S70–S72.

30 Elstein, A. S., Shulman, L. S. and Sprafka, S. A. (1990). Medical problem solving: a ten year retrospective. *Eval. Health Prof.*, **13**, 5–36.

31 Schmidt, H. G. and Boshuizen, H. P. A. (1993). On acquiring expertise in medicine. *Educ. Psychol. Rev.*, **5**, 205–221.

32 Arocha, J. F., Patel, V. L. and Patel, Y. C. (1993). Hypothesis generation and the coordination of theory and evidence in novice 'diagnostic' reasoning. *J. Med. Decision Making*, **13**, 198–211.

33 Jull, G. (1997). Management of cervical headache. *Man. Ther.*, **2**, 182–90.

34 Merskey, H. and Bogduk, N. (1994). *Classification of Chronic Pain, Descriptions of Chronic Pain Syndromes and Definitions of Pain Terms*, 2nd edn. IASP Press.

35 Kendall, N. A. S., Linton, S. J. and Main, C. J. (1997). *Guide to Assessing Psychosocial Yellow Flags in Acute Low Back Pain: Risk Factors for Long-Term Disability and Work Loss*. Accident Rehabilitation and Compensation Insurance Corporation of New Zealand and the National Health Committee.

36 Elstein, A. S. (1995). Clinical reasoning in medicine. In: *Clinical Reasoning in the Health Professions* (J. Higgs and M. Jones, eds), pp. 49–59. Butterworth-Heinemann.

11

Pain management in patients with chronic craniofacial pain

F. A. M. Winter

Introduction

In cases of craniocervical and craniofacial pain one is usually talking about a range of pain complaints. The use of the muscles involved in chewing and of the mandibular joint may be painful and lead to limited movement. Besides this there are also more general complaints about pain such as headache, facial pain, neck and shoulder pain and stiffness. Also, specific complaints are sometimes mentioned such as grinding or clenching of the teeth (bruxism), clicking or popping noises, buzzing in the ears, earache, painful nose, eyes, mouth, throat and problems with balance.

Pain complaints form a complex problem, where physical and psychosocial factors eventually affect each other. It is desirable to distinguish the different aspects which affect the complaints, so that they can be given consideration in an integrated treatment (see also Chapter 8). A case history of a whiplash patient may clarify the complexity of the problem.

Both the way the psychosocial discipline is introduced and the way, in which the psychologist goes to work determine the good outcome of an integrated treatment.

A patient has serious neck and facial pain and memory and concentration problems after a whiplash incident. She can no longer adequately perform her tasks and needs help. This change is frustrating for her and her family and the necessary adjustments to the new situation are not being made.

She can only ask for help with difficulty, but does expect that the family will sense her needs and help. This does not happen and the patient becomes rebellious and depressive. She does not understand how her family can ignore her like this, when she has always been available for everyone. However, the family responds that the only possible help can be from a psychiatrist. The patient feels this is wrong: she has no complaints as a result of psychiatric problems, the complaints are the result of a car accident, which besides physical complaints has also caused psychological problems.

After consultation with a dentist he refers her to a clinic specializing in temporomandibular dysfunction (TMD). It is apparent that a big change to her jaw has occurred. For the first time she feels she is being taken seriously. Additionally, she is prescribed earplugs, with which she can cut out much 'noise' (undesirable sounds from the surroundings) and thus is able to follow conversations better. Thanks also to discussions with a psychologist she is more able to accept her complaints, communicates adequately and paces her activities better.

An integrated therapy, where the physical and the psychosocial aspects of the problem are dealt with adequately, appears able to break through the impasse she had reached.

Introduction of the psycho-social discipline

The patient presents with a physical problem. It is only from the perspective of this primary premise and subject to this premise, that a psychologist can be engaged. A referral is doomed to failure if the conclusion is drawn that the complaints are psychological in origin, and that for this reason a referral to either a psychologist or psychiatrist is necessary. It is possible to motivate most patients towards psychological help so long as this discipline is introduced in an acceptable manner.

A medical specialist can explain that the pain cannot solely be ascribed to a clearly physical factor, but that a dysfunction has probably developed whereby different factors maintain and exacerbate the complaint. For a long time it has been supposed that a nociceptive stimulus is the only cause for primary hyperalgesia after damage or infection. It has taken many studies and much research to show that changes resulting from damage at molecular, biochemical and physiological levels lead to functional changes in the nervous system.[1] These changes generate secondary hyperalgesia, even when nociception (actual or threatening tissue damage) is no longer a consideration.

What is needed, then, is pain medication,

physiotherapy, stress management and relaxation exercises to break the pain cycle. Correctly introduced, the psychologist can legitimately look at the psychosocial situation and the stress factors which play a role in it.

A cognitive-behavioural approach

Cognitions, emotions and behaviours and their mutual feedback systems all exercise their influence on stimulus sensitivity in general and on pain in particular.

Minimization (reduction in sensitivity to stimuli) or intensification (increase in stimulus sensitivity) is not dependent on the duration and intensity of the stimuli alone. Among others, the following affect long-term craniofacial pain:

- The constitution of the person. Does he feel rested, relaxed and in a fit condition, or tired, tense and weakened?
- The situation. Does it involve isolation, loss of purpose and depression or is the person in a cheerful frame of mind?
- Cognition, the way the person interprets the situation. Does he think, 'Where will this lead? I'm becoming an invalid. I'm a burden to my family. I am powerless, the doctor has to help me' or, 'I can cope with this, I can improve my situation'.
- Behaviour. Silence, sighing, complaining, denial, avoidance, restlessness, medical shopping around, versus making needs known, taking purposeful action, alternate relaxation and effort.

There is a connection between the type of stimulus and the degree of arousal. A stimulus causes more arousal when it is unexpected, new and with emotional content.[2] Chronic pain often changes in intensity in a manner that is unpredictable for the patient (unexpected), is therefore experienced differently each time (new) and, seeing the feelings and the limitations caused by the pain, is very emotionally charged. Chronic pain, therefore, causes heightened arousal. Chronic pain is also often associated with anxiety, which causes nervous tension (arousal), leading to a heightened stimulus sensitivity (intensification, Figure 11.1).

Arntz and Peters[3] researched the connection between anxiety-generated arousal and pain in the laboratory. They found no connection between anxiety and pain. This may be for two reasons:

1 The connection between arousal and stimulus sensitivity is not a straight-line relationship. Only where there is a 'normal' level of arousal is there a straight-line relationship between the strength of the stimulus and awareness. High and also low arousal lessen the stimulus sensitivity. Low arousal is a situation of safety and trust, where one is less alert and thus observes and feels less. High arousal is a situation where intense fight/flight reactions are expected. Here one is so focused on survival rather than observation that the stimulus sensitivity is clearly reduced.

2 Besides arousal, attention especially influences stimulus sensitivity.[4] The gate theory is based on the principle that the various stimuli jostle for priority and so cannot be recognized equally well.

High arousal with attention to personal feelings increases the stimulus sensitivity, high arousal and attention focused outwards (onto situations or the environment)

lowers the stimulus sensitivity.[5]

Optimal arousal is necessary for learning and for therapy. Too low or too high arousal interrupts the learning process. Too low arousal means too little information will be absorbed due to a shortage of attention and thus a limited learning effect. Too high arousal with a lot of stress can even lead to complete amnesia, as the experience is overwhelming and traumatic. Cognitive-behavioural therapy thus serves to lower the arousal and at the same time ensures that attention is focused on elements of self and others which are stimulating and satisfying to the patient, and on tasks and challenges. Lowering of arousal takes place through relaxation exercises, good communication and the confidence that the patient receives in his own possibilities, enabling him to exert influence on the situation.

> A whiplash patient feels useless and worthless. She becomes increasingly irritable and emotional. She avoids social contacts outside the family due to anxiety that others will consider her stupid. She notices that her isolation makes her lonely. Thanks to the therapy she is better able to relax and she gets more rest. She notices that this enables her to concentrate better and that the greater inner peace further increases her concentration and her ability to listen. She absorbs information offered better and her memory improves. Her self-confidence improves as a result.
> She was very scared of being seen as a complainer, or as being weak. She learns to discuss her limitations in a balanced manner and she discovers support and understanding in place of the feared rejection. She breaks through her isolation. There are more distracting activities in her life and she functions better in her family as a result.

Whenever a pain patient concentrates exclusively on the pain, the pain is not only

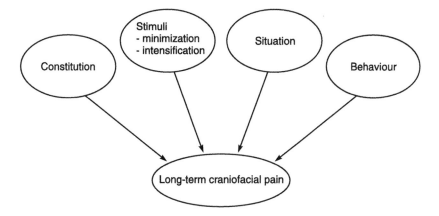

Figure 11.1 Minimization and intensification. Possible predisposing factors for long-term craniofacial pain

perceived in all its intensity, but is made even worse. Pain is worsened both by focusing attention on the pain, and by the quality of the attention. The pain is increased especially if the attention given to it is coloured by negative emotions, by feelings of anxiety, rebellion, depression and anger. Pain is reduced by positive emotions, by humour, acceptance, feelings of competence and confidence. The cognitive-behavioural approach attempts, through changing cognition and behaviour, to change the attention and emotions around the pain so that the pain cycle – pain → anxiety and attention to the pain → more pain – can be broken.

Characteristics of the cognitive-behavioural approach

With chronic pain and orofacial complaints cognitive-behavioural treatment has a number of advantages. It is an approach that focuses directly on the complaint, generally does not last too long and is reasonably straightforward to evaluate. This approach has a number of specific characteristics, such as:

- a clear goal
- attention to registration and measurement
- self-assessment
- involvement of the patient's partner in the therapy
- attention to instructions, homework assignments and the learning of skills (relaxation techniques, social skills, assertiveness, etc.)
- attention to 'healthy' behaviour.

Clear goal

The patient believes that he has a serious physical sickness/ailment or aberration/disorder. He thinks that he will only be able to restart his normal way of life when the cause of the pain has been found and removed. The patient has the same goal as the clinician: to cure the ailment that causes the complaint.

It is important that the patient also has a personal goal – to function as well as possible, despite the ailment – in addition to the clinician's goal – to cure the ailment by finding the cause (diagnosis) and then its removal (prescription).

Table 11.1 A pain activity diary

Timetable: General base level

Day scheme – Example: lying down, sitting and standing or walking

Time	Lying	Sit	St/w	Activity
8.00			X	Toilet
8.30		X		Breakfast
9.00			X	Cleaning
9.30			X	Cleaning
10.00		X		Coffee
10.30			X	Vacuum
11.00	x			Relax
11.30			X	Housework
12.00		X		Lunch
12.30	x			Rest
13.00	x			Rest
13.30			X	Walking
14.00			X	Cleaning
14.30		x		Laundry
15.00	x			Tea
15.30			X	Walking
16.00	x			Relaxation
16.30			X	Cooking
17.00		x		Cooking
17.30		x		Dinner
18.00	x			Relaxation
18.30	x			Relaxation
19.00			X	Wash
19.30		x		Coffee
20.00			X	Walking

Day scheme: how I want to do it

Time	Lying	Sit	St/w	Activity
8.00				
8.30				
9.00				
9.30				
10.00				
10.30				
11.00				
11.30				
12.00				
12.30				
13.00				
13.30				
14.00				
14.30				
15.00				
15.30				
16.00				
16.30				
17.00				
17.30				
18.00				
18.30				
19.00				
19.30				
20.00				

Day scheme: what I did

Time	Lying	Sit	St/w	Activity
8.00				
8.30				
9.00				
9.30				
10.00				
10.30				
11.00				
11.30				
12.00				
12.30				
13.00				
13.30				
14.00				
14.30				
15.00				
15.30				
16.00				
16.30				
17.00				
17.30				
18.00				
18.30				
19.00				
19.30				
20.00				

Base level specific

Activity	Mon	Tues	Wed	Thur	Fri	Sat	Sun
Walking							
Cycling							
Sport							

Measurement of pain

Measurement is particularly important, because chronic pain is difficult to locate (see also Chapter 8). There is a lot of pain without its source being clearly apparent. The clinician has to rely totally on 'subjective' information from the patient. Too often healthcare providers use the vague general term 'low pain threshold' as a euphemism for oversensitivity. The patient's complaints should be regarded as real and serious.

If pain is not allowed or is not appropriate, if pain is treated insufficiently, this causes much unnecessary anxiety and worry. The fact that pain can be and is allowed to be expressed has a calming influence on the patient.

```
   1 2 3 4 5 6 7 8 9

No Pain  I---I---I---I---I---I---I---I---I  Extreme Pain
```

Indicate what your pain was like during the last hour,

where 1 represents pain-free, 5 an average pain level

and 9 for extreme pain.

Figure 11.2 A visual-analogue scale

Regularly having the pain scored on a visual-analogue scale gives an impression of the intensity of the pain but also of the generally variable character of the pain (Figure 11.2).

Along with this a pain activity diary (Table 11.1) can be used. In this way one can note if the pain varies in intensity and which factors affect it.

Self-assessment

According to Bandura,[6] self-assessment is the best source of information leading to an expectation of self-efficacy. The concept of self-efficacy relates to the way in which individuals evaluate and direct their (psychosocial) functioning.

The patient thinks 'If I have less pain, I can do more'. His most important goal is thus to allow the pain to reduce, so that his load-bearing ability can increase. To allow the pain to reduce, he needs a doctor. This introduces him into a vulnerable, dependent situation. The behavioural-cognitive treatment tries to get the patient to think; 'If I can do more, I will have less pain'. His most important goal thus becomes to increase his load-bearing ability, so that the pain can be reduced. The patient himself can set this goal. He only needs instruction about which method will best take him towards his goal. The patient has to become his own clinician and for this reason also needs to carry responsibility for his therapy programme.

In the health service, initiative and a critical attitude from the patient is not always appreciated. Many clinicians and other medical staff believe they know what is good for their patient and therefore do not want to discuss it. Also, many patients still have a rather passive and dependent approach – the doctor is responsible for their healing and must determine what is good for them.

Partner

In a study by Funch and Gale,[7] social factors seemed to be the best predictor by far of the likelihood of continuing the therapy in instances of behavioural therapy relating to chronic craniofacial pain.

For treatment it is desirable that the partner, or other important person in the patient's life, supports the goals of treatment and is prepared to play a part. It is important to approach partners in the right manner and to motivate them to help in the therapy plan. The patient must become the clinician and the terminology that describes the essence of the partner's role is co-clinician.

It appears that partners often have difficulty in determining their own position towards the patient and, therefore, need information and guidelines. They can have all kinds of feelings, sometimes conflicting, such as powerlessness, annoyance, frustration and sympathy. If partners are given the opportunity to express and discuss these feelings, then it can also become clear how they react to the complaints and why they do so in that manner. Then one can discuss with them what the possible effects could be of their manner of reacting to the complaints.

Learning skills

If the patient wants to be his own clinician then he will need to implement a therapy programme with the necessary balance between effort, relaxation and leisure. To do this the patient must be able to adapt his environment to his abilities, or inabilities. A certain amount of assertiveness and good social skills are essential tools. A number of people are necessary to enable social skills and assertiveness to be taught. For this reason it is desirable to treat several patients at a time. Besides this practical reason, there are a number of advantages linked to treating patients in groups. The advantages of a group approach lie in the following areas:

- Efficiency. Chronic pain can take on epidemic forms. Individual treatment over long periods of time becomes too costly. Transferral of knowledge and instruction require less time when one is able to do this with more people at the same time.
- Motivation. It can be very motivational and stimulating to participate in a learning process together. This is apparent in such self-help groups as Alcoholics Anonymous (AA) and Weight Watchers. Ex-patients take care of after-care.
- Acceptance. Working in groups helps with learning to accept the connection between pain and lifestyle. For patients who have often fought alone for recognition of their complaints, it is encouraging to discover that they are not the only ones.

    Together you can brainstorm the information offered and the way to deal with it. You can practise together using role-play. You can give each other feedback. You can motivate each other and exchange thoughts about the homework assignments.

Attention to healthy behaviour

Generally, health care focuses itself on sick and unhealthy behaviour and tries to cure this. Too much attention to pain and its consequences can, however, have the wrong results. This is why it is better to determine carefully the patient's capabilities and then to build on these, rather than focusing on what he is not able to do. This means that healthy behaviour (well behaviour) by the pain patient particularly receives attention.

Traditional assistance is unfortunately still too focused on the discussion and recording of what is *not* going well, what the patient is not able to do. This leads to uncertainty. The emphasis on what the patient is able to do and on his successful experiences in systematically building on his abilities gives confidence and security.

An important aspect in this is acting at the appropriate time. Patients are inclined to allow medication, rest and assistance to be determined by the amount of pain. If they have a lot of pain they allow themselves rest, ask for attention and take their medication.

They hesitate to rest, take medication and ask for help unconnected and independent from the pain. A pain dependency develops, i.e. the pain and pain intensity determine what action is taken. It is clear that all kinds of operating mechanisms will influence the pain in this way. The patient needs to change his lifestyle, so that he himself creates a balance between effort and relaxation, and involves others in a predictable and satisfactory manner that is not dependent on pain. The family need to cooperate in this. People who are important in the patient's life in particular need to give their support and attention to the patient when things go well, and be less forthcoming when things go less well.

In many cases a multidisciplinary approach can break through the negative spiral – pain → reduced load-bearing ability → more pain etc. With chronic pain a short therapy programme can be effective. The ingredients here are gradually building up the load-bearing ability, relaxation exercises, homework assignments, including the partner in the therapy, and training in psychosocial skills. In this way the balance between load and load-bearing energy can be restored.

Therapeutic interventions

What are the loading factors with which the pain patient is confronted, and what can be done about this therapeutically?

Medical problems

Questions and uncertainty regarding diagnosis and prognosis. Anxiety and uncertainty regarding a dysfunctioning part of the body. Undesirable medical and therapy dependence.

Therapeutic intervention: through medical attendance, information about dysfunctions of the craniocervical and craniofacial area and the effects of abnormalities, fractures, dislocations, stiffness and arthritis.

Physical problems

Pain, tiredness and problems sleeping. Inability to achieve total muscle relaxation. Problems moving the neck and both mandibular joints. General loss of energy and condition.

Therapeutic intervention: relaxation exercises. Increasing the load-bearing time by gradually building energy and condition. Achieving a balance between effort and relaxation. Prevention of over/underloading.

Cognitive problems

Loss of concentration and reduced memory capacity. Habitual worrying, catastrophizing, negative self-image.

Therapeutic intervention: cognitive techniques to achieve more peace and trust. Concentration and attention exercises. Promoting a feeling of competence by developing a positive self-image. Replacing inadequate thought patterns with thinking constructively.

Emotional problems

Heightened irritability, moodiness, feelings of depression, anxiety and uncertainty. Problems with coping due to loss of work or important activities.

Therapeutic intervention: stress management and relaxation exercises with the goal of increased mental load-bearing ability.

Social and societal problems

Communication disorders, child rearing and relationship problems. Problems to do with work and finances. Benefits problems, loss of future perspective.

Therapeutic intervention: including the partner in the therapy programme, communication exercises and training in social skills. Advising patient in case of benefit problems.

Focus attention on social and recreational activities, so that the patient has more distraction and a purpose in his life.

The multidimensional approach to craniofacial pain seems to offer the best chance of reducing the complaints (Figure 11.3).

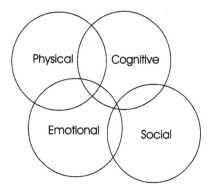

Figure 11.3 The multifactorial influences of long-term craniofacial and craniomandibular pain. Therapeutic intervention has to be of a multidimensional nature because of the overlapping of multifactorial influences

Subgroups

The character of the pain differs greatly from person to person. The question is, where does this patient have the most pain? Are tiredness and anxiety a source of tension? Are social relationships sufficiently satisfying, or is there talk of isolation, misunderstanding and hostility? What is the relationship between load and load-bearing capability? Can the patient cope with the demands that he is faced with at work or at home?

Next, the psychologist can make allowance for these various factors in the treatment. An interesting measuring instrument is the multidimensional pain inventory (MPI) (Table 11.2). This test can be part of a short test battery that gives a good picture of the way the patient experiences the pain, and what impact it has on the various life aspects.

Dworkin[8] suggests that patients with craniofacial and craniomandibular pain should, in particular, be classified on the basis of joint psychosocial and behavioural parameters. Irrespective of the somatic factors which play a role, patients can be asked how they experience their com-

plaints, how significant people in their environment react to their problems and in which way the (pain) complaints influence their daily activities. Then the clinician can adjust the treatment depending on the pattern of responses to these questions. All too often those giving the treatment start with a standard treatment which is based more or less on their own perceptions and experiences.

The MPI results in various patient profiles:

- Dysfunctional: patient indicates the pain has a major impact on daily functioning. The patient has no control over the intense, incapacitating pain. Patient has become emotionally vulnerable and can only perform a few activities.
- Interpersonally distressed: patient indicates being alone with the pain. Feels he is not understood, not supported and not helped.
- Adaptive coper: patient is managing quite well in all areas, despite the pain.
- Others: patients with characteristics of dysfunctional, interpersonally distressed, adaptive coper, and patients who cannot be classified in the three categories mentioned above.

In the therapy, the goal of the patients who are classified as dysfunctional or as interpersonally distressed is to learn skills and techniques so that they can start functioning despite the pain and can be cast as adaptive copers.

The emphasis with dysfunctional patients should be on stress management and building up the physical and mental load-bearing capacity. With the interpersonally distressed, much attention could be placed on communication skills. The way complaints are presented, the way help and understanding are requested apparently work against the patient's interests. The partner should be actively involved in the therapy.

Multimodal

If pain can be determined by a number of factors, then the pain can also be influenced in various ways. The treatment can thus consist of various active ingredients.

- Behavioural therapy helps if pain gets less attention.[9] Instead there is attention for 'well behaviour'. The benchmark level (the activity level where there is not yet any overloading) is determined as a result of accurate observation, and goals are formulated in a clear and safe manner. Daily observation charts and pain charts can play an important role here.
- Active exercise therapy helps by using light exercises to normalize the tone of the craniofacial and craniocervical regions. The patient is able to integrate the existing signals and feedback from other important parts of his body, in his consciousness. The emphasis thus lies on conscious and concentrated observation, so that the attention does not only go automatically to the pain sensations and the patient can also very consciously give other feelings a chance. This reduces pain.
- Systematic muscle relaxation and breathing therapy have a restful and pain-reducing effect. Learning systematically to relax the muscle system leads to the possibility of anxiety reduction. The fight-or-flight reactions become less and the parasympathetic nervous system can take care of building up and repair.
- Hypnosis helps if it goes together with deep relaxation and if this increases the receptiveness for suggestion focused on feelings of competence and being in control. Visualization of meaningful images in a safely administered manner can help to assimilate trauma, because they can provide a counterbalance against existing negative emotions and catastrophizing thoughts.
- Biofeedback helps when the patient gives information about muscle tension and the way in which this is induced – i.e. notices that he is able to influence the muscle tension and pain.
- Cognitive therapy helps when it shows the influence of thoughts and perceptions on emotions and behaviour. The way of thinking, the means of solving problems, can enable more peace, balance and creativity in approaching problems in general and pain problems in particular.[10]
- Stress management and improvement in communicative skills are helpful, because this is how the desirable and the possible are brought closer together and the pattern of expectations of the patient and his family becomes more realistic. This leads to a reduction in anxiety and uncertainty which has a positive effect on the experience of pain.

General advice for the clinician

- Empathy. The patient is anxious and unsure. Give the patient confidence by listening attentively.
- Control. Don't give the patient the idea that you will solve the problem.

Table 11.2 The Multidimensional Pain Inventory (MPI)

MPI questions	1	2	3	4	5

Pain severity
Rate the level of your pain at the present moment
On average, how severe has your pain been during the last week?

Interference
Since the time your pain began, how much has your pain changed
   your ability to work?
How much has your pain changed the amount of satisfaction or
   enjoyment you get from participating in social and recreational activities?
How much has your pain changed your ability to participate in
   recreational and other social activities?
How much do you limit your activities in order to keep your pain
   from getting worse?
How much has your pain changed the amount of satisfaction or
   enjoyment you get from family-related activities?
How much has your pain changed your relationship with your
   spouse, family, or significant other?
How much has your pain changed your ability to do household chores?
How much has your pain interfered with your ability to plan activities?
How much has your pain changed or interfered with your friendships
   with people other than your family?

Life control
During the past week how much control do you feel that you
   have had over your life?
During the past week how do you feel that you've been able to
   deal with your problems?
During the past week how successful were you in coping with
   stressful situations in your life?

Affective distress
Rate the overall mood during the past week
During the past week how irritable have you been?
During the past week how tense or anxious have you been?

Support
How supportive or helpful is your spouse (significant other) to you in
   relation to your pain?
How worried is your spouse (significant other) about you because of your pain?
How attentive is your spouse (significant other) to you because of your pain?

Punishing responses
Expresses irritation at me
Expresses frustration at me
Expresses anger at me

Solicitous responses
Asks me what he/she can do to help
Takes over my jobs or duties
Tries to get me to rest
Gets me some pain medications
Gets me something to eat or drink
Turns on the TV to take my mind off my pain

Distracting responses
Talks to me about something else to take my mind off the pain
Tries to involve me in some activity
Encourages me to work on a hobby

Household chores
Wash dishes
Go grocery shopping
Help with the house cleaning
Prepare a meal
Do the laundry

Outdoor work
Mow the lawn
Work in the garden
Work on the car
Wash the car
Work on a needed household repair

Social activities/activities away from home
Go out to eat
Play cards or other games
Go to a movie
Visit friends
Take a ride in a car or bus
Visit relatives
Take a trip
Go to a park or beach

Don't make the patient passive and dependent.

- Information. Explain to the patient the pain mechanisms[11] and the impact of chronic pain on functioning of muscles and joints. Give instructions, guidelines and exercises, enabling the patient to learn better to deal with his complaints.
- Controlled exercise. Let the patient exercise at fixed times and in fixed amounts – not when prompted by the pain.
- Distracting activities. Let the patient become aware of the influence of attention and emotions on the experience of pain. Create an exercise situation where the patient devotes his whole attention to the pain and painful movements, and a similar exercise situation where there is distraction.
- Well behaviour. Let the patient record when and how often he feels relatively well and has few or clearly less complaints than on average. Always start by asking what has gone well.
- Support. Let the patient find sources of support in his close environment. Invite the partner or significant other to be present at the therapy a few times.

Conclusion

It is clear that a careful pain diagnosis is the first priority in cases of pain problems relating to craniocervical and craniofacial complaints. On the basis of this diagnosis, attention can be given to different ways of combating pain and pain management. An integrated approach is required. Depending on the specific questions asked, certain forms of treatment can receive extra attention.

The common factor in the different forms of therapy is that they all contribute to restoring the balance between load and load-bearing ability. In cases of chronic pain problems it is good to plead for multiple convergence therapies, together with Melzack and Wall;[12] an integrated approach, where different disciplines work together towards recovery.

References

1 Dubner, R. and Basbaum, A. I. (1994). Spinal dorsal horn plasticity following tissue or nerve injury. In: *Textbook of Pain* (P. D. Wall and R. Melzack, eds), pp. 225–241. Churchill Livingstone.

2 Basbaum, A. I. (1996). Memories of pain. *Sci. Am. Sci. Med.*, Nov/Dec., 22–31.

3 Arntz, A. and Peters, M. (1990). Habituatie en pijnklachten. *Gedragstherapie*, **23**, 90–109.

4 Arntz, A. R. (1991). *Pain: Attention, Emotion, Prediction and Control*. Proefschrift Rijksuniversiteit Limburg.

5 James, J. E. and Hardardottir, D. (1993). *Tolerance to Acute Pain: Effects of Attention and Arousal*. 7th World Congress on Pain.

6 Bandura, A. (1977). Self-efficacy: toward a unifying theory of behavioural change. *Psychol. Rev.*, **84**, 300–321.

7 Funch, D. P. and Gale, E. N. (1986). Predicting treatment completion in a behavioural therapy program for chronic temperomandibular pain. *J. Psychosom. Res.*, **30**, 57–62.

8 Dworkin, S. F. (1995). Behavioral characteristics of chronic temporomandibular disorders: Diagnosis and assessment in temporomandibular disorders and related pain conditions. In: *Progress in Pain Research and Management*, Volume 4 (B. J. Sessle, P. S. Bryant and A. D. Raymond, eds), pp. 175–192. JASP.

9 Fordyce, W. E. (1976). *Behavioural Methods in Chronic Pain and Illness*. Mosby

10 Winter, F. A. M. (1995). Post-whiplashsyndroom, een integrale benadering. *NTTP*, **15**, 46–48.

11 Vernon, H., Steinman, I. and Hagino, C. (1992). Cervicogenic dysfunction in muscle contradiction headache and migraine: a descriptive study. *J. Manip Physiol. Ther.*, **15**, 418–429.

12 Melzack, R. and Wall, P. D. (1988). *The Challenge of Pain*. Penguin Books.

Clinimetrics for the clinician – the use of some indexes applicable in the craniocervical and craniofacial regions

G. Aufdemkampe

Introduction

During the last few decades, a wide variety of terms has been used to describe the attributes of the measurement process. According to Wright and Feinstein[1] names such as index, scale, instrument, score, factor, criteria, profile, system and stage have regularly been applied to the result that emerges from the measurement process. To avoid ambiguity, Feinstein[2] has suggested use of the term 'index', which has been preferred in clinimetrics, and this term will therefore be used throughout this chapter.

The advantage of using the term index as opposed to measurement is that an index can contain several (unrelated or related) measurements, thus providing a more complete representation of the patient's status, while the term measurement usually refers to a single variable. Technically, a single measurement can be seen as an index consisting of one variable.

Beside the terminological issue, there has been a shift towards concepts of health outcome measurement, quality of life, and quality of care measurement.[3–8] Whatever term or ideology is adhered to, two major principles appear to supersede all indexes. The first principle is how to choose an index and the second concerns the methodological or psychometric properties of the indexes. The European Research Group on Health Outcomes (ERGHO)[9] has published an ERGHO statement regarding 'Choosing a Health Outcome Measurement Instrument' which seems to apply to all indexes. It comprises five basic steps. First, match the index to your needs. This step concerns the level of observation (individual patient, group of patients or general quality and cost-effectiveness), the formulation of the aim (effect of intervention or descriptive assessment), context of interest (description of the domain of health in which there is interest), source(s) of information (patients, carers or doctors) and determination of the users of the specific information (patients, doctors or politicians etc.). Secondly, what is the aim or use of the index? The three principal uses are:

- indicator: measuring the situation at one point in time. The endpoint is descriptive

- comparison: relating differences at different points in time, such as before and after treatment
- assessment: besides measurement of outcome, the use of the information through feedback to the clinicians.

Thirdly, choose a condition-specific, dimension-specific or generic index:

- condition-specific indexes usually have a narrow focus with considerable detail in the area of interest
- dimension-specific indexes are focused on domains such as daily functioning or the disability level of the International Classification of Impairments, Disabilities and Handicaps (ICIDH)[10]
- generic indexes are directed towards general health, interactions between different conditions or populations, which may include healthy people.

Fourthly, one should consider the fact that most health measurement indexes are essentially evaluative or subjective as opposed to objective indexes such as those concerning length or gender.

Finally, one should not forget the patient. As indexes take time to complete, the quality of the information depends on the willingness of the patient to cooperate.

Methodological or psychometric properties of indexes

Several groups worldwide have established methodological or psychometric criteria to evaluate indexes.[11,12] The most commonly used criteria are internal consistency, intrarater and interrater reliability as criteria for reliability, and content/face, construct, concurrent, predictive validity and responsiveness as criteria for validity.

Internal consistency refers to the strength of the relationship between separate items in an index, and reliability refers to the repeatability of outcomes. Content or face validity refers to the theoretical concept of the index, whereas construct validity refers to the composition of the index. Concurrent validity refers to the association of outcomes of that specific index when compared to another index, usually seen as a 'gold standard'. Predictive validity refers to the capability of an index to forecast future events, and responsiveness refers to the ability to detect small changes. These criteria can be analysed by means of statistical procedures; however, these procedures are beyond the scope of this book.

Ideally, all methodological criteria of an index should be researched before it is applied in patient care or research. In reality this may not always be so. The book by Cole *et al.*[12] encompasses 60 indexes and research results concerning the reliability and validity of these indexes. Whenever possible, information concerning reliability and validity of the indexes in the following paragraphs will be given. As there appear to be a great number of indexes applicable in the craniocervical and craniofacial region and quite a few indexes specifically designed for this region, only some examples will be presented.

Condition-specific indexes

Condition-specific indexes are characterized by the fact that they concentrate on one specific condition or disease and nearly each specific condition or disease can be scored on such a specific index. Many of these condition-specific indexes can be found in Medline® or Cinahl®. For example, Benninger and Brent[13] have developed an index specifically for

Table 12.1 The Facial Disability Index

(Reformatted with permission of authors VanSwearingen and Bach, 1996, for publication and distribution)
Please choose the most appropriate response to the following questions related to problems associated with the function of your facial muscles. For each question consider your function *during the past month*.

Physical function
How much difficulty did you have keeping food in your mouth, moving food around in your mouth, or getting food stuck in your cheek while eating?

Usually did with: Usually did not eat because:
5 no difficulty   1 of health
4 a little difficulty   0 or other reason
3 some difficulty
2 much difficulty

How much difficulty did you have drinking from a cup?
Usually did with: Usually did not drink because:
5 no difficulty   1 of health
4 a little difficulty   0 or other reason
3 some difficulty
2 much difficulty

How much difficulty did you have saying specific sounds while speaking?
Usually did with: Usually did not speak because:
5 no difficulty   1 of health
4 a little difficulty   0 or other reason
3 some difficulty
2 much difficulty

How much difficulty did you have with your eye tearing excessively or becoming dry?
Usually had: Usually did not have tearing because:
5 no difficulty   1 of health
4 a little difficulty   0 or other reason
3 some difficulty
2 much difficulty

How much difficulty did you have with brushing your teeth or rinsing your mouth?
Usually did with: Usually did not have difficulty brushing or rinsing because:
5 no difficulty   1 of health
4 a little difficulty   0 or other reason
3 some difficulty
2 much difficulty

Social/well-being function
How much of the time have you felt calm and peaceful?
6 all of the time   5 most of the time
4 a good bit of the time   3 some of the time
2 a little bit of the time   1 none of the time

How much of the time did you isolate yourself from people around you?
1 all of the time   2 most of the time
3 a good bit of the time   4 some of the time
5 a little bit of the time   6 none of the time

How much of the time did you get irritable toward those around you?
1 all of the time   2 most of the time
3 a good bit of the time   4 some of the time
5 a little bit of the time   6 none of the time

How often did you wake up early or wake up several times during your nighttime sleep?
1 every night   2 most nights
3 a good number of nights   4 some nights
5 a few nights   6 no nights

10. How often has your facial function kept you from going out to eat, or participating in family or social activities?
1 all of the time   2 most of the time
3 a good bit of the time   4 some of the time
5 a little bit of the time   6 none of the time

Scoring:
Physical function
(Total score (questions 1–5) − N)/(N×100/4)
Social/well-being function
(Total score (questions 6–10) − N)/(N×100/5)
N: number of questions answered.

rhinosinusitis, the so-called Rhinosinusitis Disability Index. Another example of such a condition-specific index is the Facial Disability Index (FDI) as developed by VanSwearingen and Brach.[14,15] In their 1996 article, the authors state: 'Disorders of the facial neuromuscular system can result in marked disfigurement of the face and difficulties in activities of daily living such as eating, drinking and communicating. No systematic means of measuring the disability associated with facial nerve disorders exists'. This led VanSwearingen and Brach[14] to the development of the Facial Disability Index (Table 12.1).

The authors studied this index for internal-consistency reliability (theta reliability for physical function was 0.88 and theta reliability for social/well-being was 0.83) and construct validity of the two subscales of the FDI when compared to clinical measures and the patients' self-report of social well-being. The FDI physical function subscale correlated significantly with the clinical measures ($r_p = 0.51$, $P < 0.01$) and the FDI social/well-being subscale correlated significantly with the patients' self-report of social well-being ($r_s = 0.69$, $P < 0.01$).

The two subscales of the FDI did correlate significantly with each other ($r_p = 0.47$, $P < 0.01$).

Dimension-specific indexes

The Neck Disability Index will be described here.

The Neck Disability Index is an example of a dimension-specific index as it focuses on the disability domain of the international classification of impairments, disabilities and handicaps.

The Neck Disability Index (NDI) has been developed by Vernon and Mior[16] as a modification of the Oswestry Low Back Pain Index[17] (Table 12.2).

The face validity was ensured through peer review and patients' feedback. Internal consistency of the index appeared to be good (alpha = 0.80) and test–retest reliability was also good ($r_p = 0.89$). The construct validity appeared to be sufficient as the scores were normally distributed with the mode in the moderate category and the concurrent validity, when compared with scores on a visual analogue scale, was moderate ($r_p = 0.60$) and fair when compared with the McGill Pain Questionnaire total score ($r_p = 0.70$). Haines *et al.*[18] studied the internal consistency, which again appeared to be very good (Cronbach alpha = 0.92), and the common interitem correlation, which appeared to be moderate ($r = 0.53$). They further performed an exploratory factor analysis to determine if the NDI was unidimensional or multidimensional. The NDI appeared to be unidimensional. Finally, they performed a stepwise multiple regression to identify which variables best predicted the scores on a visual analogue scale for pain. Item 1 (multiple $r = 0.68$, $P < 0.0005$) and the total NDI score (multiple $r = 0.65$, $P < 0.0005$) best predicted the visual analogue scale scores. The NDI has been translated into several languages and has been used in several studies[19,20] which compared the NDI with the Patient-Specific Functional Scale.

Generic indexes

There are many generic indexes which could be used in the craniocervical and craniofacial and other musculoskeletal regions of the human body. Due to the large number of generic indexes, a clinician or researcher may be overwhelmed and needs to know which one to choose.

Table 12.2. The Neck Disability Index

(Reformatted with permission of authors Vernon/Hagino 1987, for publication and distribution)

This questionnaire has been designed to give the doctor information as to how your neck pain has affected your ability to manage in everyday life. Please answer every section and mark in each section only the ONE box which applies to you. We realize you may consider that two of the statements in any one section relate to you, but please just mark the one box which most closely describes your problem.

1. Pain intensity
☐ I have no pain at the moment.
☐ The pain is very mild at the moment.
☐ The pain is moderate at the moment.
☐ The pain is fairly severe at the moment.
☐ The pain is very severe at the moment.
☐ The pain is the worst imaginable at the moment.

2. Personal care (washing, dressing etc.)
☐ I can look after myself normally without causing extra pain.
☐ I can look after myself normally but it causes extra pain.
☐ It is painful to look after myself, I am slow and careful.
☐ I need some help but manage most of my personal care.
☐ I need help every day in most aspects of self care.
☐ I don't get dressed, wash with difficulty and stay in bed.

3. Lifting
☐ I can lift heavy weights without extra pain.
☐ I can lift heavy weights but it gives me extra pain.
☐ Pain prevents me from lifting heavy weights off the floor, but I can manage if they are conveniently positioned, for example on a table.
☐ Pain prevents me from lifting heavy weights, but I can manage light to medium weights if they are conveniently positioned.
☐ I can lift very light weights.
☐ I cannot lift or carry anything at all.

4. Reading
☐ I can read as much as I want to with no pain in my neck.
☐ I can read as much as I want to with slight pain in my neck.
☐ I can read as much as I want with moderate neck pain.
☐ I can't read as much as I want because of moderate neck pain.
☐ I can hardly read at all because of severe pain in my neck.
☐ I cannot read at all.

5. Headaches
☐ I have no headaches at all.
☐ I have slight headaches which come infrequently.
☐ I have moderate headaches which come infrequently.
☐ I have moderate headaches which come frequently.
☐ I have severe headaches which come frequently.
☐ I have headaches almost all the time.

6. Concentration
☐ I can concentrate fully when I want to with no difficulty.
☐ I can concentrate fully when I want to with slight difficulty.
☐ I have a fair degree of difficulty in concentrating when I want to.
☐ I have a lot of difficulty in concentrating when I want to.
☐ I have a great deal of difficulty in concentrating when I want to.
☐ I cannot concentrate at all.

7. Work
☐ I can do as much work as I want to.
☐ I can only do my usual work, but no more.
☐ I can do most of my usual work, but no more.
☐ I cannot do my usual work.
☐ I can hardly do any work at all.
☐ I can't do any work at all.

8. Driving
☐ I can drive my car without any neck pain.
☐ I can drive my car as long as I want with slight pain in my neck.
☐ I can drive my car as long as I want with moderate pain in my neck.
☐ I can't drive my car as long as I want because of moderate pain in my neck.
☐ I can hardly drive at all because of severe pain in my neck.
☐ I can't drive my car at all.

Table 12.2. The Neck Disability Index *(continued)*

9. Sleeping
☐ I have no trouble sleeping.
☐ My sleep is slightly disturbed (less than 1 h sleepless).
☐ My sleep is mildly disturbed (1–2 h sleepless).
☐ My sleep is moderately disturbed (2–3 h sleepless).
☐ My sleep is greatly disturbed (3–5 h sleepless).
☐ My sleep is completely disturbed (5–7 h sleepless).

10. Recreation
☐ I am able to engage in all my recreation activities with no neck pain at all.
☐ I am able to engage in all my recreation activities, with some pain in my neck.
☐ I am able to engage in most, but not all of my usual recreation activities because of pain in my neck.
☐ I am able to engage in a few of my usual recreation activities because of pain in my neck.
☐ I can hardly do any recreation activities because of pain in my neck.
☐ I can't do any recreation activities at all.

Scoring the Neck Disability Index (NDI)
This is a 'neck' variation of the Oswestry Low Back Disability Scale, but fashioned with modern Canadian language. Score each section out of total 10, top box gets 10, next 8, then 6, down to 0. For example:

Pain intensity
10 I have no pain at the moment.
 8 The pain is very mild at the moment.
 6 The pain is moderate at the moment.
 4 The pain is fairly severe at the moment.
 2 The pain is very severe at the moment.
 0 The pain is the worst imaginable at the moment.

This sample is constant for each section. Note that the total score is a positive 100, meaning a fully functional person with no disabilities.
Range: Severe < 50, moderate > 50, mild > 80, near normal > 90.

Beaton *et al.*[21], for instance, compared five generic indexes in workers with musculoskeletal disorders. They included the SF-36,[22] Nottingham Health Profile (NHP), Health Status Section of the Ontario Health Survey (OHS), Duke Health Profile and Sickness Impact Profile (SIP) next to a self-report of change in health between repeated tests. In subjects with reported change in health the SF-36 appeared to be the most responsive, with moderate to large effect sizes (0.55–0.97). The authors also determined the test–retest reliability of the indexes which were: for SF-36 overall, ICC = 0.85; for NHP overall, ICC = 0.95; for Duke overall, ICC = 059; for OHS overall, ICC = 0.78; and for SIP overall, ICC = 0.93. Beaton[21] also presents reliability coefficients for subscales of the indexes such as SF-36-pain and SF-36-physical function and SIP-physical function. Portney and Watkins[23] have suggested that an ICC above 0.75 is indicative of good reliability.[23] Only the Duke Health Profile overall score appeared to be of insufficient reliability in the study of Beaton.[21]

As the SF-36 and the Sickness Impact Profile are widely used in studies worldwide and in several languages, these will be elaborated upon. A wealth of information concerning the SF-36 can be found at their Internet site (www.sf36.com). According to their site: 'This comprehensive short-form with only 36 questions yields an 8-scale health profile as well as summary measures of health-related quality of life'. As documented in more than 750 publications, the SF-36 has proven useful in monitoring general and specific populations, comparing the burden of different diseases, differentiating the health benefits produced by different treatments, and in screening individual patients. Next to the SF-36 there exists the SF-12. This even shorter one-page, 2-minute survey form has been shown to yield summary physical and mental health outcome scores that are interchangeable with those from the SF-36 in both general and specific populations. This shortform, which was published in early 1995, is already one of the most widely used surveys. Translations of the SF-36 and SF-12 are being tested in more than 45 countries as part of the International Quality of Life Assessment (IQOLA) Project. Changes in SF-36 scores in response to treatments and clinically defined changes in disease severity have been reported in nearly 200 studies. Permission to reproduce and use the SF-36 and the SF-12 is routinely granted royalty-free to individuals and organizations for their own use. Via the website it is possible to try the SF-36 online. The SF-36 has been applied in several studies to examine changes in disease severity, as a measure of responsiveness relevant to craniocervical conditions; for example, by Gliklich and Hilinski[24] for ethmoid sinus surgery for chronic sinusitis and by Boline *et al.*[25] in a randomized clinical trial to determine the effectiveness of spinal manipulation for chronic tension-type headaches. Furthermore, the SF-36 has been extensively researched for all reliability and validity items showing good methodological properties.[26,27]

The Sickness Impact Profile (SIP), like the SF-36, has a long version (136 items) and shorter versions such as the SIP-68. Furthermore, the SIP has also been translated into several languages and yields satisfactory methodological properties.[28–31] The SIP has been used in clinical trials concerning the craniofacial regions.[32,33]

Many other generic health measures can be found in the literature. For international comparison of outcome studies and (randomized) clinical trials when applying generic indexes, it seems warranted that internationally acceptable generic indexes such as the SF-36, SF-12, SIP and SIP-68 are being used for broader understanding of the results of such studies. This holds for medicine in general, as well as for the specific area of craniofacial disorders.

Discussion

An important question, both for clinicians and researchers, is whether one index can be used to assess the patient or whether several indexes (such as a disease-specific and a condition-specific and a generic index) should be used to fully understand the patient's complaint.

Enloe and Shields[34] have researched this question in patients with vestibular disease.[34] They used the Dizziness Handicap Inventory (DHI[35]) as a condition-specific index and the SF-36 as a generic index to evaluate the health-related quality of life in these patients. After having established the test–retest reliability of both indexes and their subscales (which appeared to be moderate to high for both indexes and their subscales), they associated the two indexes and their respective subscale. The associations varied between $r_p = 0.11$ ($P < 0.05$) to $r_p = 0.71$ ($P < 0.05$). The highest association ($r_p = 0.71$) was between the social function score of the SF-36 and the DHI emotional score.

Enloe and Shields[34] therefore conclude that the two indexes appear to provide different information about the health status of patients with vestibular disease. An important conclusion for both clinician and researcher is that this implies that one cannot rely on a single index to fully describe these patients. In contrast, Riddle and Stratford[36] found in patients with cervical spine disorders that the NDI and the SF-36 appeared to have substantial overlap, thus inferring that the two indexes are fairly interchangeable and only one index should suffice.

There appears to be a promising field of research into the (non)interchangeability of disease- or condition-specific, dimension-specific and generic indexes in patients with diseases in the craniofacial region.

Conclusion

Much research has already been performed on a large number of indexes applicable in the craniocervical and craniofacial regions. Although some issues still need to be addressed, the applicability of indexes in this specific region of the human body seems clear. Many other indexes have not been described but can be found via Medline® or other retrieval systems or via the Internet.

Although indexes may be researched for reliability and validity issues, they are ultimately intended for clinicians and their patients, and policy makers. Clinicians should be aware of the powerful properties of indexes for evaluation of individual patients in an era where payment for therapy is no longer unlimited. Indexes are important instruments that enable the production of reliable outcome measures for the chosen therapy.

Furthermore, indexes can be used to evaluate the patients' progress during treatment periods and thus enable the clinician to adjust the amount or type of therapy given during this period.

Finally, the use of (reliable and valid) indexes can serve as a vehicle to emancipate clinicians and to convince society at large of the effectiveness and efficiency of therapies given to patients.

References

1 Wright, J. G. and Feinstein, A. R. (1992). A comparative contrast of clinimetric and psychometric methods for constructing indexes and rating scales. *J. Clin. Epidemiol.*, **45**, 1201–1218.
2 Feinstein, A. R. (1987). *Clinimetrics*. Yale University Press.
3 Blumenthal, D. (1996).Quality of health care. Part 1: Quality of care – what is it? *N. Engl. J. Med.*, **335**, 891–894.
4 Brook, R. H. and McGlynn, E. A. (1996). Quality of health care. Part 2: Measuring quality of care. *N. Engl. J. Med.*, **335**, 966–970.
5 Chassin, M. R. (1996). Quality of health care. Part 3: Improving the quality of care. *N. Engl. J. Med.*, **335**, 1060–1063.
6 Blumenthal, D. (1996). Quality of health care. Part 4: The origins of the quality-of-care debate. *N. Engl. J. Med.*, **335**, 1146–1149.
7 Berwick, D. M. (1996). Quality of health care. Part 5: Payment by capitation and the quality of care. *N. Engl. J. Med.*, **335**, 1227–1231.
8 Blumenthal, D. and Epstein, A. M. (1996). Quality of health care. Part 6: The role of physicians in the future of quality management. *N. Engl. J. Med.*, **335**, 1328–1331.
9 European Research Group on Health Outcomes (ERGHO). *Choosing a Health Outcome Measurement Instrument.* http://www.meb.uni-boon.de/standards/ERGHO/ERGHO_Instruments.html.
10 World Health Organization (1989). *International Classification of Impairments, Disabilities and Handicaps (ICIDH)*. WHO.
11 Medical Outcomes Trust. *SAC Instrument Review Criteria.* http://www.Outcomes-Trust.Org/bulletin/34sacrev.htm
12 Cole, B., Finch, E., Gowland, C. and Mayo, N. (1994). *Physical Rehabilitation Outcome Measures*, 2nd edn. Canadian Physiotherapy Association.
13 Benninger, M. S. and Brent, A. Sr (1997). The development of the Rhinosinusitis Disability Index. *Arch. Otolaryngol. Head Neck Surg.*, **123**, 1175–1179.
14 VanSwearingen, J. M. and Brach, J. S. (1996). The Facial Disability Index: reliability and validity of a disability assessment instrument for disorders of the facial neuromuscular system. *Phys. Ther.*, **76**, 1288–1300.
15 VanSwearingen, J. M. and Brach, J. S. (1998). Validation of a treatment-based classification system for individuals with facial neuromotor disorders. *Phys. Ther.*, **78**, 678–689.
16 Vernon, H. and Mior, S. (1991). The Neck Disablity Index: a study of reliability and validity. *J. Manip. Physiol. Ther.*, **14**, 409–415.
17 Fairbank, J. C. T., Couper, J., Davies, J. B. and O'Brien, J. P. (1980). The Oswestry Low Back Pain Disability Index. *Physiother. (London)*, **66**, 271–273.

18 Haines, F., Waalen, J. and Mior, S. (1998). Psychometric properties of the Neck Disability Index. *J. Manip. Physiol. Ther.*, **21**, 75–80.

19 Verhoef, M. J., Page, S. A. and Waddell, S. C. (1997). The Chiropractic Outcome Study: pain, functional ability and satisfaction with care. *J. Manip. Physiol. Ther.*, **20**, 235–240.

20 Westaway, M. D., Stratford, P. W. and Binkley, J. M. (1998). The Patient-Specific Functional Scale: validation of its use in persons with neck dysfunction. *JOSPT*, **27**, 331-338.

21 Beaton, D. E., Hogg-Johnson, S. and Bombardier, C. (1997). Valuating changes in health status: reliability and responsiveness of five generic health status measures in workers with musculoskeletal disorders. *J. Clin. Epidemiol.*, **50**, 79–93.

22 SF-36.http://www.sf36.com

23 Portney, L. G. and Watkins, M. P. (1993). *Foundations of Clinical Research. Applications to Practice.* Appleton & Lange

24 Gliklich, R. E. and Hilinski, J. M. (1995). Longitudinal sensitivity of generic and specific health measures in chronic sinusitis. *Qual. Life Res.*, **4**, 27–32.

25 Boline, P. D., Kassak, K., Bronfort, G. *et al.* (1995). Spinal manipulation vs. amitriptyline for the treatment of chronic tension-type headaches: a randomized clinical trial. *J. Manip. Physiol. Ther.*, **18**, 148–154.

26 McHorney, C. A., Ware, J. E. and Raczek, A. E. (1993). The MOS 36-Item Short-Form Health Survey (SF-36): II. Psychometric and clinical tests of validity in measuring physical and mental health constructs. *Med. Care*, **31**, 247–263.

27 McHorney, C. A., Ware, J. E., Lu, J. F. R. and Sherbourne, C. D. (1994). The MOS 36-Item Short-Form Health Survey (SF-36): III. Test of data quality, scaling assumptions and reliability across diverse patient groups. *Med. Care*, **32**, 40–66.

28 Bergner, M., Bobbit, R. A., Pollard, W. E. *et al.* (1976). The sickness impact profile: validation of a health status measure. *Med. Care*, **14**, 57–67.

29 Pollard, W. E., Bobbitt, R. A., Bergner, M. *et al.* (1976). The sickness impact profile: reliability of a health status measure. *Med. Care*, **14**, 146-155.

30 De Bruin, A. F., Diederiks, J. P. M., de Witte, L. P. *et al.* (1994). The development of a short generic of the sickness impact profile. *J. Clin. Epidemiol.*, **47**, 407–418.

31 De Bruin, A. F., Buys, M., de Witte, L. P. and Diederiks, J. P. M. (1994). The sickness impact profile: SIP68, a short generic version, first evaluation of the reliability and reproducibility. *J. Clin. Epidemiol.*, **47**, 863–871.

32 Carlsson, J., Augustinsson, L. E., Blomstrand, C. and Sullivan, M. (1990). Health status in patients with tension headache treated with acupuncture or physiotherapy. *Headache*, **30**, 593-599.

33 Hammill, J. M., Cook, T. M. and Rosecrance, J. C. (1996). Effectiveness of a physical therapy regimen in the treatment of tension-type headache. *Headache*, **36**, 149-153.

34 Enloe, L. J. and Shields, R. K. (1997). Evaluation of health-related quality of life in individuals with vestibular disease using disease-specific and general outcome measures. *Phys. Ther.*, **77**, 890–903.

35 Jacobson, G. P. and Newman, C. W. (1990). The development of the dizziness handicap inventory. *Arch. Otolaryngol. Head Neck Surg.*, **116**, 424–427.

36 Riddle, D. L. and Stratford, P. W. (1998). Use of generic versus region-specific functional status measures on patients with cervical spine disorders. *Phys. Ther.*, **78**, 951-963.

Glossary

Abnormal impulse generating sites (AIGS) Persistent sites of abnormal impulses generated by the axon. These sites may be the result of injury or further pathobiological consequences of vascular or axoplasmatic changes

Adenoidectomy An operation for the removal of unencapsulated lymphoid tissue in the nasopharynx (adenoids)

Allodynia Pain that results from a stimulus which would not normally be painful. Can be primary (from the tissue) or secondary (from the central nervous tissue)

Anomaly Deviation from the average or norm: anything that is structurally unusual or irregular or contrary to the general rule. Connection between branches of different nerves is an example of an anomaly

Antidrome impulses Impulses in a peripheral nerve in the opposite direction. Are seen in C fibres and play an important role in neurogenic inflammation

Axonal transport The mechanisms by which axoplasm is moved in the axon cylinder, including dendrites

Bone matrix Tissue in which bone and parts of bone develop

Bruxism Diurnal or nocturnal parafunctional activity including clenching, bracing, gnashing, and grinding of the teeth

CGRP (Calcitonin gene related peptide) A neurotransmitter dominantly from the peripheral nervous system which is often seen with substance P

Cleft palate Congenital fissure in the median line of the palate, often associated with cleft lip. Often occurs as a feature of a syndrome or generalized condition. Synonym: palatoschisis

Clinical pattern Collection of signs and symptoms commonly presenting together in a clinical situation

Clivus The sloping surface from the dorsum sellae to the foramen magnum composed of part of the body of the sphenoid and part of the basal part of the occipital bone

Concurrent validity Concurrent validity deals with whether an inference is justifiable at the present time

Conjunctivitis Inflammation of the conjunctiva (the mucous membrane investing the anterior surface of the eyeball and the posterior surface of the lids)

Construct validity Is based on a logical argument that supports the idea that a measurement reflects what one wants to measure

Content validity Content validity concerns the issue of whether a test reflects the variable as has been defined

Craniosynostosis Premature ossification of the cranial sutures resulting in malformation of the skull caused by abnormal stress-transducing forces

Cystectomy Excision of the urinary bladder or removal of a cyst

Diplopia Double vision

Disability Any restriction or inability (resulting from an impairment) to perform an activity in the manner or within the range considered normal for a human being. Disabilities are descriptions of disturbances in function at the level of the person (definition of the ICIDH)

Drop attacks Attacks of falling, or sudden (loss of) consciousness.

Dysaesthesiae Abnormal sensations experienced in the absence of stimulation.

Dysarthria A disturbance of speech and language due to emotional stress, to brain injury, or to paralysis, in coordination, or spasticity of the muscles used for speaking.

Dysphagia Difficulty in swallowing

Endosteum Tissue that is the border between the medullary cavity and bone matrix

ENT specialist Doctor who specializes in diseases of the ear, nose, and larynx: including diseases of related structures of the head and neck. Synonym: otorhinolaryngologist

Face validity Face validity reflects only whether a test appears to do what it is supposed to do

Fasciculation Involuntary contractions, or twitching, of groups (fasciculi) of muscle fibres, a coarser form of muscular contraction than fibrillation

Functional development Perceptible (growth) result, logically arising from successive biological processes

Genetic Determined by genes without direct influence from the environment

Gomphosis Joint in bone matrix, lined by periosteum and spanned by a fibre system, i.e. a suture of periodontium

Handicap Any disadvantage for a given individual, resulting from impairment or a disability that limits or prevents the fulfilment of a role that is normal for that individual. The classification of handicap deals with the relationship that evolves between society, culture and people who have impairment or disabilities, as reflected in people's role in life (definition of the ICIDH)

Hyperalgesia More pain than normal for a stimulus that would normally be painful. Can be primary (from the tissue) or secondary (from the central nervous system)

Hypoplasia Underdevelopment of a tissue or organ, usually due to a decrease in the number of cells or atrophy due to destruction of source of the elements and not merely to a general reduction in size.

Intraclass correlation coefficient (ICC) Index of reliability obtained through an analysis of variance

Impairment Any loss or abnormality of a psychological or anatomical structure of function. Impairments are disturbances at the level of the organ (definition of the ICIDH)

Incarnation Form capacity of tissue

Inquiry Collecting of data

Investing layer Connective tissue between bone matrix and dental crypt

Irritability A presentation in which it takes very little activity to cause the symptoms, which then take a long time to subside. High irritability is often a result of highly mechanical and chemically-sensitive changes in neural structures

Lacrimation The secretion of tears, especially in excess

Lambda The craniometric point at the junction of the sagittal and lambdoid sutures

Malfunction A functional process leading to pathological disorders

Malocclusion Occlusional variation. Unusual biological or functional relationship between the maxillary and mandibular teeth

Mitosis The usual process of somatic reproduction of cells consisting of a sequence of modifications of the cell nucleus that result in the formation of two daughter cells with exactly the same chromosome and DNA content as that of the original cell

Morphology The science concerned with the configuration or the structure of human beings, animals and plants

Mould To change in shape: denoting especially the adaptation of the fetal head to the pelvic canal

Nasion A point on the skull corresponding to the middle of the nasofrontal suture. Synonym: nasal point

Neural container The direct environment of the nervous tissue

Neuroblastoma A malignant neoplasm characterized by immature nerve cells of embryonic type

Neurodynamics The interaction between nervous system mechanics and physiology

Nocebo Therapeutic intervention has no effect anymore or makes the patient worse, mostly without the consciousness of the clinician

Nosology Assumption of a disease

Ontogeny The study of the development of the individual organism from conception

Open dissipative system An organized system that is in continuous exchange with the environment and is not thermodynamic

Otorhinolaryngologist See ENT specialist

Passive accessory intervertebral movements Manual techniques which test/restore gliding movements of one vertebra on another

Passive physiological intervertebral movements Manual techniques which test/restore physiological movement between two vertebrae

Periaqueductal grey (PAG) Region of the mesencephalon and upper pons which has a high concentration of neurons that are capable of producing powerful neurotransmitters that can greatly modulate nociceptive impulses

Periosteum Tissue that is the border between bone matrix and the surrounding tissue

Phenomenology The description of signs and symptoms: occurrences of any sort, whether ordinary or extraordinary, in relation to the pathology or clinical pattern

Photalgia Light-induced pain (usually eye pain)

Photophobia. Avoidance of light; often an expression of undue anxiety about eyes, photosensitivity and photalgia

Phylogeny Study of development of animals in an evolutionary process

Plagiocephaly An asymmetric craniostenosis due to premature closure of the lambdoid and coronal sutures on one side; characterized by an oblique deformity of the cranium

Pneumatization The development of air cells such as those of the mastoid and ethmoidal bones

Pneumatized cells Air cells developed in the mastoid and ethmoidal bones

Predictive validity The possibility to infer from a measurement outcome to the future

Prognathic Having a forward projection of both jaws beyond the established normal relationship with the cranial base

Pterion A craniometric point at the junction of the greater wing of the sphenoid, the squamous portion of the temporal, the frontal and the parietal bones

Ptosis (of the eye) A drooping of the eyelid

Retrognathia Facial disharmony in which the mandible lies posterior to the normal position

Rhinology The branch of science concerned with the nose and diseases

Rhinorrhoea A discharge from the nasal mucous membrane

Scaphocephaly Craniosynosthosis involving the sagittal suture, resulting in a long, narrow cranial vault; sometimes accompanied by mental retardation

Secondary hyperalgesia More pain than usual from a stimulus that would normally be painful, caused by the central nervous system.

Strain Stored tension by mechanical load

Stress The reaction of a body under strain

Stress transducer Tissue system that transforms strain into a mechanical load on the bordering tissues

Substance P A neurotransmitter released at the central terminals of primary nociceptive neurons that acts as a transport substance, being found at the distal terminals as well.

Suture Gomphosis between two (bone) matrix parts

Symphysis menti The fibrocartilaginous union of the two halves of the mandible in the fetus: it becomes an osseous union during the first year.

Tensor veli palatini muscle Tensor muscle of soft palate: tenses the soft palate; contributes to opening of the auditory tube

Thermorhizotomy Section of nerve branches or a spinal nerve root by a high temperature needle for the relief of pain or spastic paralysis

Tonsillectomy Removal of any collection of lymphoid tissue in the region of the larynx (tonsil)

Index

Abnormal impulse generating sites, 154, 237
Accessory movements, 33
Adaptation, 3, 18
Adenoidectomy, 237
Adrenocorticotrophin hormone (ACTH), 158
Ageing, 24, 38
Allodynia, 237
Alveolar bone, 12–14, 71
Amitriptyline, 93
Analgesic abuse, 94
Anomaly, 237
Antidromic impulses, 152–3, 237
Anxiety and pain, 150, 218
Arm
    KISS syndrome, 52
    proprioception, 49
Arousal, 217–18
Articulations, 173–4
    dysfunction, 100–1
Asymmetry, 46, 47, 48–9
    primary/secondary, 50, 53–4
    resolution, 50
    treatment, 51, 55–60
Attention, 218–19
Auriculotemporal nerve, 132
Autorhythmic firing, 136
Axolemma, 153–4
Axonal transport, 237

Babies
    asymmetry, 47, 48–9
        primary/secondary, 50, 53–4
    birth trauma, 49–50, 52–3
    colic, 52
    crying and irritable, 52, 53–4
    head control, 49, 50, 55
    neck pain, 55
    sleep problems, 52, 53–4
    techniques for use on, 55–8
Behavioural therapy, 225
Biofeedback, 225
Biological systems, 2
Biomechanics, 171–2

Birth
    cranial moulding, 75–6
    trauma, 49–50, 52–3
Body growth, 1
Bone
    adaptation, 3
    -fusion barrier, 7
    matrix, 2, 3–5, 6, 237
    medullary tissue, 9
    ossification, 24
    stress sensitivity, 2, 3
Brachycephaly, 24
Brain
    growth, 5, 6, 7, 9, 70
    passive movement effects, 29, 30–1
Brainstem
    birth trauma, 49
    growth, 10
    topography, 121
    tumours, 120
Breathing therapy, 225
Bruxism, 31, 237
Buccal nerve, 132

Calcitonin gene related peptide, 154, 237
Calvaria, 10, 22
    embryological development, 5
Cartilage, 2, 3, 5
Case studies
    cervicogenic headache, 107–14
    clinical reasoning, 194–210
    muscular torticollis, 38–40
    whiplash, 216–17, 218
Cavernous sinus, 126–8
Central sensitization, 151, 155–8
    maladaptive, 156–8
Cephalometry, 24, 26
Cerbellopontine angle, 122–6
    surgery, 124–5
    tumours, 124
Cerebrospinal fluid, 29–30
Cervical articulations, 173–4
    dysfunction, 100–1

Cervical flexion pain, 104–5
Cervical flexors, 89–90, 165
Cervical muscle anatomy, 174
Cervical rotation pain, 105–6
Cervical spine stability, 171–2, 173–4
  with arm elevation, 179–80
Cervicogenic headache, 85–115
  associated symptoms, 95–6
  case studies, 107–14
  criteria for, 86–7
  diary keeping, 97
  dietary factors, 91–2, 94, 96
  differentiation, 103–7
  joint pain, 88–9
  muscular factors, 89–90, 101, 164
  neck movements, 96
  neural pain, 89
  neuroanatomical basis for, 87–95, 164
  neurodynamics, 102–3
  neurogenic inflammation, 91–2
  pain, 90, 95
  presentation, 95–6
  radiography, 96
  relieving factors, 96
  serotoninergic system, 90, 92
  special questions, 96
  techniques, 100–7
  trigeminocervical nucleus, 87–90
Chewing, 15
  muscles, 174–6
    head posture, 169
  tooth movement, 14
'Chicken-wings', 52
Chin-tuck, 101
Chondral matrix, 6–7, 10
Cleft palate, 17, 237
Clinical patterns, 38, 237
Clinical reasoning, 188–215
  case study, 194–210
  cognition, 190–1
  cue recognition, 193
  knowledge-based, 191, 211
  metacognition, 191, 212
  strategies, 191–3
Clinimetrics, *see* Measurement indexes
Clivus, 237
Cluster headaches, 126, 128
Cognition
  clinical reasoning, 190–1
  pain response, 150
Cognitive-behavioural therapy, 217–23
Cognitive therapy, 225
Colic, 52
Collaborative reasoning, 193, 213
Communication, 192–3
Complex regional pain syndrome, 158
Compression of occipital-frontal region, 34–6
Concurrent validity, 229, 237
Conjunctivitis, 237
Connective tissue, 120–1
Consolidation of form, 2
Construct validity, 229, 237
Content validity, 229, 237
Continuum headache model, 92–3
Corticotrophin releasing factor, 158

Cortisol, 158–9
Cranial nerve
  entry zones, 121–2
  innervation, 141
Cranioneurodynamics, *see* Neurodynamics
Craniosynostosis, 24, 238
Cranium, 22
  asymmetry, 47, 48–9
    primary/secondary, 50, 53–4
    resolution, 50
    treatment, 51, 55–60
  compliance, 30
  deformity correction, 24
  moulding during birth, 75–6
  movement, 23–6, 74–5
Cue recognition, 193
Cystectomy, 238

Dental crypts, 12–13
Dermal matrix, 7, 9–11
Detoxification, 94
Diabetic neuropathy, 120
Diagnostic reasoning, 192, 212
Diary keeping, 97, 220, 221
Diet and headaches, 91–2, 94, 96
Differentiation, 103–7
Diplopia, 238
Disability, 238
Dizziness Handicap Inventory, 234
Dolichocephaly, 24
Drop attacks, 238
Drug-induced headaches, 94
Duke Health Profile, 233
Dummy use and otitis media, 72
Dura/dural attachments, 120–1
  innervation, 89
  passive movement effects, 28–9
  sensitivity, 164
  suture morphogenesis, 75
Dysaesthesia, 238
Dysarthria, 238
Dysphagia, 238

Ear
  anatomy, 65–8
  disease, *see* Otitis media
  external auditory meatus opening, 81–2
Embryology, 5–6
Emotions and pain, 150, 218
Endocrine system, 158–9
Endosteum, 3, 238
ENT specialist, 238
Environment, 1–2
Ethical reasoning, 193
Eustachian tube, 64–5, 68–9, 82
  dysfunction, 70
  obstruction, 68
Evolution, 1
Exercise therapy, 225, 227
External auditory meatus opening, 81–2
Extracranial pressure, 28–9
Eye pain, 152, 154

Face validity, 229, 238
Facet joints, 173–4

Facet joints (*cont.*)
  and headache, 101
Facial Disability Index, 230, 231
Facial nerve
  anatomy, 137, 139
  neurodynamics, 137, 139–42
  paresis, 141
Facial skull, 6
  embryological development, 5
  fusion disorders, 17
  growth, 71
  'long face', 72
  mobilization response, 23
  pain, 23
  post-birth shape changes, 6
Facial sutures, 11–12
Family, 221, 222–3
Fasciculation, 238
Food-related headaches, 91–2, 94, 96
Foramina, 128–9
Forehead on hindhead rotation, 80–1
Form consolidation, 2
Freeway space, 168
Functional development, 238
Functional movement
  biomechanics, 171–2
  disturbances, 172–3

Gate control theory, 148
Genetics, 1–2, 16, 238
Goal setting, 219, 221
Gomphoses, 3, 5, 238
Greater occipital nerve, 89
Group therapy, 222
Growth regulation, 16–18

Handicap, 238
'Hands on' and 'hands off' approaches, 32
Harelip, 17
Head
  control, 49, 50, 55
  flexion
    masticatory muscle activity, 169
    neural tissue movement, 129–31
  posture, 166–71
    craniofacial morphology, 171
    craniomandibular function, 167–8
    forward posture, 167, 168
    mandibular position, 167–8
    measurement, 165–6
    nasal airflow, 171
    occlusion, 170–1
    temporomandibular dysfunction, 165
Headache
  associated symptoms, 151
  classification, 85
  cluster-type, 126, 128
  continuum model, 92–3
  diaries, 97
  dietary factors, 91–2, 94, 96
  drug-induced, 94
  drug therapy, 93
  economic costs, 85
  intensity, 150
  manual therapy, 93, 94

patient education, 94–5
  rebound, 94
  recurrent, 150–1
  serotoninergic system, 90, 92
  sleep habits, 94
  stress-related, 94
  see also Cervicogenic headache
Healthy behaviour, 222, 227
Hearing loss, 64, 73
Helmets, corrective, 51, 52
Hyoid bone, 168
Hyperalgesia, 238
  primary, 151
  secondary, 151, 240
Hypnosis, 225
Hypoplasia, 238
Hypothesis generation, 189–90, 211
Hypoxia, 153

Impairment, 238
Incarnation, 238
Indexes, *see* Measurement indexes,
Infrahyoid muscles, 176
Inquiry, 238
Interactive reasoning, 192, 212–13
Interclass correlation coefficient, 238
Internal consistency, 229
Interviews, 96, 194–5, 197–9, 201–3, 212
Intracranial blood pressure, 9
Intracranial blood vessels, 29
Intracranial pressure, 9
Intracranial volume, 30, 31
Investing layer, 238
Irritability, 238
Ischaemia, 153

Jugular foramen, 36

KISS syndrome, 46–62
  features, 47
  outcome, 58–60
  risk factors, 51
  signs and symptoms, 52
  treatment, 55–8
Knowledge, 191, 211

Lacrimation, 128, 238
Lambda, 238
Learning, 218, 222
Lingual nerve, 132
'Long face', 72
Longitudinal movements
  nasofrontal region, 79
  petrous bone, 79–80
Longus colli weakness, 165

Malfunction, 238
Malocclusion, 15, 170, 239
Mandible
  growth, 14–15
  position
    head posture, 167–8
    muscle activity, 168–70
    temporomandibular articular mechanoreceptors,
      169–70

Mandible (*cont.*)
  rest position, 168
  upright postural position, 168
Mandibular nerve
  anatomy, 132
  neurodynamics, 133–5
  neuropathy, 135–7
Masseter muscle, 174
Mastication, 15
  muscles, 174–6
    head posture, 169
  tooth movement, 14
Mastoid
  air cells, 69, 82
  antrum, 68
  lift, 79–80
  process, 68
Mastoiditis, 70
Maxilla, sagittal rotation, 36–8
Maxillary suture, 11, 12
Measurement indexes, 228–36
  choice, 228
  condition-specific, 229–31
  dimension-specific, 229, 231, 232
  generic, 229, 231, 233–4
  reliability, 229
  uses, 228–9
  validity, 229
Mechanical stress, 2, 3, 6, 240
  transducer, 11–12, 25–6, 240
Meckel's cartilage, 14
Medullary bone tissue, 9
Meninges, 28
Meningioma, 124
Meningitis, 131
Mental nerve, 132
Metacognition, 191, 212
Mitochondria, 2
Miosis, 128
Mitosis, 239
Modularity, 2, 5
Morphology, 1, 2, 7, 10, 18, 171, 239
Motivation, 222
Motor system, 159
Mould, 239
Mouth breathing, 72
Mouth opening device, 168
Multidimensional pain inventory, 224, 226
Muscle
  activity, 168–70
  balance, 31–2
  cervical, 174
  function, influences on, 163–4
  global systems, 172
  headache-associated dysfunction, 89–90, 101, 164
  local systems, 172
  masticatory, 174–6
  pain, 31
  relaxation therapy, 225
  spasm, 164
  strength tests, 176–80

Narrative reasoning, 193, 213
Nasal airflow, 171
Nasal growth, 11–12

Nasal septum, 11, 12
Nasal wiggle, 79
Nasion, 239
Nasopharynx
  anatomy, 65
  growth, 11
Neck
  Disability Index (NDI), 231, 232, 234–5
  extensor tests, 178–9
  flexion, neural tissue movement, 129–31
  flexor tests, 177–8
  pain
    anatomical basis, 164–5
    in babies, 55
Neck–tongue syndrome, 95–6
Neonates
  asymmetry, 48–9, 53
  birth trauma, 49–50, 52–3
  brainstem trauma, 49
Nerve entry zones, 121–2
Neural containers, 116, 122, 123–4, 141, 239
Neural tissue
  blood supply, 118
  movement, 89, 117–19, 129–31
  pain generation by, 89
  passive movement effects, 31
Neuraxis, 129
Neuroblastoma, 131, 239
Neurocranium, 22
  growth, 6–11
  mobilization response, 23
  pain, 23
Neurodynamics, 102–3, 116–47, 239
  and pathology, 131
  testing, 131–41
Neurogenic inflammation, 91–2, 119
Neurogenic pain, 153–5
Neuromas, 124
Neuron plasticity, 156
Neurosurgical decompression, 118, 123
Neurotransmitters, 91, 119, 152–3, 154, 156
Nocebo, 239
Nociceptive pain, 152–3
Nose, *see* Nasal headings
Nosology, 239
Nottingham Health Profile, 233

Occipital-frontal compression, 34–6
Occipital-sphenoid region, transverse movement, 36
Occlusion
  temporomandibular dysfunction, 170
  vertical dimension of, 170
Ocular torticollis, 26
Ontario Health Survey, 233
Ontogeny, 239
Open bite, 72
Open dissipative system, 3, 239
Opisthotonos, 51
Orthodontists, 26
Orthopaedics, 47
Orthostatic position of the head and neck, 166
Ossicles, 66
Ossification, 24
Otitis media, 63–84
  aetiology, 64–5

Otitis media (*cont.*)
  age, 70, 82–3
  associated disease, 70
  defined, 63–4
  drug therapy, 74
  dummy use, 72
  Eustachian tube involvement, 64–5, 68–9
  facial changes, 71–3
  hearing loss, 64, 73
  manual therapy, 75–82, 83
  mastoid air cell size, 69
  mouth breathing, 72
  open bite, 72
  pathogenesis, 64–5
  prevalence, 64
  sequelae, 64
  surgical treatment, 73–4, 83
Otorhinolaryngologist, 237

Pain, 148–62
  attention to, 218–19
  beliefs, 212
  classification, 149–51
  cognitive response, 150
  defined, 148–9
  dependency, 222
  diaries, 220, 221
  emotional response, 150, 218
  gate control theory, 148
  group therapy, 222
  management, 216–27
  measurement, 220–1
  mechanisms, 152–5
  multidimensional pain inventory, 224, 226
  muscular, 31
  nociceptive, 152–3
  output-related, 158–9
  peripheral neurogenic, 153–5
  postoperative, 124–5
  quality differences, 23
  sensory response, 150
  suture-induced, 26–7
  sympathetically maintained, 158
  technique application, 38
  see also Headache
Pars flaccida, 66
Partners, 221
Passive movements, 27
  accessory intervertebral, 239
  physiological intervertebral, 239
  structures influenced by, 27–32
  techniques, 33–40, 77–82
Pathology, 38, 131
Patient
  education, 94–5, 227
  interviews, 96, 194–5, 197–9, 201–3, 212
  -practitioner relationship, 192–3, 221
  sharing decision making, 193, 213
Pattern recognition, 190
Peptides, 152–3, 154
Periaqueductal grey, 239
Periodontia, 3, 4, 12–13
Periosteum, 3, 9, 12, 239
Peripheral neurogenic pain, 153–5
Petrous bone, longitudinal movement, 79–80

Phenomenology, 239
Photalgia, 239
Photophobia, 239
Phylogeny, 1, 4, 6–7, 10, 239
Plagiocephaly, 24, 51, 239
Pneumatic sinuses, 11, 71
Pneumatization, 239
Pneumatized cells, 239
Postoperative pain, 124–5
Postural analysis digitizing system, 165
Posture, 165–71
  asymmetry, 47, 48–9
    primary/secondary, 50, 53–4
  flat back, 181
  kypho-lordotic, 181
  measurement, 165–6
  re-education, 180–3
  sway back, 181
Pragmatic reasoning, 193
Predictive reasoning, 193
Predictive validity, 229, 239
Processus alveolaris, 12–14, 71
Prognathic, 239
Proprioception, arm, 49
Pterion, 239
Pterygoid muscles, 174–5
Ptosis, 128, 239

Questioning, 96, 194–5, 197–9, 201–3, 212

Reasoning
  backward, 190
  collaborative, 193, 213
  diagnostic, 192, 212
  errors, 190–1
  ethical, 193
  forward, 190
  interactive, 192, 212–13
  narrative, 193, 213
  pragmatic, 193
  predictive, 193
  strategies, 191–3
  teaching as, 193, 213
  see also Clinical reasoning
Reflex sympathetic dystrophy, 158
Regeneration, 2
Retrognathia, 72, 239
Rhinology, 239
Rhinorrhoea, 240
Road traffic accidents, 173
Rotation techniques
  forehead on hindhead, 80–1
  maxillary, 36–8

Sacculus dentis, 12
Scaphocephaly, 240
Scapular control and stability, 180
Screening questions, 212
Self-assessment, 221
Self-efficacy, 221
Sensitivity, primary/secondary, 151–2
Serotoninergic system, 90, 92, 119
SF-12, 233–4
SF-36, 233–5
Sickness Impact profile, (SIP), 233, 234

Sinuses, 11, 71
Skill acquisition, 54–5
Skull base, 5, 10, 22, 70–1
Skull growth, 1–21, 70–1, 129
  embryological, 5–6
  measurement, 24, 26
  mechanical influences, 2–3
  modularity of, 2, 5
  ossification, 24
  regulation, 16–18
Sleep
  disorders in babies, 52, 53–4
  headache management, 94
  position-induced skull deformities, 26
Slump test, 102–3
Social exchange, 192–3
Special questions, 96
Spectacle wearing, 26
Sphenoid bone, 36
  transverse movement, 36, 78
Spondylometer, 165
Sternocleidomastoid muscle shortening, 48, 50
Story telling, 193, 213
Strain, 240
Stress, mechanical, 2, 3, 6, 240
  transducer, 11–12, 25–6, 240
Stress management, 94, 225
Substance P, 91, 152, 154, 156, 240
Sumatriptan, 154
Suprahyoid muscles, 176
Sutures, 3, 9, 74, 240
  ageing, 24, 38
  bone thickening along, 9
  dural control, 75
  facial, 11–12
  gap techniques, 81
  intrasutural fissure, 9
  joint-like nature, 27
  maxillary, 11, 12
  mobility, 4, 9, 24
  pain, 26–7
  premature closing, 24
Symmetry, 46, 55
Sympathetic nervous system, 90, 91, 158
Sympathetically maintained pain, 158
Symphysis menti, 240
Synchondroses, 10
Synovial joints, 3

Teaching as reasoning, 193, 213
Techniques
  use on babies, 55–8
  cervicogenic headache, 100–7
  factors affecting choice of, 38
  frequency of use, 56
  neurodynamic, 131–41
  for otitis media, 77–82
  passive movements, 33–40, 77–82
Teeth
  alveolar bone development, 12–14, 71
  chewing-induced movement, 14
  crypts, 12–13
  eruption, 14, 71, 83

  mouth breathing, 72
  freeway space, 168
Temporalis muscle, 174
Temporomandibular articular mechanoreceptors, 169–70
Temporomandibular joint
  dysfunction
    head posture, 165
    occlusion, 170
  joint space changes, 15
  pain
    on cervical flexion, 104
    on cervical rotation, 105–6
  periosteum covering, 15
Tensor veli palatini, 69, 240
Thermorhizotomy, 240
Thoracic spine manipulation for headache, 94
Thumb sucking, 71, 72, 73
Tissue regeneration, 2
Tonsillectomy, 240
Torticollis, 31, 32, 52
  case study, 38–40
  ocular, 26
Transverse movement
  occipital-sphenoid region, 36
  sphenoid bone, 78
  zygoma-maxilla junction, 79
  zygoma-temporal junction, 79
Trigeminal nerve, 91, 136
Trigeminocervical nucleus, 87–90, 92, 164
Trigeminovascular system, 90–1, 92
Trigger points, 89
Trigonocephaly, 24
Tumours, 120, 124, 131
  surgical treatment, 124–5
Tympanic membrane, 66

Upper limb
  KISS syndrome, 52
  proprioception, 49

Validity
  concurrent, 229, 237
  construct, 229, 237
  content, 229, 237
  face, 229, 238
  predictive, 229, 239
Valsalva manoeuvre, 64, 65
Vascular decompression, 118, 123
Vascular loops, 121
Vertebral canal length changes, 89
Viscerocranium, 22
Visual–analogue scale, 221
Visualization, 225

Well behaviour, 222, 227
Whiplash, 35–6, 38, 216–17, 218

Yellow flags, 212, 213

Zygapophyseal joints, 173–4
  and headache, 101
Zygoma-maxilla junction, transverse movement, 79
Zygoma-temporal junction, transverse movement, 79

Printed and bound by CPI Group (UK) Ltd, Croydon, CR0 4YY

03/10/2024

01040345-0008